Dermatology Skills
for Primary Care

CURRENT ◊ CLINICAL ◊ PRACTICE

SERIES EDITOR: NEIL S. SKOLNIK, MD

Dermatology Skills for Primary Care

An Illustrated Guide

By

Daniel J. Trozak, MD
Private Practice of Dermatology, Modesto, CA

Dan J. Tennenhouse, MD, JD
University of California–San Francisco Medical Center, San Francisco, CA

John J. Russell, MD
*Abington Memorial Hospital, Abington, PA
and Temple University School of Medicine,
Philadelphia, PA*

HUMANA PRESS ✳ TOTOWA, NEW JERSEY

© 2010 Humana Press Inc.
999 Riverview Drive, Suite 208
Totowa, New Jersey 07512

www.humanapress.com

Due diligence has been taken by the publishers, editors, and authors of this book to assure the accuracy of the information published and to describe generally accepted practices. The contributors herein have carefully checked to ensure that the drug selections and dosages set forth in this text are accurate and in accord with the standards accepted at the time of publication. Notwithstanding, as new research, changes in government regulations, and knowledge from clinical experience relating to drug therapy and drug reactions constantly occurs, the reader is advised to check the product information provided by the manufacturer of each drug for any change in dosages or for additional warnings and contraindications. This is of utmost importance when the recommended drug herein is a new or infrequently used drug. It is the responsibility of the treating physician to determine dosages and treatment strategies for individual patients. Further it is the responsibility of the health care provider to ascertain the Food and Drug Administration status of each drug or device used in their clinical practice. The publisher, editors, and authors are not responsible for errors or omissions or for any consequences from the application of the information presented in this book and make no warranty, express or implied, with respect to the contents in this publication.

This publication is printed on acid-free paper. ∞
ANSI Z39.48-1984 (American Standards Institute) Permanence of Paper for Printed Library Materials.

Cover design by Daniel J. Trozak, MD
Left Photo: Bullous Impetigo (see color photo section, Part VI)
Right Photo: Vesicle/Bulla (see p. 10, Fig. 11)

Production Editor: Robin B. Weisberg

For additional copies, pricing for bulk purchases, and/or information about other Humana titles, contact Humana at the above address or at any of the following numbers: Tel.: 973-256-1699; Fax: 973-256-8314; E-mail: orders@humanapr.com, or visit our Website: http://www.humanapress.com

Printed in the United States of America. 10 9 8 7 6 5 4 3 2 1
eISBN: 1-59259-906-0

Library of Congress Cataloging-in-Publication Data

Trozak, Daniel J.
  Dermatology skills for primary care : an illustrated guide / by Daniel J.
Trozak, Dan J. Tennenhouse, John J. Russell.
     p. ; cm. -- (Current clinical practice)
  Includes bibliographical references and index.
  ISBN 978-1-61737-598-9   e-ISBN 978-1-59259-906-6
  1. Skin--Diseases. 2. Dermatology. 3. Primary care (Medicine)
  [DNLM: 1. Skin Diseases--diagnosis. 2. Skin Diseases--therapy. 3.
Primary Health Care--methods. WR 140 T864d 2005] I. Tennenhouse, Dan J.
II. Russell, John J., MD. III. Title. IV. Series.
  RL71.T76 2005
  616.5--dc22
                                                                  2005012357

Series Editor's Introduction

The diagnosis and treatment of common dermatologic problems is a critical area of skill and knowledge for primary care physicians. According to the US Department of Health and Human Services,[1] patients present to their physicians a skin rash as their chief concern for nearly 12 million office visits each year. In 73% of these office visits, patients see their internist, family physician, or pediatrician. In this respect, astonishingly, primary care clinicians see far more skin disease in their offices than dermatologists. *Dermatology Skills for Primary Care: An Illustrated Guide* advances the targeted skill and knowledge base of primary care physicians, as well as the collaboration between dermatologists and primary care physicians, by its wise choice of organization, scope, and approach.

Dermatology Skills for Primary Care: An Illustrated Guide by Drs. Trozak, Tennenhouse, and Russell is an important addition to the dermatology literature because it has been written collaboratively by a skilled dermatologist and two excellent academic family physicians. As such, the book superbly targets the depth and scope of needs of primary care practitioners in the field of dermatology.

Dermatology Skills for Primary Care: An Illustrated Guide is unique in its approach by opening each chapter with the clinical questions that physicians must answer in approaching patients, and then giving the history, physical examination findings, differential diagnosis, therapeutic options for treatment, and finally explicitly answering the opening questions in each chapter. The book is important in scope, providing in-depth discussions of the most common skin conditions that primary care clinicians encounter.

If a physician knows the contents of this book, he or she will be able to competently take care of more than 90% of the dermatologic problems that are seen in a busy office practice.

That is an accomplishment.

Neil S. Skolnik, MD
Associate Director
Family Practice Residency Program
Abington Memorial Hospital
Abington, PA
Professor of Family and Community Medicine
Temple University School of Medicine
Philadelphia, PA

---

[1]Source: US Department of Health and Human Services, Public Health Service. Centers for Disease Control and Prevention, National Center for Health Statistics, 2002 data. Public Use data file. Table 35a. http://www.aafp.org/x24579.xml (accessed May 2, 2005).

Preface

Skin diseases are a very substantial part of any primary care practice. Unlike most internal conditions, dermatological lesions are apparent to the patient from their inception and the progression is usually readily evident. Accurate prompt diagnosis and appropriate treatment will alleviate a great deal of suffering and reinforce the patient's confidence in the practitioner's skills.

Dermatology Skills for Primary Care: An Illustrated Guide is designed to teach basic skills and to offer an inclusive approach to skin diseases so that primary practitioners can acquire the basic diagnostic and therapeutic skills used by their dermatologic colleagues. Part I reviews the basic skills and tools used in dermatologic diagnosis and also discusses basic principles of topical therapy. The ensuing five parts put these skills into practical scenarios and cover the treatment of specific skin conditions that are frequently encountered in everyday general medicine.

Although *Dermatology Skills for Primary Care: An Illustrated Guide* is not a comprehensive dermatologic reference, practitioners who master the skills in Part I and apply them to the 33 commonly encountered skin conditions in Parts II–VI should be able to practice very credible general dermatology.

Daniel J. Trozak, MD
Dan J. Tennenhouse, MD, JD
John J. Russell, MD

About the Authors

Daniel J. Trozak, MD, FAAD, is a graduate of the University of Michigan School of Medicine and completed his postgraduate training in dermatology at University of Oregon Health Sciences University. He served as a clinical associate professor of dermatology at Stanford University from 1974 to 1992. He has been a consultant in pharmacological research to the Psoriasis Research Institute (Palo Alto, CA) and a consultant in product research to Product Investigations Inc. (Conshohocken, PA). Dr. Trozak has authored and co-authored publications in the areas of melanoma, contact dermatitis, delayed cutaneous hypersensitivity, neuropeptides, and psoriasis. Dr. Trozak has been in the private practice of dermatology in Modesto, California since 1973 and is familiar on a firsthand basis with the dermatological problems that confront primary practitioners on a daily basis.

Dan J. Tennenhouse, MD, JD, FCLM, is a graduate of the University of Michigan School of Medicine and the University of California Hastings College of the Law. Dr. Tennenhouse is a nationally recognized medico-legal consultant, author, and lecturer and has 25 years experience in the practice of primary care medicine at the University of California San Francisco School of Medicine plus more than 30 years experience on the medical school faculty teaching lecture courses. He is the author or co-author of more than 30 references on risk management and medical law.

John J. Russell, MD, AAFP, is a graduate of Pennsylvania State College of Medicine and completed his postgraduate training in family medicine at Abington Memorial Hospital, Abington, Pennsylvania. Since 1993, Dr. Russell has served as assistant and associate director of the Abington Memorial Hospital Family Medicine Program. He is a clinical associate professor of family and community medicine at Temple University School of Medicine and lectures nationally on a variety of medical subjects including asthma, hyperlipidemia, and various aspects of dermatology. He serves as a contributing editor and reviewer for several primary care journals and has authored or co-authored several papers in the areas of dermatology and general medicine.

Contents

Part I: Basic Skills

INTRODUCTION

Few disciplines evoke more mystery and confusion among health care professionals than the examinations and diagnosis of skin disorders. Frequently, fellow physicians whose diagnostic abilities in other areas are sharp and accurate express a sense of absolute helplessness when faced with a common exanthem.

With the current evolutionary changes in the health care system, primary care practitioners are being called on to improve their skills in all areas of medicine including dermatologic diagnosis. Diseases of the skin are a surprisingly large part of primary care practice. The aim of this book is to improve dermatologic skills by presenting a concise, logical, stepwise approach to skin examination. Mastery of these principles will improve your diagnostic accuracy and minimize use of expensive laboratory testing. This is truly "cost-effective" medicine.

Part I is designed to provide the basic skills upon which subsequent disease-specific chapters are based. A thorough knowledge and understanding of these principles is essential.

As in other medical disciplines, accurate diagnosis of skin disorders requires a history and physical examination. After many years of practice, dermatologists become skilled at cutting through the chaff while obtaining a specific history of the immediate problem. This specific history does not replace a general medical history and may, in fact, reveal areas where the general medical history should be amplified. This book will address salient areas of the specific history.

Physical examination of skin lesions is primarily visual and to a lesser extent tactile. Accurate diagnosis is sometimes dependent on subtle changes in color and surface character. Recognizing these changes is a skill acquired over many years. Mastery of the basic information in this book will allow primary care practitioners to improve their skills in diagnosing common skin diseases. Once these principles have been incorporated into your armamentarium, you can go on to acquire a sense of more subtle aspects of dermatologic diagnosis.

Each word in the description of a skin lesion is a meaningful clue. When faced with a difficult diagnostic challenge, these are the basics that a dermatologist will return to in order to obtain a correct answer.

Ask yourself, for instance, "Is the color red, red-yellow, dusky, or bright red? Are these papules dome-shaped, flat-topped, or polygonal?" In this way you will truly begin to see the physical changes which are present—changes that allow dermatologists to distinguish one condition from another.

1 Specific History

CLINICAL APPLICATION QUESTIONS

A 75-year-old white male presents at your office with a history of tenesmus and perirectal pain. He describes extension of pain onto the left posterior thigh. He also has been aware of developing skin discoloration and surface roughness over the area of pain. Moistness and weeping have been present over some of the skin lesions.

1. Why is it important to accurately establish the date of onset of the problem?
2. Why is it important to elicit from this patient's history whether the onset was acute or chronic, or was associated with recurrent attacks and/or exacerbations?
3. What are the reasons you would elicit the sequence of the patient's subjective complaints and observations?
4. What is the reason for determining the sequence of change in specific skin lesions observed by the patient?
5. What is the reason for asking this patient what medications have been used over what time period? What information should be elicited for a thorough medication history?
6. Why would you ask this patient if he has had possible back injuries or chiropractic manipulations, radiation therapy, or chemotherapy?
7. What are the reasons you would ask this patient about prior bowel habits, rectal bleeding, recent stool tests, prior diagnoses of gastrointestinal (GI) disorders, and previous GI-related pain?

APPLICATION GUIDELINES

Onset

Establish accurately the time of onset of the problem. If it is a chronic disorder, document the frequency and duration of individual attacks, exacerbations, or recurrent episodes. Many skin problems have a fairly characteristic age of onset, gender preference, and duration. Recurrences may follow recognizable fixed patterns, which will aid in diagnosis.

Evolution of the Disease Process

Ask the patient to explain in a stepwise fashion what has happened with respect to (1) onset of symptoms, (2) extension or changes in location, (3) onset of associated symptoms (e.g., itch, pain, tenderness), and (4) correlation of the skin findings with any systemic symptoms, such as fatigue, fever, or myalgia. This will give a global view of the illness and help to determine whether this is purely a cutaneous process or is part of a larger systemic problem.

From: *Current Clinical Practice: Dermatology Skills for Primary Care: An Illustrated Guide*
D.J. Trozak, D.J. Tennenhouse, and J.J. Russell © Humana Press, Totowa, NJ

Evolution of Skin Lesions

Have the patient describe, and if possible point out, how the individual skin lesions have evolved. Start with the earliest type of lesion, as these "primary lesions" are often critical clues to the correct diagnosis. Have the patient show you the newest spots (usually the most characteristic primary lesions) and the oldest spots (which will usually have evolved secondary changes). The primary lesion and its evolution in the disease process are fundamental to correct dermatological diagnosis. The evolution of these individual lesions must be understood and considered with the evolution of the whole disease process.

Provoking Factors

Find out if the skin lesions are precipitated or aggravated by any external condition or substances such as heat, cold, sunlight, foods, or medications. This history will often offer a clue as to etiology or may be another sign supporting the diagnosis.

Self-Medication

Unlike many other medical problems, patients often feel comfortable self-treating skin disorders. There are myriad topical proprietary medications available, ranging from low-potency steroids to veterinary preparations. These home remedies or potent steroid creams (often borrowed from friends and relatives) can significantly alter the appearance of the eruption, even though they are ineffective at relieving or resolving it. Knowing what has been used will often explain unusual physical findings or, for instance, the negative potassium hydroxide preparation (*see* Chapter 3) that you expected to be positive.

Supplemental Review From General History

Frequently, clues gleaned from the specific history will point out areas in the general medical history that need to be reviewed in greater depth. For example, a 35-year-old man presents a specific history of an intensely pruritic, scaling skin disorder of 6 to 8 months' duration, suggesting the possibility of an ichthyosis. Family history for similar disturbances is negative, which rules out dominant ichthyosis vulgaris. The symptoms suggest the possibility of acquired ichthyosis, a condition that has been frequently reported with underlying systemic disease. The most common association is with Hodgkin's disease, but it has also been linked to other lymphomas, malnutrition, and occasionally other malignancies. This should prompt a supplemental review from the general history of the patient's dietary pattern, weight gain/loss, adenopathy, and a general review of systems.

ANSWERS TO CLINICAL APPLICATION QUESTIONS

History Review

A 75-year-old white male presents at your office with a history of tenesmus and perirectal pain. He describes extension of pain onto the left posterior thigh. He also has been aware of developing skin discoloration and surface roughness over the area of pain. Moistness and weeping have been present over some of the skin lesions.

1. Why is it important to accurately establish the date of onset of the problem?

Answer: If this problem started 6 days earlier, the differential diagnosis would be very different than if it started 6 weeks earlier. For example, if you were considering a diagnosis of sacral herpes zoster, an onset 6 weeks before would be inconsistent with that diagnosis.

2. Why is it important to elicit from this patient's history whether the onset was acute or chronic, or was associated with recurrent attacks and/or exacerbations?

Answer: An acute or chronic pattern characterizes certain disorders and may help rule out some diagnoses. For example, a chronic pattern in this patient would tend to support a diagnosis of chronic perianal cellulitis or perianal monilia, but not sacral herpes zoster.

3. What are the reasons you would elicit the sequence of the patient's subjective complaints and observations?

Answer: The sequence of complaints may be diagnostic. In this patient, this history can help you distinguish peri-anal cellulitis from sacral herpes zoster.

For example, the history revealed initial tenesmus followed by perirectal pain radiating down one thigh. Four days later, skin lesions were observed to localize in the areas of pain. This sequence is most consistent with sacral herpes zoster. Perianal cellultis can cause tenesmus and local perianal dermatitis, but the pain and skin lesions do not radiate in a segmental fashion. Perianal monilia is usually pruritic and tender but does not cause radiating pain or dermatitis.

4. What is the reason for determining the sequence of change in specific skin lesions observed by the patient?

Answer: On physical examination you should attempt to distinguish among primary lesions, primary lesions with secondary change, and secondary lesions. Determining the sequence of change observed by the patient will assist you in this process.

In addition, the sequence of change may suggest a pattern characteristic of a specific disease process. For example, this patient describes the following sequence of skin changes:

    a. Red discoloration 4 days after the onset of pain.
    b. Surface roughness 48 hours after redness appeared.
    c. Moistness and weeping 12 hours after surface change.

Based on the above sequence, a diagnosis of sacral herpes zoster would be likely.

5. What is the reason for asking this patient what medications have been used over what time period? What information should be elicited for a thorough medication history?

Answer: Antibiotics are a common provoking factor for perianal monilia. Also, when you examine this patient the appearance of the lesions may have been altered by the use of medication. Your history should include over-the-counter (OTC) medications, which often have as great an impact on the morphology of lesions as do prescription medications. You should inquire about use of topical as well as systemic products and treatments borrowed from friends or relatives.

6. Why would you ask this patient if he has had possible back injuries or chiropractic manipulations, radiation therapy, or chemotherapy?

Answer: Back injuries, chiropractic manipulations, radiation therapy, chemotherapy, or other sources of immunosuppression could precipitate herpes zoster. Such provoking factors are not associated with perianal cellulitis.

7. What are the reasons you would ask this patient about prior bowel habits, rectal bleeding, recent stool tests, prior diagnosis of GI disorders, and previous GI-related pain?

Answer: This history will help you unearth previous complaints referable to the GI tract to be certain you do not miss a primary GI problem that might explain the current findings, such as a malignancy or a perianal cellulitis. Bleeding and mucus discharge are common symptoms with perianal cellulitis.

2 Dermatologic Physical Examination

The four components of the dermatologic physical examination are (1) primary lesions, (2) secondary lesions, (3) distribution, and (4) configuration. Because primary and secondary lesions are rather constant with most dermatitides, they should be relied on heavily to lead to the correct diagnosis. The two other basic components of the physical exam, distribution and configuration, are used for support and confirmation. Some skin disorders lack a distinct distribution or configuration. Occasionally, however, these latter components can be so characteristic for certain diseases that they are by themselves diagnostic. When the distribution and configuration are confusing or fail to support a diagnosis, it is wise to rely most heavily on the information and clues from the primary and secondary lesions.

Learn to internalize what you are observing. It is easy to look at a skin rash but not really see it. Look for and think about each of the distinguishing characteristics of the lesion.

Develop skills in:
1. Recognizing primary lesions.
2. Recognizing secondary lesions.
3. Recognizing distribution.
4. Recognizing configuration.
5. Diagnostic aids.

CLINICAL APPLICATION QUESTIONS

You are asked to evaluate a 60-year-old female patient who is obtunded and cannot give a history. Widespread skin lesions are present; however, family members are not helpful as to the onset or evolution of the lesions.

1. Why do you need to be able to distinguish the various types of primary skin lesions from secondary skin lesions?
2. What is a secondary skin lesion, and how does it assist your diagnostic process?
3. You notice that although there are scattered lesions elsewhere, the patient's eruption is concentrated on the palms and dorsum of the hands, dorsal wrists, and distal dorsal forearms. Why is this information useful for assisting a diagnosis?
4. Scattered lesions on this patient's palms and dorsal hands show an iris configuration. How can this information help you to make a diagnosis?

From: *Current Clinical Practice: Dermatology Skills for Primary Care: An Illustrated Guide*
D.J. Trozak, D.J. Tennenhouse, and J.J. Russell © Humana Press, Totowa, NJ

APPLICATION GUIDELINES

Recognizing Primary Lesions

The earliest constant recognizable lesions in a skin disease are called the *primary lesions*. Although some dermatitides have primary lesions that are transient and rarely seen, in most conditions the primary lesion is an important clue to the correct diagnosis. Types of primary lesions include the following:

Macule: A circumscribed alteration in skin color, 1 cm or less in size, without any elevation or depression in relation to the adjacent skin (*see* Figs. 1,2; Photos 1,2).

Patch: A circumscribed alteration in skin color greater than 1 cm in size, without any elevation or depression in relation to the adjacent skin (*see* Figs. 3,4; Photos 3,4).

Papule: A solid lesion elevated above the adjacent skin less than 1 cm in diameter (*see* Figs. 5,6; Photos 5,6).

Nodule: A palpable solid lesion usually greater than 1 cm in diameter, which may or may not be elevated above the level of the adjacent skin (*see* Figs. 7,8; Photos 7,8). The term *nodule* implies a lesion with depth. The term *tumor* is sometimes used to denote a large nodule. Because of the associated implication of malignancy we will avoid its usage here.

Plaque: An elevation, solid and fixed, above the level of the adjacent skin. The diameter is large in relation to its degree of elevation. Plaques may have a smooth surface or, if they arise from a confluence of papules, the surface may be pebbly (*see* Figs. 9,10; Photos 9,10).

Vesicle: A circumscribed fluid-filled lesion less than 0.5 cm in diameter, usually elevated above the level of the adjacent skin. Vesicles may be intraepidermal or subepidermal (*see* Fig. 11; Photo 11).

Bulla: A circumscribed fluid-filled lesion greater than 0.5 cm in diameter elevated above the level of the adjacent skin. Bullae may be intraepidermal or subepidermal (*see* Fig. 11; Photo 11).

Pustule: A circumscribed fluid-filled lesion usually less than 0.5 cm in diameter in which the fluid consists of purulent exudate. Pustules may or may not be elevated. Pustules may be intraepidermal or adnexal in location. Adnexal pustules are those that occur within the ostium of an adnexal skin structure such as a hair follicle or sweat gland (*see* Figs. 12,13; Photos 12,13).

In certain skin disorders, some of the preceding primary lesions may occur as a late event, superimposed on otherwise characteristic primary lesions; for example, vesicles and bullae may occur as a secondary event on the characteristic primary plaque lesions in urticaria. Primary and secondary lesions are not always mutually exclusive.

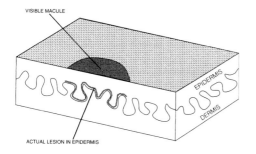

Figure 1: Macule

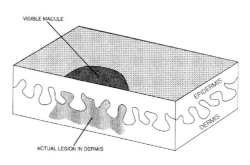

Figure 2: Macule

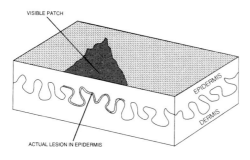

Figure 3: Patch

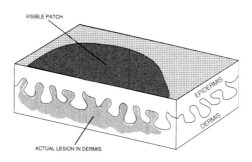

Figure 4: Patch

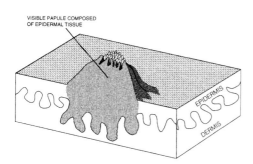

Figure 5: Papule

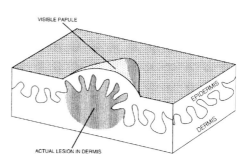

Figure 6: Papule

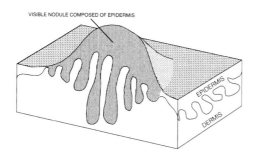

Figure 7: Nodule

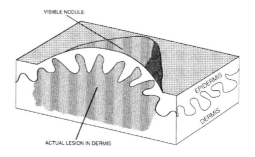

Figure 8: Nodule

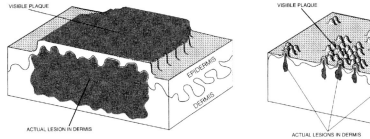

Figure 9: Plaque   Figure 10: Plaque

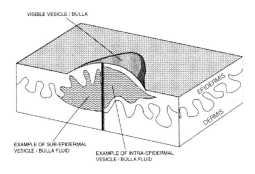

Figure 11: Vesicle/Bulla

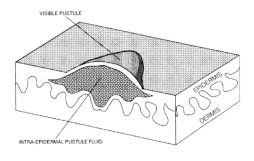

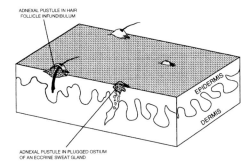

Figure 12: Intra-epidermal pustule   Figure 13: Adnexal pustules

Recognizing Secondary Lesions

Secondary lesions are those that develop as the disease process matures. These secondary lesions may evolve from and replace the primary lesion (e.g., a vesicle may be replaced by crust and scale) or, in other instances, the secondary changes may occur while the primary lesions remain. Under certain conditions, lesions normally considered as primary may in fact be secondary lesions. For example, a group of vesicles become pustular when secondarily infected.

Types of secondary lesions include the following:

Scale: The normal maturation process of the epidermis is called *ortho-keratinization*. Small fragments of the outer stratum corneum are continually shed into the environment in an unnoticed fashion. A scale is a grossly visible piece or plate of stratum corneum; the presence of scale signals an alteration of the process of epidermal maturation. The character of the scale usually offers a clue to the correct diagnosis.

1. **White or brown adherent scale:** An adherent scale is usually a sign of hyperkeratosis, which is a microscopic change in the epidermis indicating excessive maturation and retention of the stratum corneum. Hyperkeratosis is typically seen in certain disorders such as dominant ichthyosis, lichen planus, and discoid lupus erythematosus (*see* Photos 14,15).

2. **Silvery loosely adherent scale:** This distinctly white or silvery scale occurs in disorders with enhanced epidermal turnover, where the upper layers of skin show a disordered, incomplete maturation. This process is termed *parakeratosis* when viewed under the microscope. The silvery snow-white color is due to air spaces between the loose, poorly stacked cells of the upper epidermis. This type of scale is seen in many skin conditions but is especially characteristic of psoriasis (*see* Photo 16).

3. **Seborrheic scale:** This yellow, greasy, loose scale is most often associated with seborrheic dermatitis and microscopically shows changes of parakeratosis similar to silver scale. The altered color and consistency are due to heavy sebum secretion; one could draw an analogy to light flakes of pie crust soaked with cooking oil (*see* Photo 17).

Erosion: A moist circular or oval shallow depression caused by loss of the epidermis. Erosions heal without scar formation and often occur at the base of vesicles, bullae, and pustules. This secondary change is very common with impetigo and cutaneous monilia (*see* Fig. 14; Photo 18).

Necrosis: Literally, this means "a condition of death." In the gross sense, it refers to death of parts or portions of skin lesions, not total death of the whole.

Crust: An accumulation of exudate and/or blood (*see* Fig. 15; Photo 19).

Impetiginization: A superficial honey-colored or purulent exudate. Usually a sign of superficial infection, this change is a characteristic finding in cases of bacterial impetigo. It is seen as a secondary change in many other dermatitides (*see* Photo 20).

Sclerosis:	An alteration in the dermis due to an abnormal accumulation of fluid, connective tissue, or metabolite. This change is best recognized by palpating the affected skin between the thumb and forefinger. The dermis has an inelastic feel, which varies from doughy to rock-hard consistency. Normal surface wrinkling during palpation is reduced or absent. Surface changes that suggest an area of sclerosis include white macule, white patch or white plaque formation, epidermal atrophy, peau d'orange effect, coarse telangiectases, and blotchy hyperpigmentation. Surface change may be entirely absent and sclerosis, which is strictly a dermal process, can be fully appreciated only by touch. Sclerosis is typically seen with morphea and other forms of scleroderma but can also occur in a large number of unrelated skin disorders (*see* Fig. 16; Photo 21).
Excoriations:	A self-excavation usually limited to the epidermis (*see* Photo 22). Excoriations imply the presence of itching, except in dermatitides with heavy psychosomatic overlay or overt delusions. In the latter instances, such changes are deeper and more destructive.
Fissures:	Cleavages or splits in the epidermis that have occurred spontaneously without trauma. Painful fissures are an indication that the split has exposed the underlying dermis. This event usually occurs in very thick or dry epidermis and suggests altered maturation, poor water holding capacity, or both (*see* Fig. 17; Photo 23).
Papillomatosis:	A pebbly epidermal surface caused by a tight grouping or confluence of papules. Papillomatosis may be of epidermal origin or due to an infiltrate filling the papillary dermis (*see* Figs. 18,19; Photos 24,25).
Hypertrichosis:	Excessive hair growth. This change may be generalized or focal. When generalized it suggests a metabolic alteration of the dermis. When focal it is often associated with a focal lesion, scar, or alteration in dermal vasculature.
Hypotrichosis:	Diminished hair growth. This change may be generalized or focal. When generalized it suggests a metabolic alteration of the dermis or widespread fibrosis. When focal it is often associated with a focal lesion or scar. Manipulation of hair can produce breakage or premature epilation, which simulates hypotrichosis.
Lichenification:	An epidermal thickening with a surface pattern of accentuated skin lines. Lichenification is caused by chronic repeated low-grade rubbing or scratching and implies the presence of severe pruritus or dysesthesia. It is characteristically, but not exclusively, found in cases of atopic dermatitis (*see* Photo 22).

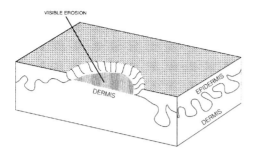

Figure 14: Erosion

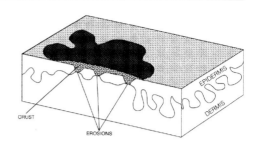

Figure 15: Crust

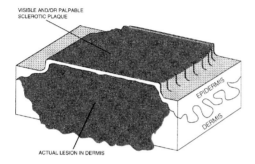

Figure 16: Sclerosis

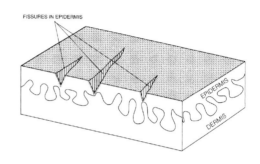

Figure 17: Fissure

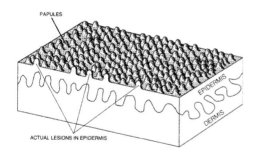

Figure 18: Papillomatosis

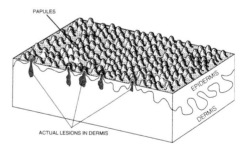

Figure 19: Papillomatosis

Vegetation: A surface alteration caused by tightly packed projections or elevations forming papillary masses. Vegetations may be dry and scaly, soft and smooth, or moist, depending on the underlying cause (*see* Fig. 20; Photo 26).

Eschar: An area of crust and tissue necrosis that will heal with residual scarring (*see* Fig. 21; Photo 27).

Purpura: Discoloration of skin ranging from bright red to deep dusky purple, which is due to extravasation of red blood cells into the skin. Purpura does not blanch with pressure (*see* description diascopy in Diagnostic Aids section).

Atrophy: Loss of tissue by resorption or compression.
1. **Epidermal atrophy:** There is thinning limited to the epidermis, which imparts to the skin surface a translucent, shiny, ironed-out appearance. When the skin is gently pinched between the examiner's fingers, fine, closely aligned wrinkles appear, much like those one would see stretching a cigarette paper (*see* Fig. 22; Photos 4,7,23).
2. **Dermal atrophy:** When limited to the fibrous dermis, this secondary change may or may not be visible. The change is felt by the examiner's finger as a soft area surrounded by a ring of dermis (*see* Fig. 23; Photo 28).
3. **Subcutaneous atrophy:** Usually seen in conjunction with epidermal and dermal atrophy, this atrophy produces a deep visible depression. Vascular structures are often visible at the base of the lesion through the thinned skin layers (*see* Fig. 24; Photo 29).

Ulceration: A loss of epidermis and dermis. Skin ulcers always heal with some residual scar formation (*see* Fig. 25; Photos 30,31).

Scar or Cicatrix: A permanent alteration of normal tissue—in this instance, skin—as a result of injury or disease. Scar formation in skin implies some degree of injury to the dermis with an alteration of the normal connective tissue, which may result in both dermal and epidermal changes.

Gangrene: A sharply demarcated area of tissue death, which usually involves all three skin layers. There are two types of gangrene:
1. **Wet gangrene**, usually due to bacterial infection (*see* Photo 31).
2. **Dry gangrene**, usually due to some vascular event (*see* Photo 32).

Hyperpigmentation: Increased color usually due to deposits of melanin pigment. Hyperpigmentation may be due to enhanced melanin production with storage in the basal epidermis, or to deposits of free melanin or foreign pigment in the dermis following injury or an inflammatory process that disrupts the lower epidermis, releasing basal cell melanin into the dermis (*see* Figs. 26,27; Photos 33,34).

Hypopigmentation: Diminished but not absent melanization due to impaired pigment transfer or enhanced epidermal turnover (*see* Fig. 28; Photo 35).

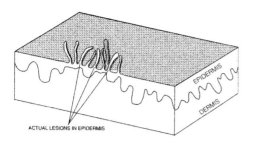

Figure 20: Vegetation

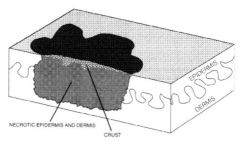

Figure 21: Eschar

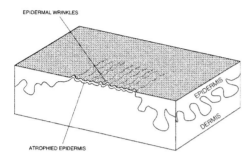

Figure 22: Epidermal atrophy

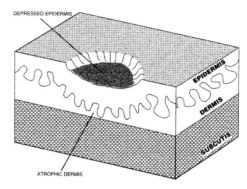

Figure 23: Dermal atrophy

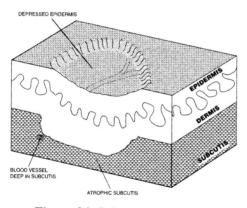

Figure 24: Subcutaneous atrophy

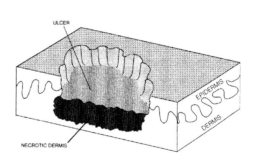

Figure 25: Ulcer

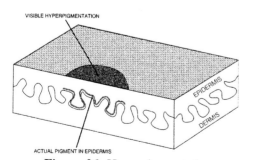

Figure 26: Hyperpigmentation

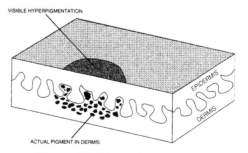

Figure 27: Hyperpigmentation

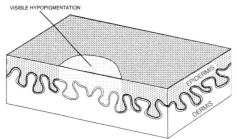
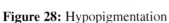

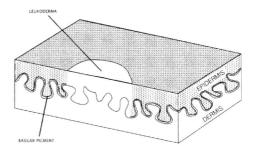

Figure 28: Hypopigmentation   **Figure 29:** Leukoderma

Telangectasia:	Visibly enlarged or dilated small capillaries or slightly larger terminal vessels visible on the skin surface.
Leukoderma:	Total depigmentation. A change characteristic of, but not limited to, vitiligo (*see* Fig. 29; Photo 36).
Calcinosis:	A pathologic condition in which abnormal amounts of calcium are deposited in a tissue where it does not belong—in this instance, areas of damaged skin.
Poikiloderma:	A constellation of secondary features consisting of pigmentary change (hyper, hypo, or both), atrophy, and telangectasia (dilated surface blood vessels). Poikiloderma is a feature of several skin disorders. Its presence, however, directs the dermatologist toward certain specific diagnoses (*see* Photo 37).
Cutaneous horn (cornu cutaneum):	A focal area of hyperkeratosis that takes the shape of a miniature horn. These are almost always associated with premalignant or malignant lesions.

Recognizing Distribution

Distribution refers to specific anatomic sites of predilection on the body at which a particular eruption tends to occur. Distribution should be considered in two ways.

Microanatomic distribution:	Some skin disorders affect or localize around specific structures, e.g., hair follicles or eccrine or apocrine glands. This can produce specific, recognizable patterns that are diagnostic. Examples are:

1. **Herpes zoster:** Follows the course of specific cutaneous sensory nerve trunks; hence a distribution along sensory dermatomes or in the face and scalp, sites that coincide with cranial nerve distribution (*see* Fig. 30).
2. **Hidradenitis supporativa:** This is a disease of apocrine gland-bearing hair follicles and is found in body regions where these structures are located, such as axillae, groin,

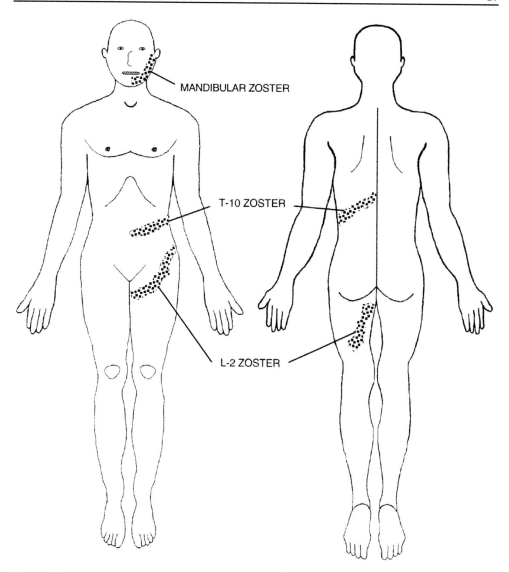

Figure 30: Herpes zoster. Example of microanatomic distribution along neural structures.

inframammary, gluteal, and buttock regions. The examiner must always keep these accessory and adnexal structures in mind and determine whether there is a microanatomic distribution of lesions (*see* Fig. 31).

Macroanatomic distribution: Where on the general skin surface is the eruption? Is it on flexural or on extensor surfaces? Are the lesions grouped around joints or does the rash occur in intertriginous regions? These are important supporting clues to establishing a correct diagnosis.

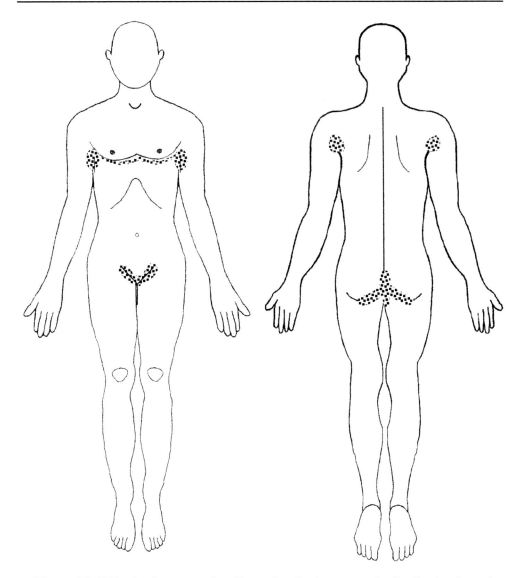

Figure 31: Hidradentis supporativa. Example of microanatomic distribution in region of apocrine glands.

Recognizing Configuration

Configuration is the external form or arrangement of specific skin lesions. When present, configuration may be diagnostic or may point to a very limited list of diagnostic possibilities.

Annular: Round, like a ring. This is one of the more common configurations, and the term is incorporated into the name of several diseases (*see* Photo 38). Other types of annular lesions include the following:

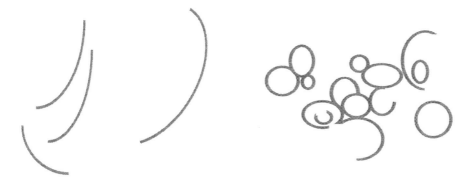

Figure 32: Arciform configuration.   **Figure 33:** Polycyclic configuration.

1. **Arciform:** Shaped in curves or incomplete circles (*see* Fig. 32; Photo 39).
2. **Polycyclic:** Multiple rings or incomplete circles either contained within one another or overlapping. These latter two variations of annular configuration are uncommon and decidedly limit the number of diagnostic possibilities (*see* Fig. 33; Photo 40).

Iris: This configuration alludes to a many-colored lesion of concentric rings, which may show within itself varied surface morphology. A classic example is the target or iris lesion that is pathognomonic of erythema multiforme. When the margins of such a lesion are vesicular it is referred to as the herpes iris of Bateman (*see* Fig. 34; Photo 41).

Serpiginous: This term applies both to the shape of individual lesions and to the way they evolve and multiply. The term means serpentine or snakelike, and can refer to lesions that have the shape or curl of a resting snake. Serpiginous can also refer to a dermatosis where the individual lesions progress by crawling along in a linear pattern (*see* Fig. 35; Photo 42).

Linear: A dermatosis that occurs along a stripe or line. Linear lesions are quite striking because they often extend across physically diverse skin regions. Keep in mind that linear lesions may have skip areas; one should always look distal and proximal to the main lesion to be certain of the full extent of the problem (*see* Fig. 36; Photo 43).

Zosteriform: Refers to the shape or form of a girdle. This is a classic configuration of herpes zoster. Here is an example of how the various elements of the dermatologic physical exam fit together: Grouped (configuration) vesicles (primary lesions) on an

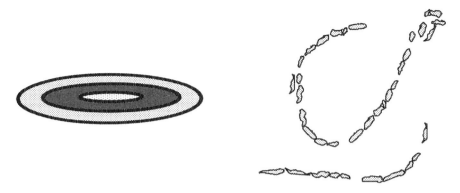

Figure 34: Iris configuration.   **Figure 35:** Serpiginous configuration.

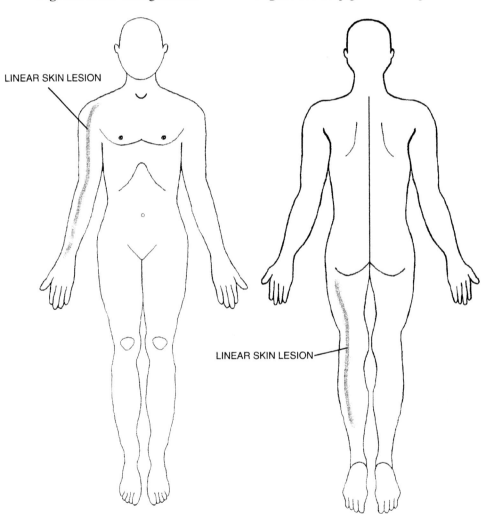

Figure 36: Linear configuration.

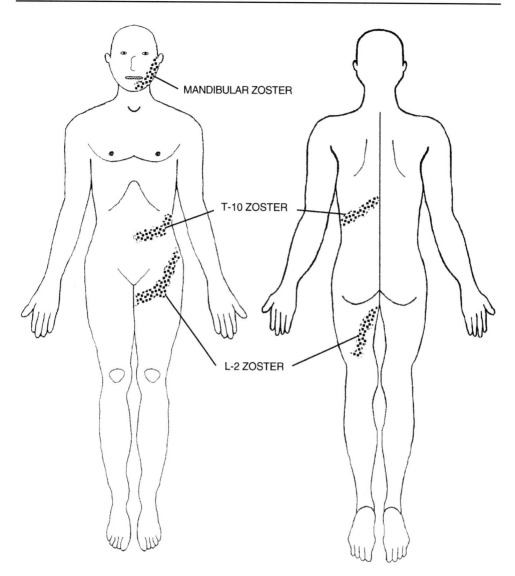

MANDIBULAR ZOSTER

T-10 ZOSTER

L-2 ZOSTER

Figure 37: Zosteriform configuration.

urticarial plaque (second primary lesion) following a unilateral, zosteriform pattern (distribution and second configuration) is diagnostic. Many other dermatitides show a zosteriform configuration but other elements of the examination are different (*see* Fig. 37; Photo 44).

Grouped: This configuration is almost self-explanatory and refers to similar skin lesions that occur in proximity to one another to form a distinct larger entity. Grouping is quite common and must be

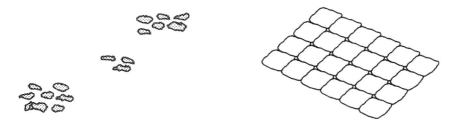

Figure 38: Grouped configuration.   **Figure 39:** Retiform configuration.

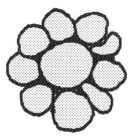

Figure 40: Corymbiform configuration.

	combined with the other elements of the exam so that a diagnostic picture can emerge (*see* Fig. 38; Photo 45).

Retiform: Shaped like a net, this is an uncommon configuration that, when present, greatly narrows the diagnostic possibilities (*see* Fig. 39; Photo 46).

Corymbiform: Resembling a cluster of flowers. This configuration is rare, and is characteristic of certain lesions of secondary syphilis. It can also occur occasionally with mosaic types of verrucous warts (*see* Fig. 40; Photo 47).

Diagnostic Aids

The following are some simple diagnostic aids and tips that are peculiar to the dermatologic examination:

Color examination: In addition to the features noted above, the color of an eruption is often a critical clue.
1. Bright to dusky red color usually indicates enhanced blood flow due to hyperemia or flow through ectatic (dilated) vessels. If intravascular, the color should blanch with diascopy.
2. Dark blue to purple-black color suggests a stagnant low blood flow condition. If the color fails to blanch with diascopy (*see* later text), consider extravascular deposits

such as red blood cells (purpura or hematoma), melanin, graphite, or other pigments free in the tissue.

3. Brown discoloration is caused by melanin or hemosiderin deposits. As melanin is deposited more deeply in the dermis the physics of color contrast, light reflectance, and the absorption of wavelengths change the color from tan to brown to dark brown, then blue to blue-black.

4. White color can signify diminished melanin content or absent melanin, as seen in vitiligo. It may also indicate intense local vasospasm, a metabolic dermal infiltrate, or dermal fibrosis. Melanin disturbances can be distinguished on physical exam using diascopy and Wood's lamp exam. They do not change with diascopy; however, they are usually accentuated by Wood's lamp exam. The white color of vascular spasm, metabolic infiltrates, and fibrosis will disappear with diascopy and are not accentuated with the Wood's lamp (*see* later text).

5. Intense yellow-white color is usually due to deposits of lipids or altered connective tissue.

6. Yellow to orange color is caused by the presence of bile or carotene.

7. Gray, blue-gray, to black stains are usually due to deeply deposited melanin, heavy metals, graphite, silica, or the metabolites of certain medications (e.g., desipramine)

Magnification: Use of magnification with a simple handheld magnifier during the visual exam serves two purposes. It may reveal features that are not evident with the naked eye, and the act of using the lens often enhances the examiner's concentration.

Lighting: Proper examination of the skin requires a good color-balanced light source that can be moved around the subject and can be positioned to provide side lighting from various angles. Some skin lesions such as actinic keratoses are visible only by this means. In addition, good lighting is important when assessing surface characteristics such as papillomatosis or a subtle depression. We recommend ceiling-mounted tungsten incandescent lights with a 9-inch reflector. These are shielded with a color-balanced, blue-tinted, quartz shell. This allows the light to be used in varied positions and at different distances. Light sources that are dull, glaring, or overly blue or yellow will obscure findings and make the exam more difficult.

Tactile examination:

1. Skin surface temperature by feel gives a clue as to the degree of blood flow. An inflammatory skin condition such as an eczema is red due to vasodilation but is not warm like

the marked hyperemia of a cellulitis. Diminished temperature can confirm a clinical impression of local vascular insufficiency or intense vasospasm.

2. Light touch, accomplished by lightly sliding fingertips over the skin surface, will often reveal lesions that are not readily visible. This is especially true of actinic keratosis.

3. Palpation done gently over lesions will reveal subtle changes such as the outlines of a plaque or nodule or an area of dermal atrophy that is not visible on the surface. One can also determine the consistency of a lesion, whether soft, firm, hard, or fluid-filled, or whether it is pulsatile or compressible.

4. Pinching—that is, gently palpating the skin from side to side between the fingers—allows the examiner to assess the condition of the dermis for thickening or sclerosis and at the same time observe the wrinkle pattern on the surface —if accentuated like a stretched cigarette paper, this suggests epidermal atrophy.

5. Stroking the skin surface firmly with either a fingernail or a blunt instrument will reveal features such as the exaggerated triple response of Lewis seen in immediate dermographism or white dermographism, which is characteristic of atopic dermatitis. The same maneuver applied to most lesions of cutaneous mastocytosis elicits a wheal response referred to as Darier's sign.

Diascopy: This simple technique is performed by compressing the skin surface with a glass microscope slide or a clear plastic stent. Most vascular lesions will empty and will partially or totally disappear, while solid or pigmented lesions remain unchanged (*see* Photos 46,48). This technique can differentiate, for instance, a large venous ectasia on the ear from a developing melanoma. It will distinguish vascular ectasia (intravascular blood) from purpura (extravascular blood) and by subtracting dusky erythema it may reveal dermal hemorrhage that is not otherwise evident. Light pressure over vascular lesions will often reveal arterial pulsations, giving an additional clue as to the true anatomic structure. Diascopy of papular lesions composed of dense granulomatous or lymphoid infiltrates will accentuate the lesions and impart an amber-yellow or so-called "apple jelly" color. This change is seen in granuloma annulare, cutaneous sarcoid, some forms of cutaneous tuberculosis, and certain benign and malignant lymphocytic infiltrates.

Wood's lamp   A long ultraviolet lamp or so-called "black light" has a number
examination: of uses and is a helpful clinical screening tool. Inexpensive battery-powered Wood's lights are available.

1. Certain microsporum fungi (canis, audouini, distortum and ferruginium) produce pigments that give a brilliant green fluorescence when exposed to this light. Once a major screening tool for tinea capitis, black-light exam's usefulness has diminished as *M. audouini* has been replaced by other nonfluorescent species. Favus, an indolent form of tinea capitis caused by *T. schoenleinii,* gives off a dull gray-green color.

2. *Pseudomonas pyocyanea* secretes pyocyanin, which emits a yellow-green color, while the organisms of erythrasma emit a porphyrin, which fluoresces a brilliant coral pink. Similar coral-pink fluorescence is seen in some cases of trichomycosis axillaris.

3. Wood's lamp light will also cause a pink-red to orange-red color in urine and fecal samples of some patients with porphyria cutanea tarda (*see* Photo 49).

4. Wood's lamp examination is also useful in the evaluation of pigmentary disturbances. It helps to distinguish partial pigment loss (hypopigmentation) from absolute pigment loss (leukoderma) and also helps to delineate the extent of the disturbance. Conditions such as tinea versicolor and pityriasis alba accentuate as lighter areas. Tinea versicolor with scale may also show pale yellow fluorescence. Vitiligo, where there is complete pigment loss, has a stark white appearance.

5. In conditions in which there is hyperpigmentation, Wood's lamp exam helps to locate the depth and extent of the pigment and, to some degree, predicts the relative success of therapy. Melanin in the epidermis or high dermis is accentuated and appears as dark areas. Pigment in the mid- and deep dermis is not accentuated.

Basic Equipment List for Dermatologic Exam

1. A movable tungsten balanced light source so that the skin can be evaluated at various angles.
2. A simple hand lens or magnifying glass.
3. A small caliper for measuring lesions.
4. A glass slide or clear plastic stent for diascopy.
5. A Wood's lamp (inexpensive battery powered models are available and convenient)

ANSWERS TO CLINICAL APPLICATION QUESTIONS

History Review

You are asked to evaluate a 60-year-old female patient who is obtunded and cannot give a history. Widespread skin lesions are present; however, family members are not helpful as to the onset or evolution of the lesions.

1. Why do you need to be able to distinguish the various types of primary skin lesions from secondary skin lesions?

Answer: Examination of this obtunded woman reveals red macules 3 mm to 1 cm in size, erythematous papules, small and large erythematous plaques up to several centimeters in size, and occasional intact vesicles and bullae filled with clear amber fluid. These are primary, not secondary, lesions. The presence of several different types of primary lesions within the same eruption strongly suggests erythema multiforme. Vesiculobullous drug eruptions, pemphigus vulgaris, bullous pemphigoid, and other major blistering disorders may have a similar appearance but rarely show discrete papular lesions. Blistering viral exanthems usually contain vesicles of uniform size. The presence of bullae in this eruption suggests something other than a viral exanthem.

2. What is a secondary skin lesion, and how does it assist your diagnostic process?

Answer: Secondary skin lesions are changes that evolve from a maturing primary lesion. They are the result of varying degrees and types of injury to the skin. If you cannot distinguish secondary from primary lesions, you cannot identify the primary lesions that are usually essential to the diagnosis. In addition, secondary lesions often offer a clue as to the degree of skin damage, which may alter treatment options.

Erosions may be secondary to epidermal damage caused by vesicle and blister formation. Purpura may occur when there is a significant amount of vascular injury. Necrosis and ulceration can follow severe vascular injury. The presence of secondary lesions such as purpura, erosions, necrosis, and ulceration can assist in identifying the degree of injury in erythema multiforme and in supporting the diagnosis.

3. You notice that although there are scattered lesions elsewhere, the patient's eruption is concentrated on the palms and dorsum of the hands, dorsal wrists, and distal dorsal forearms. Why is this information useful for assisting a diagnosis?

Answer: Many skin disorders have a typical pattern of macrodistribution, which may assist in making a diagnosis. In some conditions, the distribution may be pathognomonic. The pattern of distribution in this patient makes a diagnosis of pemphigus and bullous pemphigoid unlikely. They are usually more generalized. The macrodistribution pattern in this patient suggests erythema multiforme.

4. Scattered lesions on this patient's palms and dorsal hands show an iris configuration. How can this information help you to make a diagnosis?

Answer: Some skin disorders have a typical configuration that may assist or confirm the diagnosis. With the other physical findings, the iris configuration in this patient is pathognomonic for erythema multiforme.

3 Indicated Supporting Diagnostic Data

Examination of the skin remains a discipline that relies heavily on the basic clinical skills of vision and touch. If this information is combined with the practitioner's knowledge of the disease process, the correct diagnosis can be determined with a minimum of expensive laboratory testing. The dermatologist usually orders labwork to confirm a diagnosis or to stage the disease process rather than using it to seek a diagnosis. After all, the disease process is evolving before your eyes. In addition to the standard testing that is done to support or confirm a clinical diagnosis, there are certain special tests that are common in a dermatologic evaluation.

1. Potassium hydroxide exam (KOH test).
2. Tzanck preparation.
3. Ectoparasite exam (scabies preparation).
4. Skin biopsy.

CLINICAL APPLICATION QUESTIONS

A 25-year-old woman requests evaluation for symmetric white macules and patches on her neck and upper torso. She has recently read about vitiligo on the internet and is terrified of permanent disfigurement. Examination reveals oval thumbprint-size white macules and larger confluent patches with smooth margins. Gentle scraping of a lesion raises a loose white scale.

1. Would a KOH examination be of value for this patient, and if so, why?
2. Would a Tzanck preparation be of any value for this patient, and if so, why?
3. Would biopsy be of any value for this patient, and if so, why?

A patient presents with an irregular erythematous scaling patch 1.7 cm in size on the dorsum of the right foot extending into the first interdigital web. The lesion has been present for 2 years, has gradually enlarged, and itches occasionally. In addition to the other features, examination reveals a thready, slightly raised, translucent margin.

4. Would a KOH examination be of value for this patient, and if so, why?
5. Would biopsy be of any value for this patient, and if so, why?

APPLICATION GUIDELINES

Potassium Hydroxide Exam (KOH Test)

This test is done most often to confirm the presence of a dermatophyte fungus, candida, or the organisms of tinea versicolor. The skin surface of the affected area is swabbed

From: *Current Clinical Practice: Dermatology Skills for Primary Care: An Illustrated Guide*
D.J. Trozak, D.J. Tennenhouse, and J.J. Russell © Humana Press, Totowa, NJ

with alcohol and scale is gently scraped from the advancing edge of the lesion, or in the case of a vesicular tinea, an inverted blister roof makes an excellent specimen. The scale or inverted blister roof is placed on a glass microscope slide and a cover slip is placed on top. Using the edge of the cover slip for capillary action, 20% potassium hydroxide solution with 37% DMSO is slowly flooded around the scale. The specimen is then gently heated over an alcohol lamp short of the boiling point. Gentle compression on the cover slip over the scale (smashing) will distribute the solution and speed clearing of the specimen. Within 3 to 5 minutes most specimens can be read. The degree of separation of the epidermal cells will tell you if adequate clearing has occurred.

Experience is essential for reliable reading of a KOH skin preparation. Today, the average clinical laboratory lacks personnel who are adept at this exam. It is best for the practitioner to personally acquire this skill. Prior treatment with topical antifungals or even a small amount of ointment base on the area can cause a false-negative exam.

Examples:

1. Dermatophyte fungi will show long or short branched hyphae, depending on the organism (*see* Photo 50).
2. In tinea versicolor, the hyphae are plump, short, and not branched. In addition, clusters of round spores like grapes on a vine are also present (*see* Photo 51).
3. Candida will show short pseudohyphae and round spores, with and without budding (*see* Photo 52).

Tzanck Preparation

This simple test can give a very rapid confirmation of the presence of infection by either herpes simplex or herpes zoster (varicella) virus. A typical fresh blister is gently unroofed and the blister base is scraped short of producing bleeding. The material obtained is smeared on a glass microscope slide and is stained with giemsa, toluidine blue, or Wright's stain. A positive smear will show epidermal keratinocytes with ballooning nuclei (a marked increase of nuclear-to-cytoplasmic ratio), and large syncytial multinucleated giant cells (most characteristic) (*see* Photo 53). Although this confirms the presence of a herpetic infection, it cannot distinguish one herpesvirus from the other.

Other viruses have been occasionally reported to have positive findings on Tzanck preparation, and it has also been used in the initial evaluation of certain of the major blistering diseases. These are beyond the scope of this book.

Ectoparasite Exam (Scabies Preparation)

This test is done in the same way as the KOH exam. Look for track lesions or early blisters around the fingers, wrists, or ankles. Scrape or very superficially shave them. The slide should be examined in its entirety for the presence of adult mites, nymphs, ova, or egg casings (*see* Photo 54). Any of these elements confirms the diagnosis.

Skin Biopsy

Tissue examination is undertaken for the following four main reasons:

1. As a diagnostic tool for a lesion or an eruption that is vexing to the practitioner.
2. To confirm a clinical impression.

3. To stage a tumor and therefore determine how aggressive the surgical approach needs to be.

4. To confirm what was already removed.

Whenever tissue is excised, it should be submitted for microscopic confirmation. **Failure to do this in the present medical-legal climate is an invitation to disaster.**

Dermatologists biopsy common skin conditions only when there is a question as to the actual diagnosis, or when there is a meaningful differential diagnosis requiring exclusion. Biopsy is an expensive and invasive procedure that leaves a permanent scar. It should be done only when there are clear indications and there is a reasonable possibility that the test will provide worthwhile data.

Performing skin biopsies to compensate for clinical inadequacies is inappropriate, costly, and not in the patient's best interest. As with any other test, the benefits depend on the skill of the practitioners who are involved. A skin biopsy must be adequately performed and the tissue should be examined by someone skilled in dermatopathology.

Because dermatologists have extensive training in skin pathology, many read their own biopsy tissue, and their ability in this sphere exceeds that of most general pathologists. There are also dermatologists and pathologists who have a separate board certification in skin pathology. It is strongly recommended that skin biopsies be read by a person with special competency. Biopsy may be incisional or excisional.

Incisional biopsy: Partial or incisional biopsies are performed to establish a diagnosis or to remove a lesion with a minimum of scarring while acquiring an adequate specimen to evaluate the histology. The four types of incisional biopsy are punch incision, shave incision, saucerization, and elliptical incision.

1. **Punch incision biopsy:** The most common type of skin biopsy performed. Under a local infiltration anesthetic, a dermal punch is applied and with a rotating motion the cutting edge is driven through the epidermis and dermis into the subcutaneous fat. The disk of skin is then atraumatically elevated with toothed forceps and is snipped as deep as possible at the base of the specimen. Cutting the disk superficially may miss the important histologic changes. Hemostatis is then achieved by electrocautery, aluminum chloride solution, Monsel's solution, or suturing (*see* Fig. 41).

   The size punch used depends on the site and the purpose of the biopsy. In cosmetically sensitive areas small 2- to 3-mm punches are preferred provided they are judged large enough to obtain the desired information. Larger specimens 4- to 8-mm in size may be needed to obtain enough tissue for the diagnosis of certain eruptions or when the intention is complete removal of a small lesion. Disposable elliptical punches in graded sizes are also available for removal of small benign lesions, which then allows the resulting wound to be sutured like a small elliptical excision. Suturing small punch biopsies of 2- to 3-mm is of no benefit and may accentuate scarring on the nasal skin. Suturing at other sites is at the discretion of the physician but is usually done when the punch is done for cosmetic removal of a benign lesion or when biopsying a cosmetically sensitive area.

   The specimen should be taken from the most representative part of the dermatosis or lesion. With annular lesions, the active margin usually shows the most representative change. In blistering diseases, a biopsy of a whole, intact new

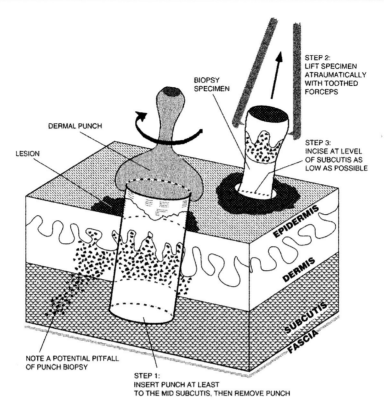

STEP 2:
LIFT SPECIMEN
ATRAUMATICALLY
WITH TOOTHED
FORCEPS

BIOPSY
SPECIMEN

DERMAL PUNCH

LESION

STEP 3:
INCISE AT LEVEL
OF SUBCUTIS AS
LOW AS POSSIBLE

EPIDERMIS

DERMIS

SUBCUTIS

FASCIA

NOTE A POTENTIAL PITFALL
OF PUNCH BIOPSY

STEP 1:
INSERT PUNCH AT LEAST
TO THE MID SUBCUTIS, THEN REMOVE PUNCH

Figure 41: Punch incision biopsy.

blister is usually best. If none are present, then a specimen from the interface at the edge of a blister should be taken. In an inflammatory disorder with papules, biopsy should include an intact papular area. With other inflammatory disorders, try to biopsy the most developed or infiltrated portion. It is best to avoid necrotic, traumatized, crusted, or ulcerated sites, as these usually yield little information. Also try to avoid sites that have been modified by treatment. The specimen is then placed in fixative and is submitted with a careful description of the anatomic site and the lesion from which it was taken.

Because punch biopsy usually obtains only a partial specimen, the limitations of the technique must be kept in mind. For instance, this type of biopsy is not recommended for the diagnosis of melanoma because the small specimen may not be representative of the full depth of invasion just a few millimeters away. Common basal cell cancers often have skip areas. If a biopsy is negative on a very suspect lesion, a repeat biopsy should be done.

2. **Shave incision biopsy:** A superficial partial removal that is done by literally shaving the lesion flush with the adjacent epidermis and is completed by very gently blending the edges with light electrocautery and a sharp dermal or ear curette. This type of biopsy is reserved for raised, presumably benign lesions occurring on sites that are cosmetically sensitive.

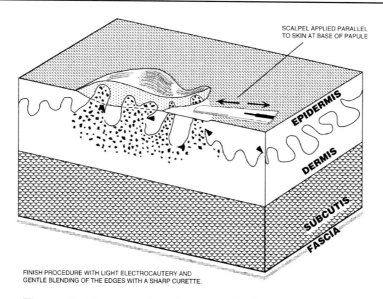

SCALPEL APPLIED PARALLEL
TO SKIN AT BASE OF PAPULE

EPIDERMIS

DERMIS

SUBCUTIS

FASCIA

FINISH PROCEDURE WITH LIGHT ELECTROCAUTERY AND
GENTLE BLENDING OF THE EDGES WITH A SHARP CURETTE.

Figure 42: Shave incision biopsy of a benign papular lesion.

Shave biopsy should be avoided on suspect melanomas or common skin cancers. The procedure destroys the interface at the base of the tumor and interferes with depth staging, which is critical in treating a melanoma. In common tumors, it obscures the lateral margins, making definitive excision margins more difficult to judge (*see* Fig. 42).

3. **Saucerization biopsy:** A technique used by some dermatologists to remove pigmented lesions for evaluation. It is basically a shave biopsy that is carried into the dermis to the depth of the dermal subcutaneous interface. This technique should be discouraged. Not only is there the risk of missing or destroying important histology, but the procedure also usually leaves wide, unattractive scars (*see* Fig. 43).

4. **Elliptical incision biopsy:** Performed to obtain a representative section of a lesion that cannot be easily biopsied by complete excision. This may be indicated by the lesion's large size or because it is in a critical anatomic location. It should be considered when the practitioner finds or expects a punch biopsy to be inadequate. This type of biopsy is performed by taking an ellipse 2 to 3 mm wide across the center of the lesion from one interface to the other. The specimen should extend well into the subcutaneous tissue, preferably to the superficial fascia. Closure is accomplished with suture. The specimen should then be sectioned parallel to its long axis and read (*see* Fig. 44).

When possible, avoid incisional biopsies from the following:

1. Cosmetically critical sites.
2. Ankle and pretibial areas, especially when there is an established circulatory disorder.
3. Shoulder, upper arm, upper chest, and back, which are areas of thick scarring.

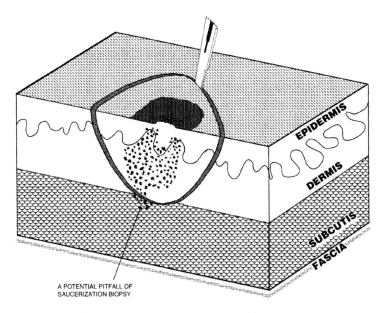

A POTENTIAL PITFALL OF
SAUCERIZATION BIOPSY

Figure 43: Saucerization biopsy of a pigmented nevus.

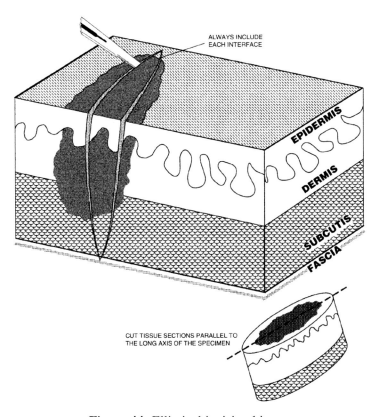

ALWAYS INCLUDE
EACH INTERFACE

CUT TISSUE SECTIONS PARALLEL TO
THE LONG AXIS OF THE SPECIMEN

Figure 44: Elliptical incision biopsy.

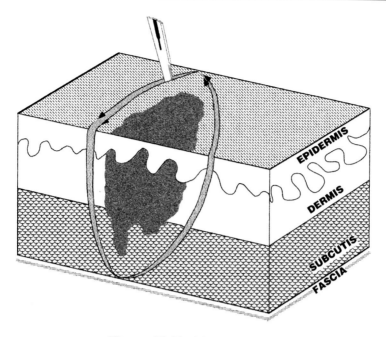

Figure 45: Excisional biopsy.

Absolutely avoid incisional biopsies from the following unless they have been thoroughly evaluated and immediate adequate surgical backup is available:

1. Compressible lesions.
2. Pulsating lesions.
3. Midline lesions of the face and scalp.
4. Scalp lesions that overlie suture lines or fontanels, are by history congenital, or occur at a site of cranial trauma or surgery.

Excisional biopsy: Performed whenever the patient desires removal of the lesion and the scar is an acceptable tradeoff. This is also the preferred method of biopsy for suspect pigmented lesions where melanoma enters into the differential diagnosis. The margins of the excision are determined by the site and the nature of the lesion removed, but should be generous enough to accomplish complete removal (*see* Fig. 45).

ANSWERS TO CLINICAL APPLICATION QUESTIONS

History Review 1

A 25-year-old woman requests evaluation for symmetric white macules and patches on her neck and upper torso. She has recently read about vitiligo on the Internet and is terrified of permanent disfigurement. Examination reveals oval thumbprint-size white macules and larger confluent patches with smooth margins. Gentle scraping of a lesion raises a loose white scale.

1.   Would a KOH examination be of value for this patient, and if so, why?

Answer: KOH examination should be performed when you suspect a yeast infection such as tinea versicolor (*Pityrosporum obiculare*) or monilia (*Candida* species). When combined with physical findings, a positive test is diagnostic.

If a KOH examination of this patient reveals short plump, non-branched hyphae and clusters of round spores, this would confirm a diagnosis of tinea versicolor. The pigmentary change in this disorder resolves with adequate treatment of the yeast infection.

2.   Would a Tzanck preparation be of any value for this patient, and if so, why?

Answer: No. A Tzanck preparation is used primarily to diagnose herpetic skin infections.

3.   Would biopsy be of any value for this patient, and if so, why?

Answer: If the patient has a repeatedly negative KOH exam and has not recently received any effective treatment for tinea versicolor, biopsy may be indicated. In this rare circumstance, the decision regarding biopsy and special pigment stains should be made by a dermatologic consultant.

History Review 2

A patient presents with an irregular erythematous scaling patch 1.7 cm in size on the dorsum of the right foot extending into the first interdigital web. The lesion has been present for 2 years, has gradually enlarged, and itches occasionally. In addition to the other features, examination reveals a thready, slightly raised, translucent margin.

4.   Would a KOH examination be of value for this patient, and if so, why?

Answer: A KOH examination should be performed on a sample from the active margin of the lesion. If this is tinea pedis, KOH examination is an inexpensive and noninvasive test. A positive examination that shows long branching hyphae would confirm the presence of a dermatophyte fungal infection.

5.   Would biopsy be of any value for this patient, and if so, why?

Answer: If the KOH examination is negative, biopsy would be indicated for this patient. The biopsy specimen should be taken from the thready advancing margin. Biopsy in this case may show a superficial spreading basal cell carcinoma, *in situ* squamous cell carcinoma (Bowen's disease), or a subacute eczema.

4 Therapy

Dermatologic treatment usually involves the use of topical therapy, which is a discipline unto itself. This form of treatment was primarily an art until about 20 years ago. Since then science has begun to unravel the biology of the epidermis, making it a more scientific process. Much of topical therapy is simply not written down and it is more complicated than the old bromide, "If it's wet, dry it; if it's dry, wet it." This discussion will cover some basic principles of topical therapy, but is by no means exhaustive. As with any form of treatment, there are rules to follow and precautions to take.

This chapter will discuss the following topics:

1. Percutaneous absorption.
2. Vehicles.
3. Occlusion.
4. Topical steroids.
5. Emollients.
6. Enhancers.
7. Other topical agents.
8. Systemic steroid therapy.
9. Intralesional steroid therapy.
10. Antihistamines.

CLINICAL APPLICATION QUESTIONS

An 11-month-old infant presents at your office with an intensely pruritic generalized atopic dermatitis with multiple areas of excoriation and lichenification in some flexor locations. The eruption spares only the diaper area, the palms, and the soles. Most skin regions are dry and fissured.

1. Should you treat this patient with topical steroids, and if so, what type of topical steroids?
2. Should you treat this patient with systemic steroids, and if so, what type of systemic steroids?
3. Should you apply occlusive dressings in this patient over the affected areas, and if so, what type of occlusive dressings?
4. Should you treat this patient with an emollient, and if so, why?
5. Is this patient an appropriate candidate for antihistamines, and if so, why?

From: *Current Clinical Practice: Dermatology Skills for Primary Care: An Illustrated Guide*
D.J. Trozak, D.J. Tennenhouse, and J.J. Russell © Humana Press, Totowa, NJ

Percutaneous Absorption

The stratum corneum is the major barrier to any substance applied to the skin surface. Removing this layer increases permeability by a factor of 10^4. The skin surface shows marked variation in permeability and can be divided into four separate regions (*see* Fig. 46).

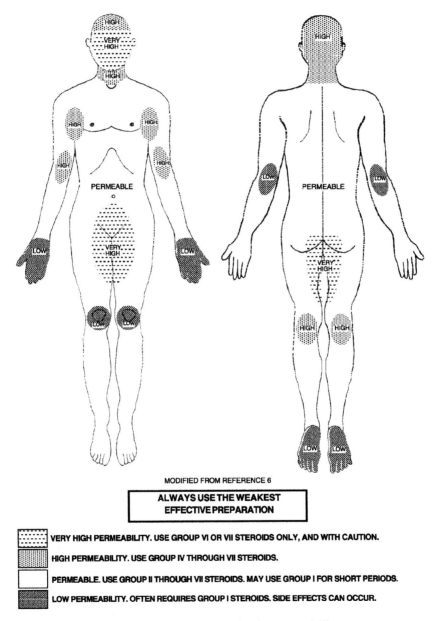

MODIFIED FROM REFERENCE 6

ALWAYS USE THE WEAKEST EFFECTIVE PREPARATION

VERY HIGH PERMEABILITY. USE GROUP VI OR VII STEROIDS ONLY, AND WITH CAUTION.

HIGH PERMEABILITY. USE GROUP IV THROUGH VII STEROIDS.

PERMEABLE. USE GROUP II THROUGH VII STEROIDS. MAY USE GROUP I FOR SHORT PERIODS.

LOW PERMEABILITY. OFTEN REQUIRES GROUP I STEROIDS. SIDE EFFECTS CAN OCCUR.

Figure 46: Regions of skin permeability.

Regions of low permeability will be most resistant to the effects and side effects of topical agents. Those with high permeability will respond more readily to treatment, but are more prone to complications.

Because the epidermis is the major barrier, abraded or damaged skin will be more susceptible to the effects and side effects of topically applied substances. Atopic dermatitis, exfoliative eruptions, and skin that is fissured or ulcerated exhibit enhanced absorption of applied substances because of alterations and breaks in the barrier. Typical plaque psoriasis has an absorptive capacity similar to normal skin; however, thick scale or crusting will markedly decrease the absorptive capacity.

Other factors that affect penetration include the molecular structure of the active medication, the vehicle, occlusion, and additives such as urea and salicylic acid.

A warning regarding topical therapy in infants and children is warranted. Although most studies show similar barrier function in children and adults, children show greater percutaneous absorption of topical agents such as corticosteroids. This is explained by the child's increased skin-surface-to-weight ratio and the occlusive effect of diapers and plastic pants when medication is applied to the diaper area.

All these factors should be considered when prescribing a topical agent.

Vehicles

The delivery of a compound to the stratum corneum is a complex interaction between the vehicle and the active moiety. In general, gel and ointment vehicles are more effective in this regard than are creams and lotions. "Optimized" vehicles have altered this old rule so that some steroid preparations now have cream and ointment bases of equivalent potency. The vehicle also affects treatment by the degree of patient acceptance and, therefore, compliance.

Gels: Apply easily and disappear without a visible residue. Unfortunately, most have a high propylene glycol content and burn or sting when applied to abraded or intertriginous skin. They are most useful on the scalp and hair-bearing regions of the trunk where the epidermis is thick.

Ointments: Are composed primarily of petrolatum and tend to be simple vehicles. They have the drawback of leaving a distinct residue that imparts a greasy feel and a shiny appearance. They also discolor clothing worn over the site. Ointments are best used on dry scaling lesions. They seldom burn or sting and restore moisture and flexibility to the surface. They are also valuable in patients who are allergic to the more complex cream bases. Do not use them to treat macerated, moist, or oozing lesions.

Creams: Are the most popular topical vehicles because they feel cool and soothing when applied and disappear shortly after application. Except for the products with optimized vehicles, most creams are weaker than their ointment counterparts. They have high patient acceptance and can be used in most locations except dense hairy areas and ear canals, where an unacceptable accumulation of base occurs. Creams with high propylene glycol content will sting when applied to abraded sites.

Lotions: Are liquid preparations that leave a minimal residue. The base may be predominantly alcohol, propylene glycol, or an oil-in-water emulsion. Alcohol-based lotions are dispensed in dropper bottles and are most effective in the scalp, where they leave no residue and do not alter the hair texture or manageability. Because of their drying effect and irritancy, usage is limited. Propylene glycol-based lotions are also used primarily in thick hair-bearing regions and seem to penetrate thick scale more effectively. Unfortunately they give the hair a matted, shiny appearance, which makes compliance a problem. Oil-in-water emulsion bases are soothing and disappear rapidly without visible residue. They are usually employed in moist macerated sites or on exposed skin such as the face. They have high patient acceptance.

Foams: Are the newest vehicles available and have been devised to replace older spray products that have been phased out because of their banned propellants. These foam products rapidly melt at skin temperature into a liquid form with minimal residue and are particularly useful in dense hair-bearing areas such as the scalp. Foams appear similar to gel vehicles in their ability to release the active ingredient. Those currently available sting when applied to open or abraded areas, however.

Occlusion

Occlusive therapy with impermeable wraps can greatly enhance the penetration of topical corticoids but is associated with increased side effects and complications. Because of the increased efficacy of topical steroids, occlusive therapy is no longer commonly used. A dermatosis that requires this type of treatment is best referred to a dermatologist.

Topical agents are *not* innocuous. Be familiar with all the characteristics of the topical agent prescribed.

Topical Steroids

These are available in an extensive array of vehicles and potencies. Side effects, both local and systemic, have been well documented; the incidence increases with potency or with use of an inappropriate compound on an area of high permeability, or usage over large surface areas. For these reasons, topical corticoids should be carefully monitored regarding the quantity used and the total surface area of application. This is particularly true in infants and children, for the reasons cited earlier in this chapter.

There are several questions that should be asked when choosing a topical steroid:

1. How steroid-responsive is the condition to be treated?
2. How permeable is the skin region afflicted; therefore, how susceptible is it to local side effects?
3. What percent of body surface area is involved; hence, what is the risk of systemic effect?
4. What vehicle should be used? This is usually dictated by skin region, condition of the skin surface, and to a lesser degree by patient preference.
5. What is the overall cost of treatment? Sometimes a more expensive product is less costly due to rapid effect. In other situations, an inexpensive generic may be all that is needed. The vehicle has a profound effect on these agents and studies have shown marked variation in biological potency among products with the same concentration of active ingredient. All topical steroids are not created equal; the practitioner must be familiar with the activity of the specific product prescribed, whether it is brand-name or generic.

Topical corticoids are divided according to potency into seven groups, from the group I "superpotent" products to the weakest group VII preparations. Some of the latter are available over the counter. All practitioners should be conversant with this system and should also be familiar with which products contain a fluorinated versus a nonfluorinated active ingredient (*see* Table 1).

Fluorinated steroids have special side effects when applied to facial skin, genital, and intertriginous regions. Dermatologists try to avoid their use in these areas.

Areas of very high skin permeability include the face and anogenital regions. For such areas, use nonfluorinated group VI or VII products with active ingredients such as desonide, aclometasone, or higher concentrations of hydrocortisone. Use them with caution. Twice-daily application is usual.

The scalp, neck, axillae, and flexures of the extremities have high permeability, and group IV through VII preparations are best. Always use the weakest effective product. An exception is on the scalp when there is thick scale present. Then, potent lotions such as clobetasol proprionate or betamethasone diproprionate may be needed.

The skin of the trunk and outer extremities is less permeable. Here group II through group VII steroids are recommended, and group I superpotent products can be used for short periods of time.

Palms, soles, elbows, and knees have low permeability and often require group I super-potents to achieve an adequate effect. Brand-name or generic products containing betamethasone diproprionate, clobetasol proprionate, or diflorasone diacetate in special optimized vehicles are currently the only true group I preparations. Weaker products should be used whenever possible. Application is usually BID except for the palms, where activity and washing during active hours will require more frequent use. On palm and sole lesions with thick scale, enhancers such as urea or salicylic acid may be required.

In order to minimize side effects, become familiar with the pitfalls of these agents and consider these general rules:

1. Use a topical steroid of sufficient potency to control the disease, but aim for the weakest effective preparation.
2. In skin regions of high and very high permeability, use group VI or VII steroids only, and then only with caution.
3. When the disease is controlled, shift to bland lubrication or the weakest corticoid for maintenance. If possible, try to use intermittent therapy with rest periods.
4. With children, exercise caution with all groups of corticoids, especially when used in the diaper area. When possible use 1 to 2.5% hydrocortisone acetate, which, except for instances of gross abuse, has a long safety record.
5. When control of the disease is lost, assess the situation. A complicating infection or side effect of the corticoid may be present.

With use of superpotent corticoids, the following guidelines are recommended:

1. Use daily in short courses of 2 weeks or less and limit total dose to 45 to 50 g/wk.
2. Avoid use in children or in pregnant or lactating patients.
3. Do not use in regions of high or very high skin permeability.
4. After 2 weeks switch to intermittent therapy or to a weaker product.

Table 1
Potency of Topical Steroids

This listing is not all-inclusive and is based on potency as measured by vasoconstrictor assay. Group I compounds are referred to as "super-potent" products. Temovate and Ultravate are considered more potent than the others in group I. The remaining groups are arranged in descending order of potency and products with these groups are biologically and clinically equivalent.

Group	Brand / Vehicle	Generic Name	Conc.%
I	**Superpotency**		
a	Temovate cream	Clobetasol proprionate	0.05
	Temovate ointment		
	Temovate gel		
	Olux foam		
	Ultravate cream	Halobetasol proprionate	0.05
	Ultravate ointment		
	Vanos cream	Fluocinonide	0.1
a	Diprolene ointment	Betamethasone diproprionate	0.05
a	Psorcon ointment	Diflorasone diacetate	0.05
a	Cordran tape	Flurandrenolide	4 mg/cm^2
II	**High potency**		
a	Aristocort-A cream	Triamcinolone acetonide	0.5
	Cyclocort ointment	Amcinonide	0.1
a	Diprolene AF cream	Betamethasone diproprionate	0.05
a	Diprolene gel		
a	Diprolene lotion		
b	Elocon ointment	Mometasone furoate	0.1
		Fluocinonide	0.05
		(cream, ointment, solution, gel)	
	Maxiflor ointment	Diflorasone diacetate	0.05
	Topicort cream	Desoximetasone	0.25
	Topicort gel		0.05
	Topicort ointment		0.25
III	**High potency**		
a	Aristocort-A ointment	Triamcinolone acetonide	0.1
	Cutivate ointment	Fluticasone proprionate	0.005
	Cyclocort cream	Amcinonide	0.1
	Cyclocort lotion		0.1
	Diprosone cream	Betamethasone diproprionate	0.05
	Diprosone lotion		0.05
	Maxiflor cream	Diflorasone diacetate	0.05
	Topicort LP cream	Desoximetasone	0.05
		Betamethasone valerate ointment	0.1
IV	**Medium potency**		
		Triamcinolone acetonide ointment	0.1
b	Elocon cream	Mometasone furoate	0.1
b	Elocon lotion		0.1
	Luxiq foam	Betamethasone valerate	0.12
b,c	Pandel cream	Hydrocortisone buteprate	0.1
	Capex shampoo	Fluocinolone acetonide	0.01

Continued

Table 1 *(Continued)*

Group	Brand / Vehicle	Generic Name	Conc.%
V	**Medium potency**		
	Cutivate cream	Fluticasone proprionate	0.05
[b]	Dermatop cream	Prednicarbate	0.1
[b]		Desonide ointment	0.05
		Triamcinolone acetonide lotion, cream	0.1
		Triamcinolone acetonide ointment	0.25
[b,c]	Locoid cream	Hydrocortisone butyrate	0.1
[b,c]	Locoid ointment		0.1
[b,c]	Locoid solution		0.1
		Betamethasone valerate cream	0.1
[b,c]		Hydrocortisone valerate (cream, ointment)	0.2
VI	**Low potency**		
[b]	Aclovate cream	Aclometasone	0.05
[b]	Aclovate ointment	Aclometasone	0.05
[b]		Desonide cream	0.05
		Triamcinolone acetonide cream	0.025
VII	**Very low potency**	Topicals, which contain hydrocortisone acetate[b] in 1.0% and 2.5% concentrations. Also topicals with dexamethasone[b], prednisolone[b] and methylprednisolone[b].	

[a] Optimized (augmented) vehicle contributes to the product's potency. Some generic products now have augmented vehicles. Generics without augmentation should not be expected to have the same biological or clinical potency as augmented generic or augmented brand-name preparations.

[b] Nonfluorinated steroid preparations.

[c] Hydrocortisone products with side chains that enhance potency. These should not be confused with group VII products of hydrocortisone acetate.

Brand-name products are listed in Table 1 because these were used in the original vasoconstrictor assays. Although generic equivalent products may show the same biological and clinical equivalency, studies of some generic products have shown as little as 25% of expected potency.

Modified from Stoughton RB, Cornell, RC. Semin Dermatol 6:72–76, 1987, and from refs. *4,6,9.*

5. With prolonged use consider periodic monitoring of the hypothalamic–pituitary axis.
6. Do not use group I products under occlusion.
7. Maintain careful control of quantities prescribed.
8. Beware of enhanced systemic risks in persons with liver disease, diabetes, glaucoma, or prior tuberculosis.
9. Beware of enhanced systemic toxicity due to interactions in persons concurrently taking sulfonamides and nonsteroidal anti-inflammatory drugs (NSAIDs).

Emollients

The role of emollients in the treatment and maintenance of the epidermal barrier cannot be overemphasized. Proper use of hydrating agents will maintain comfort, improve appearance, control itching, and reduce the overall need for active medication. The emollient base must have enough occlusive property to help the skin surface retain water content. At the same time, it must be cosmetically acceptable. Two products valuable for general use on dry skin are Original Formula Eucerin® Cream and Cetaphil® Moisturizing Cream. These are available also in lotion form. Initially, patients should start with the more lubricating cream base. Later, when the skin is hydrated, the lighter lotions can be introduced for daytime use. These should be applied in a general fashion and over any topical steroids after the shower, then once or twice more during the day.

Enhancers

Salicylic acid 3 to 6% in petrolatum or in a hydrophilic cream base can be used to remove heavy scale that otherwise impedes topical treatment. Systemic absorption with extensive use could lead to salicylism in children, persons on salicylates, or persons with compromised renal function. Combined use with topical steroids can increase absorption of the steroid by two- to threefold. This is probably mediated by the keratolytic action.

Urea containing creams and lotions are also available in 10 to 40% concentrations both by prescription and over the counter (OTC). Urea can double the penetration of some topical corticoids such as hydrocortisone. This effect is unreliable however, and some steroids are markedly inhibited.

Other Topical Agents

Discussion of other topical medications such as topical antibiotics, retinoids, and macrolactams is covered in other chapters under the specific diseases they are used to treat. A discussion about antipruritic ingredients, however, may be of value here.

A plethora of OTC preparations are marketed for the symptomatic relief of pruritus. Most of these products contain either a topical caine anesthetic or a topical antihistamine that acts as a local topical anesthetic. The most common active ingredients are benzocaine and diphenhydramine, both of which have a fairly high sensitizing potential when used on abraded or dermatitic skin. Even more important than the potential local reaction is the fact that benzocaine is capable of inducing broad cross-sensitivity to hair, fabric, and leather dyes, sulfonamide-based medications, and sunscreen agents.

Hypersensitivity to topical antihistamines will often result in a generalized delayed-type reaction upon systemic administration, and with topical sensitization to antihistamines of the ethylenediamine group (pyribenzamine, antistine, phenergan) generalized cross-reactions with aminophylline are reported. Use of these for symptomatic relief of pruritus is not recommended.

Pramoxine, a local anesthetic that has proven to have very low sensitizing potential with topical use, is available OTC in cream, lotion, gel, and spray preparations. Also available by prescription are a 2.5% hydrocortisone cream and lotion with pramoxine in the formulation.

Also recently marketed by prescription is a cream product that contains 5% doxepin hydrochloride. Use of this product should be limited to local areas, and caution is especially important if there is any interruption of the epidermis. Significant percutaneous absorption may occur, with attendant drowsiness and anticholinergic side effects. Use in infants and preadolescents is not recommended.

Finally, there are time-tested antipruritics, including menthol and camphor, which can be compounded with most topical steroids and most bases. These additives act as counter-irritants to relieve the itch. Menthol is usually added in a concentration of 0.025%, while camphor is typically used in 0.05 to 1.0% concentrations.

Systemic Steroid Therapy

Systemic steroid therapy will be discussed under specific disease entities. There are however some general concepts and precautions that should be mentioned.

1. Never commit a patient to systemic steroids without a firm diagnosis, especially if a referral is anticipated. This can make a dermatologist's task virtually impossible.
2. Once a decision is made to use systemic corticoids, use enough to get the job done. There is lower risk with higher doses that achieve rapid control, rather than prolonged administration of low doses while chasing after the disease process.
3. Systemic steroids can result in severe withdrawal flares in some cases of psoriasis and atopic dermatitis. In psoriasis, these can, on rare occasion, be life-threatening. Because both diseases are chronic and are only temporarily improved by corticoids, avoid their use and defer to a dermatologic consultant.
4. Use short-acting oral steroids whenever possible.

Intralesional Steroid Therapy

Injection of dilute solutions of corticosteroids into local skin lesions can result in complete clearing for months or years. This treatment is valuable for management of limited stable psoriasis, lichen simplex chronicus, alopecia areata, and focal lesions of hypertrophic lichen planus, to mention a few.

The authors recommend triamcinolone acetonide exclusively. Other preparations tend to cause more skin atrophy. Whenever possible, dilute the solution to 2.5 mg/cc with physiologic saline, as higher concentrations increase the risk of side effects. Injections should be done only with a control syringe using a 30 gage needle, withdrawing each time to prevent intravascular or lymphatic injection. Injections should be made into the high dermis, which raises a wheal. Deeper injections are less effective and increase the risk of subcutaneous atrophy. Injections into the scalp should be done with great caution because of possible embolization of this crystalline drug to the retinal artery with resulting blindness. Limit patients to a total of 10 mg of triamcinolone acetonide in any given 1-month period and try to keep the injections to an absolute minimum to minimize systemic side effects.

Antihistamines

Antihistamines are of only moderate value compared with topical medications and are mainly used for their sedative effect, except in the treatment of urticaria and related disorders of histamine release. Systemic use of antihistamines will be covered in depth in the section on urticaria.

Mastery of these basic elements will make you more confident and accurate in diagnosing and treating common skin conditions.

ANSWERS TO CLINICAL APPLICATION QUESTIONS

History Review

An 11-month-old infant presents at your office with an intensely pruritic generalized atopic dermatitis with multiple areas of excoriation and lichenification in some flexor locations. The eruption spares only the diaper area, the palms, and the soles. Most skin regions are dry and fissured.

1. Should you treat this patient with topical steroids, and if so, what type of topical steroids?

Answer: Atopic dermatitis is highly responsive to topical steroids.

Use the lowest-potency preparation that is effective for this patient. Begin with group VII preparations such as 1 to 2.5% hydrocortisone acetate in an emollient cream base. If this is ineffective, a trial of the next higher potency class is indicated. Because children have a high ratio of skin surface area to weight, higher-potency steroids are more likely to produce systemic effects such as growth retardation or adrenal suppression.

2. Should you treat this patient with systemic steroids, and if so, what type of systemic steroids?

Answer: No. Topical steroids are effective treatment with much less risk of growth retardation or adrenal suppression. If low-potency topical steroid treatment is not effective, dermatologic consultation is indicated.

3. Should you apply occlusive dressings in this patient over the affected areas, and if so, what type of occlusive dressings?

Answer: No. Occlusive dressings markedly increase systemic absorption of topical steroids and create a special risk to infants with generalized dermatitis. Also, occlusive dressings promote secondary infection, which may aggravate the eczema.

4. Should you treat this patient with an emollient, and if so, why?

Answer: Dry skin can precipitate flares of atopic dermatitis. Proper use of emollients has a steroid-sparing effect. Often emollients will make a lower-potency steroid more effective and prevent relapse of the eczema in areas that have cleared with treatment.

5. Is this patient an appropriate candidate for antihistamines, and if so, why?

Answer: Antihistamines appear to have little effect on the primary disease process. Their main role is to provide sedation, which will reduce the response to pruritus and improve sleep. Only sedating H-1 antihistamines are indicated (example: diphenhydramine).

REFERENCES for Part I

1. Champion RH, Burton JL, Ebling FJG: Textbook of Dermatology. 5th. ed. Oxford: Blackwell Scientific Publications, 1992, pp. 157–167.
2. Braun-Falco O, Plewig G, Wolff HH, Winkelmann RK: Dermatology. Berlin-Heidelberg: Springer-Verlag, 1991, pp. 1–12.
3. Leider M, Rosenblum M: A Dictionary of Dermatological Words, Terms and Phrases. New York-Toronto-London-Sydney: McGraw-Hill, 1968.
4. Drug Facts and Comparisons. St. Louis: Wolters-Kluwer Co., 2003 ed., pp. 1844-1853.
5. Baldwin HE, Berck CM, Lynfield YL: Subcutaneous nodules of the scalp: Preoperative management. J Amer Acad Dermatol 1991;25:819–830.
6. Trozak DJ: Topical Corticosteroid Therapy in Psoriasis. Cutis 1990;46:341–350.
7. Lerner MR, Lerner AB. Dermatologic Medications, 2nd. Ed. Chicago: The Yearbook Publishers, 1960, pp. 32–36.
8. Reisfeld RL. Blue in the skin. J Amer Acad Dermatol 42:597-605.
9. Physicians Desk Reference. Thomson. 57th ed., 2003.
10. Wolverton SE. Comprehensive Dermatologic Drug Therapy. W.B. Saunders, 2001.

From: *Current Clinical Practice: Dermatology Skills for Primary Care: An Illustrated Guide*
D.J. Trozak, D.J. Tennenhouse, and J.J. Russell © Humana Press, Totowa, NJ

Part II: Papular, Papulosquamous, and Papulo-Vesicular Skin Lesions

Learn to internalize what you are observing! It is easy to look at a skin rash but not really see it. Look for and think about each of the distinguishing characteristics of the lesion.

IMPORTANT ABBREVIATIONS USED IN THIS PART:

AIDS	Acquired immunodeficiency syndrome
HIV	Human immunodeficiency virus
LE	Lupus erythematosis
LP	Lichen planus
MC	Molluscum contagiosum
OTC	Over the counter
PV	Psoriasis vulgaris
PR	Pityriasis rosea
SD	Seborrheic dermatitis
VV	Verruca vulgaris

5 Molluscum Contagiosum *(Dimple Warts)*

CLINICAL APPLICATION QUESTIONS

A 16-year-old male high school student presents with a large number of papular lesions of recent onset in the right thoracic and axillary region. There is a second grouping of similar lesions on the right knee. The patient is on the wrestling team, desires removal of the lesions, and was sent to you by his wrestling coach to find out if they might be contagious. You suspect this is molluscum contagiosum.

1. What are the primary lesions you would expect to find in molluscum contagiosum?
2. What is the prognosis for molluscum contagiosum?
3. How do you answer the patient's question about whether this condition is contagious?
4. How do you confirm your diagnosis of molluscum contagiosum?
5. If this is molluscum contagiosum, how will you treat it?

APPLICATION GUIDELINES

Specific History

Onset

Molluscum warts occur characteristically in small children and in young adults, although they may be seen occasionally in any age group. They present as single or grouped papules, and parents will often indicate there was a single lesion present for some time. The incubation period after exposure has been estimated to vary from 14 days to 6 months. Molluscum contagiosum (MC) virus is a member of the poxvirus family and is not related to human papilloma virus, the cause of common verrucous warts.

Evolution of Disease Process

The infection usually starts with single or a small number of lesions and, if left untreated, will gradually spread to the point where hundreds of papules may develop. In small children, the face, neck, and upper trunk, especially the axillae and antecubital creases, are sites of predilection. Young adults more often present with lesions on the lower abdomen, pubic escutcheon, or inner thighs contracted during sexual transmission. The presence of MC lesions in the pubic area occurs from autoinoculation in small children and should not be considered a sign of sexual abuse unless there is other evidence. Molluscum warts are very common in human immunodeficiency virus (HIV) disease and occur typically on the face and beard areas.

In children, and occasionally in young adults, eczematous patches will develop within the regions of activity. The eczema is identical to patches of atopic dermatitis and, if left untreated, the resultant excoriations can lead to dissemination of the MC infection.

From: *Current Clinical Practice: Dermatology Skills for Primary Care: An Illustrated Guide*
D.J. Trozak, D.J. Tennenhouse, and J.J. Russell © Humana Press, Totowa, NJ

Whether this represents an exacerbation of latent atopic disease or a delayed immune response to the virus is uncertain. Atopic dermatitis patients do seem to have an increased incidence of MC.

Although spontaneous remissions occur, untreated MC can last for years. During this time, the victim remains a potential source of infection to others.

Evolution of Skin Lesions

Although single lesions occur, most often these warts appear in groups and localize within the presenting anatomic area. On the trunk they are usually unilateral; on the pubic areas and inner thighs, involvement is usually on both sides. Parents or patients will often point to lesions that have involuted or are inflamed and involuting. Involution occurs even as new lesions continue to form. Solitary MC papules may exceed 1 cm in size. In acquired immunodeficiency syndrome (AIDS) and certain other states of immunosuppression, the lesions may be unusually profuse and large or may be atypical and simulate other infectious or malignant conditions.

Provoking Factors

Molluscum warts are spread by close physical contact and by fomites. The physical nature of play among preschool children predisposes them, and outbreaks often occur within family and day-school classroom units. In school-aged children, common swimming pool facilities, communal shower facilities, and contact sports have been implicated. Sexual contact is the most common mode of transmission in young adults.

Immunosuppression predisposes patients to MC, which is the most likely reason for the increased frequency in atopics and in HIV victims and accounts for their unusual virulence in patients with HIV, sarcoid, and leukemia, and patients on chemotherapy. Multiple, atypical, or therapeutically resistant MC are a sign of HIV infection and correlate with disease progression.

Self-Medication

Self-treatment is not a problem in MC.

Supplemental Review From General History

The presence of widespread, large, or atypical MC lesions should prompt a general review searching for systemic diseases such as HIV infection, sarcoid, or underlying malignancy.

Dermatologic Physical Exam

Primary Lesions

1. Dome-shaped umbilicated papules (*see* Photo 1).
2. Dome-shaped umbilicated nodules (rare).
3. Plaques of tightly grouped papules (rare).

Pinhead-sized dome-shaped firm flesh-colored papules gradually enlarge to reveal a central dimple or umbilication. As the wart matures, a thin ridge or scale may be seen at the edge of the pit (*see* Photo 2). More mature lesions may become yellow or pink in color, and lesions that are ready to involute are usually a deep dusky red (*see* Photo 3). Solitary mature lesions may, on rare occasions, exceed 1 cm in diameter.

Secondary Lesions

1. Crust formation on involuting lesions.
2. Excoriations of some papules.
3. Mild scarring.

As lesions evolve, some will enlarge rapidly, become edematous and dusky red, and form a yellow or dark crust. In patients with associated eczema, excoriations are usually present and may cause mild scarring, as can overly exuberant treatment. Solitary large lesions are rare and may simulate a keratoacanthoma, squamous cell carcinoma, or basal cell carcinoma. These are more common in HIV disease. In HIV-positive patients, lesions of disseminated cryptococcosis, histoplasmosis, or cutaneous coccidioidomycosis can resemble MC lesions, but develop central necrosis as they enlarge.

Distribution

Microdistribution: None.

Macrodistribution:
1. Face, neck, upper trunk, axillary, cubital, and genital regions in small children (*see* Fig. 1).
2. Lower abdomen, pubic escutcheon, and inner thighs in young adults (*see* Fig. 2).
3. Face and beard area with HIV disease (*see* Fig. 3).

Configuration

1. Grouped, usually within the region of onset (*see* Photos 1,2,4).
2. Occasionally linear following inoculation by excoriation (autoinoculation).

Indicated Supporting Diagnostic Data

Typical MC is clinically diagnostic. No supporting data are indicated.

Atypical lesions (large or necrotic) and lesions that are unusually refractory to therapy or are seen in the context of HIV disease need laboratory confirmation.

1. **Molluscum smear:** This simple test can be performed by gently squeezing or curetting a lesion and examining the central contents. The unstained contents of MC will show anucleate homogeneous ovoid molluscum bodies, which are diagnostic (*see* Photo 5).
2. **Skin biopsy:** MC has very characteristic histology. When the clinical findings are confusing and a smear is negative, a biopsy is diagnostic.

Therapy

Avoidance

Patients should avoid sources of reinfection if these can be identified from the history. They also should avoid communal swimming pools, baths, and use of fomites such as common towels and shared clothing items.

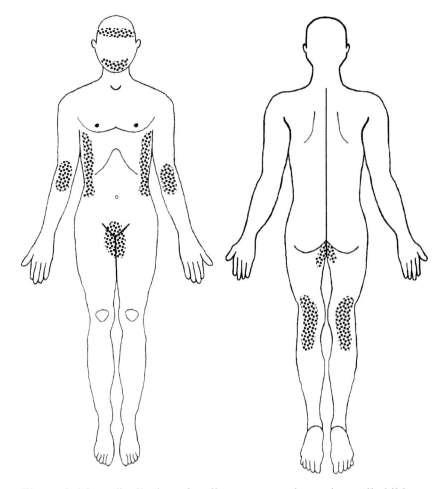

Figure 1: Macrodistribution of molluscum contagiosum in small children.

Cryotherapy

Light freezing with liquid nitrogen (LN_2) is effective and nonscarring. This is most effective in adult cases and must be repeated every 10 to 14 days until clear. The authors strongly recommend use of a cotton swab rather than cryospray application. These lesions require only a short blanch to accomplish destruction. With cryospray it is very easy to cause permanent scars, especially on the facial skin. Small children will usually not tolerate the discomfort of LN_2.

Vesicants

Treatment of small children is best accomplished by applications of 0.7% cantharidin in a film-forming adhesive base. The applications are done very carefully to the tops of visible lesions every 14 days until clear. The wooden applicator is not threatening, the

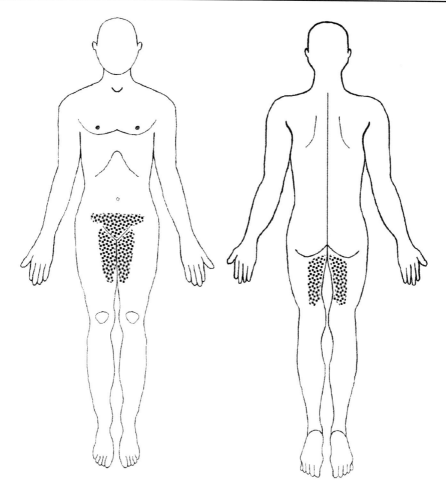

Figure 2: Macrodistribution of molluscum contagiosum in young adults.

applications are painless, and long-term there is minimal risk of scarring. The application is left in place until the evening bath. Occlusion is not required.

Irritants

An alternative but somewhat less effective method is the application of an aqueous solution containing 2% iodine and 2.4% sodium iodide. The solution is applied with a flat toothpick and is gently introduced into the central pore or dimple. This solution is available without prescription; however, because of potential toxicity with an accidental ingestion, application in the practitioner's office is strongly recommended.

Curettage

Curettage with or without fulguration has been used, but is tedious with a large number of lesions and can lead to unacceptable scarring. Today this technique is mainly used to obtain tissue for histology when the diagnosis is uncertain.

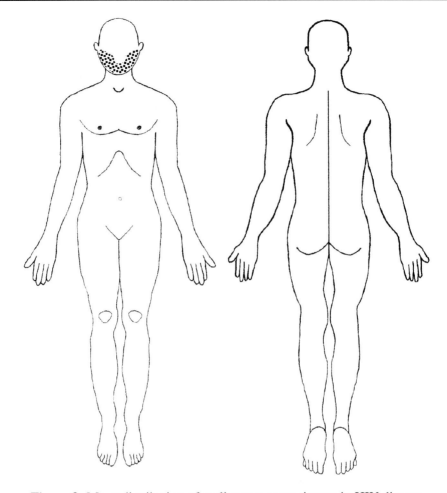

Figure 3: Macrodistribution of molluscum contagiosum in HIV disease.

Conditions That May Simulate Molluscum Contagiosum

Basal Cell/Squamous Cell Carcinomas, Keratoacanthoma

Solitary MC lesions can simulate any of these nodular lesions. All three tend to arise on heavily sun-damaged skin, but each may have a central dell or keratotic pit. A molluscum smear or a biopsy will differentiate them.

Cryptococcosis and Other Deep Fungi

Cutaneous lesions of cryptococcosis and other deep fungi can occasionally simulate giant molluscum lesions. Both conditions favor the facial skin and occur in advanced HIV disease and other states of profound immunologic suppression. With cryptococcal lesions the central core has a more gelatinous quality and saline exam shows large budding yeast cells rather than molluscum bodies. India ink examination will demonstrate the character-istic clear capsule. Histoplasmosis and coccidioidomycosis can also produce similar lesions. Biopsy with stains for fungi are indicated if routine histology fails to show typical molluscum bodies. Cutaneous cryptococcosis, histoplasmosis, and coccidioidomycosis are all a sign of disseminated systemic infection.

ANSWERS TO CLINICAL APPLICATION QUESTIONS

History Review

A 16-year-old male high school student presents with a large number of papular lesions of recent onset in the right thoracic and axillary region. There is a second grouping of similar lesions on the right knee. The patient is on the wrestling team, desires removal of the lesions, and was sent to you by his wrestling coach to find out if they might be contagious. You suspect this is molluscum contagiosum.

1. What are the primary lesions you would expect to find in molluscum contagiosum?

Answer: Grouped dome-shaped umbilicated papules; less commonly, umbilicated nodules.

2. What is the prognosis for molluscum contagiosum?

Answer: Although spontaneous involution can occur, it is more common for the lesions to multiply and spread unless treated.

3. How do you answer the patient's question about whether this condition is contagious?

Answer: Molluscum warts are highly contagious by both direct contact and fomite transmission. This patient should not be wrestling until the lesions are completely resolved, and the coach should be warned to clean mats and other equipment with which the wrestlers come in contact.

4. How do you confirm your diagnosis of molluscum contagiosum?

Answer: Express the contents from the center of a papule. Perform a molluscum smear.

5. If this is molluscum, how will you treat it?

Answer: Cryotherapy or vesicant application is appropriate. There are some studies that show that topical Imiquimod may also be effective.

6 Verruca Vulgaris *(Common Warts)*

CLINICAL APPLICATION QUESTIONS

A 7-year-old girl was seen by her pediatrician with a single wart on her right index finger. Her mother was told that treatment was unnecessary because the wart would resolve by itself. Six months later the child presents at your office with 30 warts over both hands, around and beneath several fingernails.

1. List the reasons why immediate treatment is indicated.
2. What preparation is required before active treatment begins?
3. What treatment approach is appropriate in this situation?
4. What will you tell the mother about prognosis and possible recurrence?

APPLICATION GUIDELINES

Specific History

Onset

Common warts are caused by human papillomavirus infection; clinical lesions develop after a latent period of weeks to several months. They have a peak incidence in late childhood and adolescence and then the occurrence sharply declines. They may, however, be found in all age groups. Usually patients will recall a single lesion, which is often interpreted at first as a splinter or thorn.

Evolution of Disease Process

The clinical course is variable. Some will develop only a few lesions over years, while others will be covered within a few months. Conventional wisdom is that given time all verrucae (VV) will spontaneously involute. Unfortunately this is not a universal occurrence and in children, uncontrolled spread can lead to social disfigurement and infection of playmates and other family members. In one longitudinal study of the natural history of common warts, only 40% of patients were clear 2 years later.

Evolution of Skin Lesions

The initial lesion may be indolent for years but most often expands in size while satellite lesions emerge.

Provoking Factors

1. Natural sunlight or ultraviolet light in the UVA and UVB spectra.
2. VV is spread by close physical contact and fomites and is especially common in some occupations such as butchering, where chronic cuts and abrasions afford a

From: *Current Clinical Practice: Dermatology Skills for Primary Care: An Illustrated Guide*
D.J. Trozak, D.J. Tennenhouse, and J.J. Russell © Humana Press, Totowa, NJ

portal of entry. Warts occur frequently on the soles of persons who go without footwear in locker rooms and public bath facilities.

3. In immunosuppressed patients, pregnancy, and persons in active stages of HIV disease, warts tend to be more aggressive and more refractory to treatment.

Self-Medication

Multiple proprietary wart medications are available at any pharmacy. The marginal efficacy of these products can be measured by the number that are on the shelf. On occasion, patients will have some success but in general most of these products are variations of keratolytics that have been in use since the early part of the last century. Self-treatment is a problem mainly when delay leads to widespread lesions or when applied to lesions that have been inappropriately diagnosed.

Supplemental Review From General History

In unusually widespread or therapeutically refractory lesions, obtain history for possible sources of immunosuppression. Warts in the genital and perianal areas of small children have been reported in the literature as an indication of sexual abuse. In clinical studies where this has been investigated, the relationship to abuse has been unreliable. The practitioner should, however, be wary and look for other corroborating history or physical findings.

Dermatologic Physical Exam

Primary Lesions

1. Tiny firm flesh-colored papules that interrupt skin lines or dermatoglyphic lines when on palms or soles (*see* Photo 6).
2. Filiform (threadlike) papules, especially on the eyelid and facial areas (*see* Photo 7).

Secondary Lesions

1. Raised dome-shaped papules with a grey-white scaling surface and black pinpoint blood vessels (*see* Photo 8).
2. Large nodules with multiple tightly grouped filiform papules, the tips composed of gray scale or tipped by black thrombosed vessels (*see* Photo 9).
3. Tightly clustered round papules often with minimal or no elevation (corymbiform pattern) frequently at sites of compression such as plantar surface of foot (*see* Photo 10).

Distribution

Microdistribution: None.

Macrodistribution:

1. Dorsum of hands, fingers, periungual tissue, and knees in children (*see* Fig. 4; Photos 11,12).
2. Beard area and neck in young adult men (*see* Fig. 5; Photo 13).
3. Periungual warts are usually associated with nailbiting. This habit must be controlled for successful treatment of the warts.

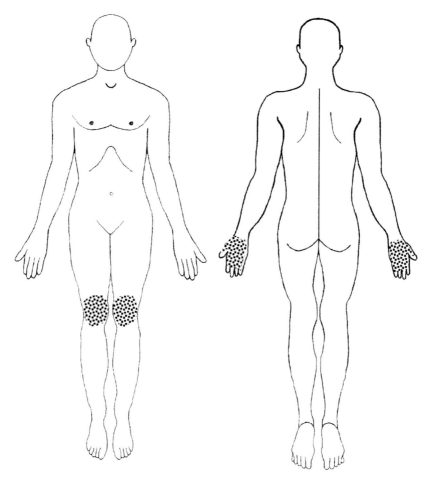

Figure 4: Macrodistribution of verrucous warts in children.

    4. Common warts may occur at virtually any site on the skin or mucous membranes.

Configuration
    1. Grouped (*see* Photos 12,13).
    2. Corymbiform (*see* Photo 10).

Indicated Supporting Diagnostic Data
    1. Typical VV is clinically diagnostic. No supporting data are indicated.
    2. On very rare occasions VV may be clinically indistinguishable from keratoacanthoma or squamous cell carcinoma.

Skin biopsy: VV has characteristic histology. Skin biopsy will distinguish VV from other tumors and growths.

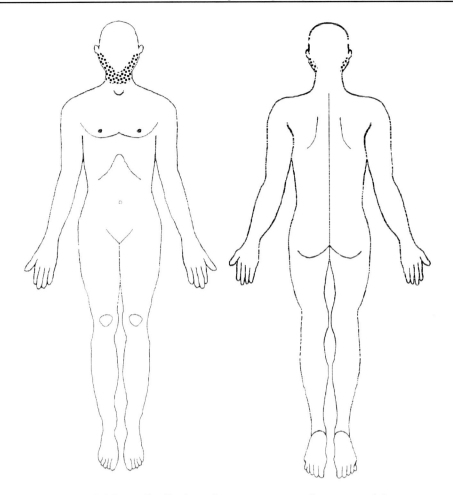

Figure 5: Macrodistribution of verrucous warts in young adult men.

Therapy

Avoidance

Patients with active infection should avoid sharing of clothing, towels, footgear, sporting equipment, and tools with others. Untreated persons are a source of new infection or reinfection which is a very common occurrence among playmates and immediate family members.

Cryotherapy

Liquid nitrogen is at present the most effective treatment modality. In experienced hands it is safe and nonscarring; however, there is some discomfort involved. With proper preparation, children will usually tolerate treatment of a small number of lesions. The authors recommend application with large cotton swabs rather than a cryospray unit. The swabs offer greater control over the rate and depth of freeze with less risk of injury to deep structures. Severe peripheral motor and sensory nerve injuries and tendon damage have occurred with overly aggressive LN_2 treatment. Areas of greatest risk are the ulnar nerve at the elbow, the digital sensory nerves, and the dorsal tendons of the hands. These injuries can be avoided by moving or elevating the skin away from the deep structure and controlling the depth of freeze. LN_2 therapy must be repeated every 2 weeks until all warts are clear. Single applications are rarely curative. This is especially true with palmar and plantar verrucae.

Vesicants

Vesicants should be limited to the treatment of periungual and subungual warts. Cantharidin 0.7% in flexible colloidin or a similar base is quite effective when applied for 48 hours and kept dry under plastic tape occlusion. After 48 hours, the tape should be soaked off, as the involved digit will be quite tender at that time. Stronger cantharidin preparations are available but should be applied very cautiously to avoid permanent nail injury. These products should be applied by the practitioner and are not recommended for home use. Treatment of warts on other locations with these agents is not recommended and may actually spread the lesions. As with cryotherapy, follow up and repeat treatment should be on a 2-week basis until the lesions are clinically resolved.

Curettage With or Without Fulguration

This modality has a lower overall cure rate than LN_2. In addition, it carries the disadvantages of scarring and the need for local anesthesia. Today, curettage is generally reserved for the treatment of solitary warts that have proven resistant to other less or non-scarring techniques. This method of removal should never be used on a palm, sole, or the primary sensory area of a digit. Permanent, painful, disabling scarring may occur. Despite many early claims, laser therapy has about the same utility and disadvantages as curettage and fulguration. In addition, the equipment is costly to purchase and maintain. The authors have seen some very severe scarring as a result of inappropriate laser treatment of warts.

Keratolytics, Caustics, and Cytostatic Agents

These agents have been used singly or in myriad combinations for the treatment of common warts. Salicylic acid and lactic acid are the most commonly used keratolytics and can be compounded or purchased already made either by prescription or OTC. The plain keratolytics are quite safe, but only modestly effective. They must be used with gentle surface debridement and can be recommended for home use. Parents should be warned to return promptly if the warts are spreading. Combinations of keratolytics with vesicants (cantharidin) or cytostatics (podophyllin) produce products that can cause intense inflammation and limited tissue necrosis. These should be administered by the practitioner and carefully followed up. These preparations are most effective with periungual and subungual warts, and when used in other skin locations tend to cause annular spread of verrucae.

Caustics, such as mono-, di-, and trichloroacetic acid, are both keratolytic and virucidal. These acids produce almost immediate tissue coagulation and must be handled with extreme caution. They should be applied only to limited areas with either a flat toothpick or the tip of a broken cotton swab. The adjacent skin should be protected with a border of petrolatum. If use is undertaken around the eye, be prepared to flush with water or sodium bicarbonate immediately in the event of contact with the eye. The action of these acids is self-limiting and adequately treated areas will turn an intense white color. Treatment is associated with a moderate amount of pain, that is usually transitory. Other caustics which are virucidal include formaldehyde and glutaraldehyde. Formaldehyde is sometimes formulated extemporaneously with the keratolytics and used under occlusion with daily debridement. Glutaraldehyde 10% buffered with sodium bicarbonate is particularly useful in the treatment of extensive plantar warts and for patients unable to tolerate cryotherapy. The solution is applied morning and evening and the warts are lightly debrided by the patient with pumice stone or callus remover daily after showering. More vigorous debridement should be done in the office on a 2-week basis until VV is cured.

Patient compliance is easily monitored by the distinct orange-brown color produced at the treatment site. This side effect unfortunately limits the use of this regimen to the feet. Silver nitrate preparations are not recommended because of staining and toxicity.

Podophyllum resins are cytostatic agents that inhibit cell division in metaphase. They are used mainly in the treatment of moist warts located on mucous membrane areas and thin skin. They can cause serious and potentially fatal toxicity if ingested or if there is substantial absorption from extensive application or use on areas of raw skin. In animal studies, they are abortifacients and are contraindicated during pregnancy. They should be applied only by the treating practitioner. Patient application is not recommended.

Alternative Therapies

Topical immunotherapy, intralesional bleomycin, and the use of systemic retinoids all fall within the realm of the dermatologist and are either expensive, fraught with potentially significant complications, or still considered experimental. Intralesional and systemic interferon therapy using both natural and recombinant interferons has been reported, with markedly variable results in patients with condylomata. There is no body of evidence to support the use of these agents in the therapy of common warts. Interferon therapy is very expensive.

Conditions That May Simulate Verruca Vulgaris

Plantar Calluses

The distinction between warts and plantar calluses is sometimes difficult and is important because the latter can be treated with keratolytics and debridement alone and do not require the more destructive therapies used on verrucae. The difference can be determined by paring the lesion down with a scalpel blade. Warts will show a single or sometimes multiple cores that interrupt normal skin lines. They also exhibit dark red or black speckles, which are the thrombosed ends of the feeder vessels. Calloses show neither of these changes.

Basal Cell Carcinomas, Squamous Cell Carcinomas, and Keratoacanthoma

Large, keratotic VV that arise on sun exposed skin can simulate these nodular lesions. The differentiation can usually be made with a skin biopsy. The specimen should be read by a dermatologist or dermatopathologist.

Verrucous Carcinoma of Skin (Epithelioma Cuniculatum),
and Squamous Cell Carcinoma of the Nail Bed

These rare lesions can simulate VV both clinically and histologically. The distinction is important because both are capable of metastasis. More often they cause local invasion which necessitates amputation or deforming surgery. Verrucous carcinomas are sizable fungating lesions, often on the soles. These should be referred to a dermatologist for management. Any subungual warty lesion that does not respond promptly to therapy should be referred to a dermatologist for evaluation. This is especially true in an adult patient or when there is a history of prior radiation exposure.

ANSWERS TO CLINICAL APPLICATION QUESTIONS

History Review

A 7-year-old girl was seen by her pediatrician with a single wart on her right index finger. Her mother was told that treatment was unnecessary because the wart would resolve by itself. Six months later the child presents at your office with 30 warts over both hands, around and beneath several fingernails.

1. List the reasons why immediate treatment is indicated.

Answer:
a. The warts are continuing to spread.
b. Some of the warts are split and tender and they interfere with manual activities.
c. Warts are contagious and the child is a source of infection for playmates and family members.
d. The child may become a social outcast due to the disfiguring appearance of these lesions.

2. What preparation is required before active treatment begins?

Answer: Before treatment begins, the mother and child must understand that treatment will require an indeterminate number of regular visits which must be followed through until the warts are gone. They must also understand there will be some discomfort.

3. What treatment approach is appropriate in this situation?

Answer: Combined therapy using cantharone under occlusion for the periungual and subungual warts, and cryotherapy with liquid nitrogen for the others.

4. What will you tell the mother about prognosis and possible recurrence?

Answer: With regular follow-up, the prognosis for cure is excellent. However, recurrences are possible and should be treated promptly.

7 Seborrheic Dermatitis *(Dandruff)*

CLINICAL APPLICATION QUESTIONS

A somewhat irascible 70-year-old woman with a highly stylized bouffant hairdo complains of intolerable scalp pruritus. You notice white flakes on the shoulders of her black sweater. You suspect seborrheic dermatitis.

1. What history should you attempt to elicit from this patient?
2. When you examine this patient's scalp, what primary and secondary lesions would support your diagnosis of seborrheic dermatitis?
3. Where else on this patient's body should you look for active dermatitis?
4. How should you approach treatment in this patient?
5. What should you tell this patient is the prognosis for seborrheic dermatitis?

APPLICATION GUIDELINES

Specific History

Onset

Seborrheic dermatitis (SD), and its diminutive scalp variant, dandruff, first appear at puberty, exhibiting a peak incidence in the third and fourth decades. A significant number of cases also occur in elderly patients, where there is an association with chronic neurologic disease, especially Parkinsonism. The disease begins insidiously and patients often delay for long intervals before seeking assistance. Major complaints are usually referable to appearance rather than physical discomfort.

Infantile seborrheic dermatitis, which occurs during the first 6 months of life, is controversial and may represent a distinct entity. An extensive discussion is beyond the scope of this book. The disease occurs in otherwise healthy infants and usually remits spontaneously within 2 to 3 months after onset. Scalp lesions clear with Johnson's Baby Shampoo® and other skin lesions respond to topical treatment with a group VII steroid or a topical macrolactam. Progressive, persistent, or widespread disease opens a large differential which includes infantile psoriasis, atopic dermatitis, Langerhan's cell histiocytosis, acrodermatitis enteropathica, and several primary immunodeficiency diseases. Under these circumstances a dermatologic consult is advisable.

Evolution of Disease Process

Adult SD classically affects the scalp, creases, and hair-bearing areas of the face and ears. On the scalp and other heavy hair-bearing regions, flaking or dandruff is usually the initial complaint. Elsewhere, the appearance of the dermatitis evokes the patient's attention. Sometimes there is an associated seborrheic blepharitis with complaints of mattering, redness, and chronic eye irritation. Infrequently, extensive lesions develop on the

From: *Current Clinical Practice: Dermatology Skills for Primary Care: An Illustrated Guide*
D.J. Trozak, D.J. Tennenhouse, and J.J. Russell © Humana Press, Totowa, NJ

upper torso and in the body flexures. On rare occasions SD may progress to an extensive erythroderma. Diffuse scalp involvement can cause reversible hair shedding, and some authorities believe SD can hasten the onset and extent of genetic pattern hair loss.

Evolution of Skin Lesions

Lesions of SD are usually persistent, but will vary in intensity and extent. Despite years of activity, there is no scarring. Cosmetic effects are usually the overriding concern. Scalp lesions can cause significant pruritus, however, and the blepharitis is associated with itching, crusting, and burning irritation.

Provoking Factors

Infrequent shampooing, inadequate body hygiene, and climate conditions, especially long spells of wet weather, exacerbate existing cases and precipitate latent disease. Severe emotional stress, as well as focal and general neurologic conditions, also cause flares. When neurologic injury is focal, the flare of SD is sometimes confined to the distribution of the neurologic deficit. Extensive SD that can be refractory to therapy is very common in HIV disease. It occurs in the context of AIDS-related complex and full-blown AIDS. In these settings, the disease can have an acute and explosive onset.

Self-Medication

Self-medication is common and can significantly alter SD. Obtain a history regarding the frequency of shampooing and the use of medicated shampoos. Both of these treatments can resolve areas of scalp involvement, which is helpful in establishing a firm diagnosis. If a patient shampoos frequently, ask why. Often the answer is, "My head itches and flakes if I don't." Also ask why the patient is using a medicated shampoo preparation. Ask the patient about the use of topical creams. Fluorinated corticosteroids prescribed for other conditions or obtained from friends will initially improve facial seborrhea. With continued use, however, they exacerbate the disease and eventually cause atrophy and a sunburned appearance, which hides the true nature of the problem.

Supplemental Review From General History

SD is limited to the scalp and facial skin in the vast majority of patients. When it is associated with neurologic disease, it occurs as a secondary phenomenon and the neurologic problem is usually quite evident. When SD occurs in an explosive fashion, is refractory to therapy, or occurs in the context of opportunistic infection, an in-depth history for high-risk behavior and other signs and symptoms of HIV infection is indicated. HIV-associated SD can be an early symptom and herald overt AIDS by as much as 2 years.

Dermatologic Physical Exam

Primary Lesions

1. Dull to yellow-red patches, usually sharply demarcated (*see* Photo 14).
2. Trunk lesions may begin as red-brown follicular papules that evolve into patches (uncommon).
3. Patches of erythema develop, may remain discrete or become confluent, but tend to be sharply demarcated.

When seborrhea becomes quite inflammatory, the margins smudge, making the distinction from an eczema more difficult. In most locations, these patches rapidly develop a scale, which aids in the diagnosis.

Secondary Lesions

Scale is most commonly loose, easily dislodged, yellow, or yellow-tan, and has an oil-soaked appearance (*see* Photo 15). Scale that is white but not silvery, always loose, and easily dislodged is common contrary to textbook descriptions (*see* Photo 16).

Scale is particularly heavy in hair-bearing regions such as the scalp and beard. Sometimes the simple act of shaving a beard area is sufficient to promote clearing. Intertriginous seborrhea is sometimes an exception. The scale may be minimal or marginal, making the clinical distinction from monilia and erythrasma difficult.

Fissuring is common in intertriginous regions.

Distribution

Microdistribution: Follicular papules may be present with early truncal involvement. These usually evolve into patches but can remain present at the margin of larger lesions or as satellites on the adjacent skin (this is usually a subtle feature).

Macrodistribution:
1. Hair-bearing areas: scalp, axillae, eyebrows in both men and women, beard, and presternal area in men (*see* Fig. 6).
2. Creases and folds: nasolabial folds, perialar creases, glabellar creases, postauricular creases, intertriginous creases in both men and women, and inframammary creases in women (*see* Fig. 6).
3. Pinna, concha, and the outer third of the external auditory canal.
4. Eyelid margins.
5. Upper back, shoulders, and chest, usually in the form of large patches, or may be confluent over the whole region in men (*see* Fig. 6).
6. Generalized erythrodermic form (rare).

Involvement of the scalp alone, or combined scalp, ear, and facial SD, are the most common patterns. Eyelid and ear canal involvement is infrequent but not rare. Patch lesions over the upper trunk may simulate pityriasis rosea or pityriasis (tinea) versicolor. These distributions are distinctly uncommon. Confluent activity on the face or upper torso may be very difficult to distinguish from atopic dermatitis. Erythrodermic SD is fortunately very rare and must be separated from other causes of erythroderma.

Configuration

Petaloid (shaped like petals on a plant) configuration is seen when SD occurs on the central and lateral chest (*see* Photo 17).

Follicular lesions may be seen with early activity on the scalp, brows, and shoulders. These may also be noted at the periphery of large truncal patches.

Indicated Supporting Diagnostic Data

Common presentations of SD are clinically diagnostic. No supporting data are indicated.

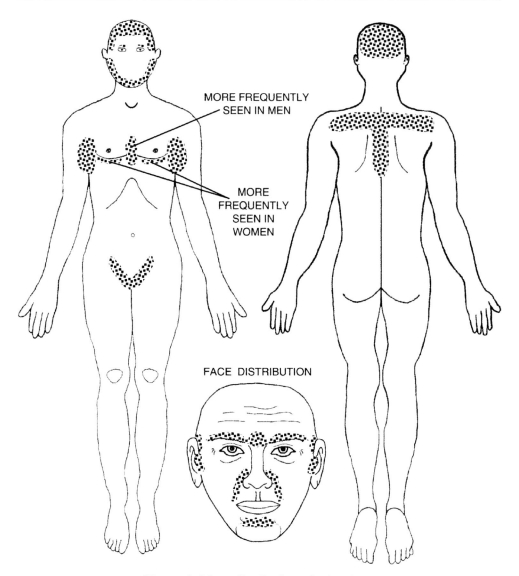

Figure 6: Macrodistribution of seborrhea.

Less common presentations of SD may simulate atopic dermatitis, pityriasis rosea, psoriasis vulgaris, lichen simplex chronicus, intertrigo, intertriginous monilia, and pityriasis versicolor.

1. Woods lamp examination: SD has a negative examination.
2. KOH preparation of scales: SD has a negative examination.
3. Skin biopsy: As noted above, SD can simulate several other inflammatory dermatitides. Unfortunately, the histology of SD can also show features of each of these disorders. For this reason, biopsy of SD is not a definitive procedure and

should not be undertaken routinely. If the disease is atypical, extensive, or refractory to treatment, it should be referred to a dermatologist, who can best decide whether this expense is cost-effective.

Therapy

It is important to stress to SD patients that treatment of this condition is not curative and, at present, is an ongoing process.

Hygiene

Proper cleansing and shampooing are sometimes sufficient to control mild SD. These simple measures are often overlooked. This is especially true with older female patients who have their hair done professionally and therefore shampoo infrequently. Determine each patient's hair care and skin practices and get a feel for how much they are willing to modify this behavior. Once informed, some patients would rather change behavior, while others prefer to maintain their current styling practices and depend entirely on medication for control.

Medicated Shampoos

Several types of medicated shampoos are available and effective. Most of these products contain zinc pyrithione, selenium sulfide, sulfur, parachlorometaxylenol, or tar derivatives. These are available without prescription and share common ingredients that inhibit growth of *Pityrosporum ovale*, a yeast inhabitant of the skin implicated in the etiology of SD. Other products that contain salicylic acid are mainly keratolytic. Ketoconazole, which specifically supresses *P. ovale*, is available as an OTC shampoo and in a more concentrated prescription preparation. Also available by prescription is Loprox® shampoo containing the broad-spectrum antifungal and anti-yeast ingredient ciclopirox. The choice of shampoos is dictated by both effectiveness and cosmetic acceptance. These products should be used initially on a daily or alternate-day basis. The scalp should be lathered with the preparation of choice, which should be left in place for 3 to 5 minutes, then thoroughly rinsed. Most of these shampoos leave the hair coarse and unmanageable; therefore, have patients follow rinsing with an application of conditioner. The conditioning application does not seem to decrease efficacy. Patients should be instructed to guard their eyes during the shampoo rinse-off, as most of these agents are quite irritating to the ocular mucous membranes.

After long periods of control, a product will often lose its punch. At this point it is best to rotate the patient to a shampoo with a different active ingredient. Later, one may return to the original product, which will have regained its effectiveness. Disinfecting hair-care tools with a 5-minute application of the medicated shampoo is also recommended on a weekly basis.

Keratolytics

Pure keratolytic lotions and ointments will remove scale of SD. This disease has such loose scale and is usually so responsive to treatment that keratolytic products are seldom needed.

Topical Steroids

Steroids dramatically improve the treatment of SD. They provide safe, effective, and inexpensive therapy when prescribed appropriately. Facial and truncal seborrhea should be treated with the weaker nonfluorinated steroids in potency groups VI and VII. Products that contain hydrocortisone, desonide, and aclometasone are very effective. These are available in acceptable vanishing cream and lighter lotion bases. The composition of the base is often as critical as the active ingredient. Over-the-counter hydrocortisone preparations often have irritating bases that can override the clinical effect of the steroid. Fluorinated steroid products should be shunned on the facial skin because they can rapidly cause atrophy and induce telangectasia. Although this is uncommon with the weaker products, vigilance is still necessary. Fluorinated steroids have been reported to exacerbate facial seborrhea after an initial period of improvement.

For resistant disease, 0.5 to 1% precipitated sulfur can be added to the steroids to enhance effectiveness. Ketoconazole cream compounded with 1 to 2.5% hydrocortisone powder is also very effective and cosmetically more acceptable.

Scalp lesions respond well to foam and lotion preparations that contain potency group VI and VII steroids. These products add to the expense of therapy and should be considered adjunctive treatment to proper hygiene and a medicated shampoo. With older female patients who are unwilling to shampoo regularly, steroids may add needed control in between grooming. Although aerosol foams are more expensive, the ease and precision of application makes them cost-effective. Most seborrhea patients prefer products with a foam or alcohol lotion base. Products that contain betamethasone valerate, triamcinolone acetonide, fluocinonide, or clobetasol proprionate are used most often. On rare occasions where heavy scale persists, 1 to 2% salicylic acid can be added to the nonaerosol products for keratolytic effect and to enhance potency.

Intertriginous seborrhea usually has an inflammatory and bacteriological component. Ketoconazole cream compounded with 1 to 2.5% hydrocortisone is particularly effective. Iodochlorhydroxoquin 3% with 1% hydrocortisone is also effective, but it stains clothing a bright yellow color.

Topical Antifungal Agents

Ketoconazole cream 2% has been demonstrated effective and has been approved for treatment of SD. Loprox® and Oxistat® preparations are equally effective.

Systemic Therapy

Systemic agents are indicated only in extensive or extremely refractory disease and only after other entities have been ruled out. Antifungal agents of the azole group can be used in pulse doses to temporarily reduce skin colonization by the yeast *P. ovale*. Either 200 mg/day fluconazole once weekly or 100 mg itraconazole BID for 1 week out of four until improved should be effective when combined with standard topical measures. Systemic ketoconazole is also effective but has a greater risk of serious side effects. Systemic steroids and retinoids have also been reported effective; however, disease of this severity should be referred to a dermatologic consultant.

Treatment of Seborrheic Blepharitis

This is a special and uniquely irritating facet of SD that is often ignored. The lid margins are red and scaly and there is often an associated conjunctivitis, which is very symptomatic. This blepharitis usually responds rapidly to short courses of 10% sodium sulamyd ophthalmic solution or ointment administered BID. Chlortetracycline and tetracycline ophthalmic ointments are also effective. These preparations need be used only intermittently on a symptomatic basis. Products that contain steroids should be avoided, as the steroid is not essential and could mask or exacerbate other unrelated eye conditions.

Conditions That May Simulate Seborrheic Dermatitis

Psoriasis Vulgaris

Psoriasis vulgaris (PV) of the scalp, face, and ears may be clinically and microscopically indistinguishable from SD. Biopsy is often of no value, as at this point both diseases can show similar findings. Family history and follow-up will usually separate the two. The lesions of PV develop a deeper color, are more raised, and develop a silvery rather than yellow scale. In addition, PV lesions tend to be more fixed and circumscribed than SD lesions. In the absence of other lesions, the presence of linear nail pitting points to a diagnosis of PV.

Bacterial Intertrigo

This condition is caused by flexural infection with corynebacteria. It can be difficult to distinguish from flexural SD. Wood's lamp exam will show a distinct coral-red fluorescence with bacterial intertrigo, which is due to a porphyrin secreted by the bacteria.

Intertriginous Monilia

Monilia of the inframammary creases, axillae, groins, and external genitalia can develop scale and can simulate intertriginous SD. Satellite lesions, moist fissures, and pustules favor monilia. A KOH preparation that demonstrates spores and/or pseudohyphae is definitive (*see* Part I, Photo 52).

Pityriasis (Tinea) Versicolor

Petaloid SD and pityriasis versicolor can have a substantial resemblance to each other. The distribution of SD is usually more limited to the central truncal regions and the scale is evident. Pityriasis versicolor scale usually is evident only after gentle scraping, and the white spotting effect seen after solar exposure does not occur with SD. A KOH preparation revealing grouped spores and short hyphae in pityriasis versicolor distinguishes the two (*see* Part I, Photo 51).

Pityriasis Rosea

Resemblance of generalized SD to pityriasis rosea is fairly superficial. SD lesions have a duskier yellow-red hue and a looser, greasier scale, which does not form a defined collarette. SD lesions also tend to become confluent, whereas PR lesions remain discrete. In addition, SD has a slow gradual onset, and lacks a herald plaque.

Nummular Eczema

This common problem should be clinically separable from SD. The lesions of nummular eczema are less numerous and differ in morphology. The wet form has a beefy-red moist surface and the dry form has a fissured surface often compared to the crackle finish on oriental pottery. Both variants of nummular eczema are widely distributed rather than central truncal. Pruritus is intense.

Atopic Dermatitis

Inflammatory diffuse facial SD can be difficult to distinguish from atopic dermatitis. Both affect the scalp and face with diffuse erythema. SD tends to produce more scaling, is associated with less pruritus, and does not show the circum-oral pallor or white dermographism of atopic dermatitis. Personal and family histories for other atopic problems are helpful.

Lichen Simplex Chronicus

This condition, which occurs frequently in adult women, can be confused with SD when it is localized to the posterior scalp. Patients complain of unremitting itching and the lesions show thickening, lichenification, and excoriation, which are normally absent with SD.

Secondary Syphilis

Although this is at present a relatively rare disease, the incidence of syphilis is again rising and it is an important differential diagnosis with any of the papulosquamous diseases. Secondary-stage lues can simulate the facial and petaloid chest lesions of SD. Normally the onset is more abrupt and victims have constitutional symptoms and generalized lymphadenopathy. Usually, other skin lesions are present on the mucous membranes, palms, or soles. Suspicion should prompt a history for high-risk behavior and a syphilis serology. Serologies in this stage are almost universally positive. If negative in the face of strong suspicion, ask the lab to dilute the serum looking for the prozone effect, which can give a false-negative test in patients with very high titers. Negative syphilis titers with active infection have also been reported on rare occasions in HIV infection.

Pediculosis Capitis

This differential occurs most often in adult patients who present with severe pruritus and may have minimal scalp finding or concurrent SD. Always look at the hair for evidence of nits. The itching with pediculosis is usually much more severe than that of SD.

ANSWERS TO CLINICAL APPLICATION QUESTIONS

History Review

A somewhat irascible 70-year-old woman with a highly stylized bouffant hairdo complains of intolerable scalp pruritus. You notice white flakes on the shoulders of her black sweater. You suspect seborrheic dermatitis.

1. What history should you attempt to elicit from this patient?

Answer:
a. How frequently does she shampoo?
b. With what does she shampoo her hair?
c. Does she frequently wear wigs?

2. When you examine this patient's scalp, what primary and secondary lesions would support your diagnosis of seborrheic dermatitis?

Answer:

a. Dull, sharply demarcated red patches.

b. Loose, easily dislodged yellow or white scale.

3. Where else on this patient's body should you look for active dermatitis?

Answer:

a. Post-auricular folds.

b. Concha of the ears.

c. Eyebrows.

d. Mid-glabella.

e. Perinasal, nasolabial, and mental creases of the face.

f. Mid-chest and inframammary creases.

g. Upper back.

4. How should you approach treatment in this patient?

Answer: Treatment approach depends on the patient's willingness to alter hair style and hygiene practices. The best approach is daily use of an antidandruff shampoo with adjuvant use of a topical steroid when required. Patients who refuse to shampoo regularly will require a topical steroid as primary therapy with use of an antidandruff shampoo.

5. What should you tell this patient is the prognosis for seborrheic dermatitis?

Answer: Seborrhea usually responds promptly to treatment. It is however, a life-long condition subject to exacerbations, and will require lifelong maintenance treatment.

8 Pityriasis Rosea

CLINICAL APPLICATION QUESTIONS

A 25-year-old woman comes to you with a 1-week history of nonpruritic lesions on the upper right inner arm. Examination reveals three annular lesions with central scale. Treatment for tinea corporis is prescribed in the form of a topical antifungal agent. The patient returns 14 days later complaining of a generalized moderately pruritic eruption from the neck to the upper hips.

1. List the disorders that should be considered in this patient.
2. Is tinea corporis still part of the differential diagnosis, and if not, why not?
3. What are the primary lesions of pityriasis rosea?
4. What are the secondary lesions of pityriasis rosea?
5. What should you tell the patient about the prognosis for pityriasis rosea?

APPLICATION GUIDELINES

Specific History

Onset

Pityriasis rosea (PR) is a common dermatitis that acts like a viral exanthem. Peak incidence is during the second and third decades, although it can occur at any age. Onset is acute and usually consists of the sudden appearance of a single skin lesion, referred to as the *herald plaque* or *patch*. About 5% of cases have a prodrome with mild constitutional symptoms, sore throat, GI complaints, and/or cervical adenopathy. In a significant number of patients, the initial lesions are overlooked or occur in hidden locations; therefore, it presents as an acute generalized eruption. Outbreaks often cluster in an epidemic fashion during the spring and fall. This supports speculation of a viral etiology. Cause, however, remains unproven and concurrent cases within family units are rare.

Evolution of Disease Process

The typical case of PR occurs in three phases. During the primary phase, a solitary lesion or a small group of lesions appears abruptly, usually on the chest or upper torso; however, they can be virtually anywhere, including mucous membranes. These are almost always asymptomatic. This herald plaque enlarges for an average of 7 to 14 days, at which point patients enter the secondary (generalized or exanthematous) phase. This phase lasts an average of 10 to 14 days, during which time smaller versions of the initial lesions develop predominantly over the upper torso and neck along skin cleavage lines. Pruritus may be absent (occasionally), mild (typically), or severe (rarely). The tertiary (regression) phase begins as the progression of new lesions ceases. Over the ensuing 2 weeks, the lesions fade in color, desquamate, and disappear. PR may leave

From: *Current Clinical Practice: Dermatology Skills for Primary Care: An Illustrated Guide*
D.J. Trozak, D.J. Tennenhouse, and J.J. Russell © Humana Press, Totowa, NJ

temporary hypopigmentation in some cases, but does not scar and has no permanent sequelae. Recurrent cases are very rare and in most instances an attack confers lifelong protection.

Evolution of Skin Lesions

The name *pityriasis rosea* is descriptive and refers to the rosy-red color of early lesions and the fine branny scale that evolves in the later phase. All PR lesions evolve in a similar way. The earliest lesions, especially the herald plaque, tend to be larger than the later ones (3–4 cm vs 1–2 cm). Early lesions and the herald plaque are usually out of phase with the smaller secondary lesions, and their more advanced morphology aids in the diagnosis. A typical lesion runs its course over a 3- to 4-week period. At onset, lesions start as bright rosy-red papules or plaques that resemble wheals of urticaria. As each lesion approaches its full size, the center darkens and a fine scale occurs. When the central scale loosens, a collarette of white scale is left at the periphery with its free edge characteristically turned toward the center of the lesion. Next the color changes to a dull salmon-pink, the plaque flattens, scales develop over its entire surface, and it disappears.

Provoking Factors

Musty garments, insect bites, atopic genealogy, and pregnancy are among predisposing factors cited in the older literature. Recent studies, however, fail to confirm these associations.

Self-Medication

Patients frequently interpret the herald plaque as a ringworm lesion, so use of proprietary antifungal agents is common. Recently, self-treatment with proprietary hydrocortisone creams has increased. Fortunately neither has any significant effect and does not interfere with the diagnosis.

Supplemental Review From General History

Intensely pruritic lesions resembling PR, or unusually extensive disease, may signal a PR-like drug eruption rather than actual PR. Associated constitutional symptoms or widespread adenopathy may be a clue that this is really a PR-like syphilid of secondary syphilis. A long-lasting fixed eruption simulating PR has been reported with advanced HIV infection. Under any of these circumstances, a complete general history review is essential.

2. Dermatologic Physical Exam

Primary Lesions

1. Rosy-red papules (*see* Photo 18).
2. Rosy-red plaques (*see* Photo 19)

The earliest lesions are not diagnostic until the central epidermal changes occur. Fortunately few patients come in this early and careful observation will almost always reveal a few with central scale or a peripheral collarette. Small papular primary lesions are more common in pregnant women, young children, and African Americans.

Secondary Lesions

1. Fine, branny, easily dislodged central scale that leaves, as it separates, a characteristic collarette with its free edge pointed to the center of the lesions (*see* Photo 20).
2. Some patients develop transient hypopigmentation at the lesion sites when resolution is complete.
3. Late lesions desquamate and change from rosy-red to salmon-pink in color.

It is not unusual to see the spectrum of lesions in a single patient.

Distribution

   Microdistribution: None.

   Macrodistribution: Can be quite variable. Classic distribution involves the neck,
back, chest, abdomen, proximal arms, hips, and proximal thighs. Face, forearms, palms,
and distal lower limbs are usually spared (*see* Fig. 7).

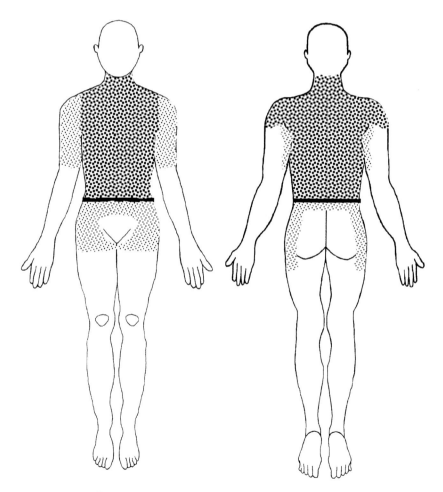

Figure 7: Macrodistribution of pityriasis rosea.

PR is suppressed by sun exposure; during intense solar exposure lesions may be limited to non-sun-exposed skin only (such as areas beneath bathing trunks or bikinis).

Configuration

PR has a "Christmas tree" configuration (*see* Photo 21). When viewed from a distance, the oval lesions of PR classically line up in a linear fashion with their long axes following skin tension lines. Hence, the lesions assume a linear descending pattern much like the drooping branches of a pine tree.

Indicated Supporting Diagnostic Data

Syphilis serology should be done in all sexually active patients. The lesions of PR and the lesions of secondary syphilis are not clinically distinguishable.

When a solitary scaling plaque or small group of plaques are present, a KOH preparation may be needed to rule out tinea corporis.

Therapy

There is no specific therapy. PR is essentially a benign self-limiting disease that resolves without sequelae. Treatment is symptomatic.

Patients with moderate or severe itching should be instructed to avoid overheating, take warm but not hot showers, keep bed clothing lighter than usual, and temporarily avoid activity that raises body temperature.

Ultraviolet light suppresses and shortens the duration of the general eruption. Patients who are distressed with extensive lesions can be helped with modest amounts of natural sunlight or ultraviolet B exposure.

A medium potency group IV or V steroid cream or lotion (*see* Chapter 4, Table 1) is helpful when there is significant itching. Menthol 0.025% can be added for additional relief. The steroid will have no effect on the appearance or duration of the lesions.

Conditions That May Simulate Pityriasis Rosea

PR-Like Drug Eruptions

Barbiturates, captopril, clonidine, gold, isotretinoin, metronidazole, and penicillamine are among the medications most commonly implicated as causes of eruptions with PR-like morphology. These agents are not exclusive and this possibility should always be considered, especially if the eruption is in any way atypical. The following all suggest a drug eruption:
1. Intense pruritus.
2. Absent herald plaque.
3. An active urticarial component with immediate dermographism.
4. Heavy scale.
5. Evolution of some lesions toward lichen planus-like appearance.
6. Persistence beyond the usual 6- to 8-week course.

Early Eruptive Psoriasis

Eruptive psoriasis vulgaris (PV) can, in its early stages, be indistinguishable from early PR. This differential must always be considered in a patient with a positive family history for PV. In general, PV will progress unless treated and as the lesions mature they develop the deeper color and loose silvery scale typical of that disease. This differential diagnosis should always be considered with fixed PR. Usually PV lacks a herald plaque and the classic Christmas tree pattern. At this stage, the biopsy findings are generally inconclusive. A short period of observation will usually spare the victim the discomfort, scar, and expense of biopsy.

Tinea Corporis

Early PR with a herald plaque or early cluster of lesions can be difficult to separate from tinea corporis. A simple KOH preparation will distinguish the two, provided the area has not been premedicated with proprietary antifungals.

Seborrheic Dermatitis

Generalized SD bears some resemblance to PR. The slow onset, limited lesions, loose scale, and central truncal rather than Christmas tree distribution should serve to distinguish between the two.

Nummular Eczema

This common problem should be clinically separable from PR. The lesions of nummular eczema are less numerous and differ in morphology. The wet form has a beefy-red moist surface and the dry form has a fissured surface often compared to the crackle finish on oriental pottery. Neither variant of nummular eczema has the Christmas tree distribution. Itching is intense.

Secondary Syphilis

This is an important differential in all sexually active persons. Both eruptions can be similar and both can undergo spontaneous resolution. Patients with syphilis usually have associated constitutional symptoms of fatigue, fever, and myalgias. In addition, there are often palmar lesions, mucous membrane lesions, and a generalized adenopathy. A syphilis serology with the same precautions noted above is definitive.

HIV Disease

There have been rare reports of a persistent PR-like eruption in cases of late HIV infection. In a single patient observed by one of the authors, the eruption was of gradual onset, had persisted longer than 1 year, and had fixed lesions. Otherwise it simulated the morphology and classic distribution of PR.

ANSWERS TO CLINICAL APPLICATION QUESTIONS

History Review

A 25-year-old woman comes to you with a 1-week history of nonpruritic lesions on the upper right inner arm. Examination reveals three annular lesions with central scale. Treatment for tinea corporis is prescribed in the form of a topical antifungal agent. The patient returns 14 days later complaining of a generalized moderately pruritic eruption from the neck to the upper hips.

1. List the disorders that should be considered in this patient.

Answer:

a. Pityriasis rosea.

b. Pityriasis rosea-like drug eruption.

c. Seborrheic dermatitis.

d. Early eruptive psoriasis.

e. Secondary syphilis.

f. Nummular eczema.

2. Is tinea corporis still part of the differential diagnosis, and if not, why not?

Answer: Tinea corporis enters the differential diagnosis when single or small numbers of lesions are present; however, tinea corporis does not spread at this rate and does not produce large numbers of individual lesions. Also, topical antifungal agents are usually effective over a 2-week treatment period.

A negative KOH preparation would have ruled out tinea corporis at the time of the initial visit and prevented unnecessary antifungal therapy.

3. What are the primary lesions of pityriasis rosea?

Answer: Rosy-red papules and rosy-red plaques.

4. What are the secondary lesions of pityriasis rosea?

Answer: Central branny scale develops on the plaques, and as the scale desquamates, the free edge is turned in toward the center of the lesion.

5. What should you tell the patient about the prognosis for pityriasis rosea?

Answer: Pityriasis rosea is a self-limited exanthem that usually clears in a 6- to 12-week time period. It heals without permanent scars or marks, and recurrence is rare.

9 Psoriasis Vulgaris

Psoriasis is an incredibly diverse condition in its onset, progression, course, and response to treatment. A common malady, it afflicts 1 to 3% of the world population. This chapter will cover only the most common presentations.

CLINICAL APPLICATION QUESTIONS

A 32-year-old man comes to your office complaining of a thick crusted flaking scalp dermatitis of 6 weeks' duration. You suspect psoriasis vulgaris.

1. What history should you elicit from this patient to support your suspected diagnosis and rule out other possibilities?
2. What are the primary lesions of psoriasis vulgaris?
3. What are the secondary lesions of psoriasis vulgaris?
4. What distribution of lesions on the head would support your suspected diagnosis of psoriasis vulgaris?
5. Where else on the patient's body should you look for evidence of psoriasis vulgaris?

APPLICATION GUIDELINES

Specific History

Onset

Peak onset is in the second and third decades; however, first activity has been reported at birth and as late as the tenth decade. The most common onset consists of the gradual development of raised scaling papules and plaques over the pressure points of joints and other loci of chronic skin friction or trauma. Common trigger sites include the posterior scalp, the skin of the presacral and upper gluteal cleft regions, and the glans penis. These are typical locations for stable plaque psoriasis.

The other common presentation is eruptive exanthematic, or so-called "guttate" psoriasis. Hundreds of scaling papules arise suddenly on large body areas over a period of weeks. Rare and atypical forms such as pustular, acral, and nail psoriasis will not be discussed here.

Evolution of Disease Process

Untreated, stable plaque psoriasis can remain static for years. Some of these patients may experience acute exacerbations when they encounter exogenous or endogenous provoking factors. With treatment, chronic plaque lesions may resolve permanently or for months or years. There is a tendency, however, for lesions to gradually recur at old sites or appear at new sites.

From: *Current Clinical Practice: Dermatology Skills for Primary Care: An Illustrated Guide*
D.J. Trozak, D.J. Tennenhouse, and J.J. Russell © Humana Press, Totowa, NJ

Eruptive exanthematic psoriasis has a more variable course. These cases may evolve into stable plaque disease but are more often subject to subacute or acute exacerbations, and are even more affected by exogenous trauma and factors that provoke the disease process. There is an overall tendency for psoriasis to worsen with time and to become increasingly refractory to therapy. It is therefore important to use the mildest effective regimens for as long as possible in a given patient.

Evolution of Skin Lesions

The earliest lesions of PV are erythematous scaling papules a few millimeters across, which enlarge in a centrifugal fashion. The papules may singly enlarge or coalesce with other plaques to produce solid plaques that cover large areas. Lesions may vary in color, thickness, and degree of scale but tend to resemble one another on a given patient.

Provoking Factors

All of the following have been reported to exacerbate PV:

1. **Emotional stress.**
2. **Obesity.**
3. **Hypocalcemia.**
4. **Heavy ethanol use.**
5. **Cold weather.**
6. **Trauma:** Local trauma to the skin of any sort sufficient to injure the epidermis and upper dermis can induce active lesions at the site of injury. This is known as the Koebner phenomenon and is common in cases of eruptive exanthematic PV. It is considered a supporting diagnostic feature.
7. **Sunlight:** Sunlight improves most cases, but 5% of patients are worsened and this must be taken into account prior to starting treatment. Severe sunburn can dramatically flare PV even in patients who have been responding to heliotherapy.
8. **Pregnancy:** Most psoriatics improve during pregnancy, and then flare during the postpartum period. There are many exceptions and the effect of pregnancy is erratic, even during succeeding pregnancies in the same patient.
9. **Intercurrent infections:** Streptococcal pharyngitis has been recognized as a specific trigger factor for the onset of eruptive exanthematic PV. Upper respiratory infections frequently precipitate intercurrent flares. Staphylococcal infections have been documented in association with rare pustular forms. When suspected, these infections should be documented and treated. Preexisting PV has been noted to flare when seen in conjunction with HIV infection.
10. **Medications:** Many modern medications have been reported to aggravate PV. The most frequently implicated are lithium, quinine derivatives, 4- and 8-amino-quionolone compounds, β-adrenergic blocking agents, and systemic corticosteroids. These drugs can exacerbate existing disease or provoke latent cases into activity. The flares following withdrawal of systemic steroids can be so severe as to be life-threatening, and use of these agents in a psoriatic for treatment of PV or other conditions must be weighed very carefully as to the potential benefits. Less severe flaring of PV has been documented after withdrawal of potent group I topical steroids and with ocular administration of β-blockers for glaucoma.

Nonsteroidal anti-inflammatory drugs (NSAIDs) have been variously reported to flare or improve psoriasis. Because of their extensive use, a decision should be made in each case based on history of disease activity relative to the indication for the NSAID. A psoriatic patient starting one of these agents should be warned to report flaring promptly.

Self-Medication

Self-treatment is seldom a problem in PV.

Supplemental Review From General History

When PV occurs in an explosive fashion, becomes refractory to therapy, or occurs in the context of opportunistic infection, an in-depth history for high-risk behavior and other signs and symptoms of HIV infection is indicated.

Dermatologic Physical Exam

Primary Lesions

The earliest lesions of PV are erythematous, scaling papules 1 to 2 mm across, which enlarge in a centrifugal fashion (*see* Photo 22). The papules may enlarge singly or coalesce with other papules to produce solid plaques that cover large areas (*see* Photo 23). Color can vary from pink, to bright or dusky red. Color fades visibly as lesions go into remission. Thickness also varies, and increased thickness correlates directly with disease activity.

Secondary Lesions

1. Scale is loose and silvery, often referred to as "micaceous" or mica-like (*see* Photo 24).
2. Fissures are seen on occasion with intertriginous psoriasis.
3. Hyperpigmentation often occurs as lesions resolve and takes the shape of the resolving plaque (*see* Photo 25).
4. Hypopigmentation may also occur with resolution. Usually it has the shape of the resolving lesion.

Degree of scale varies dramatically from barely visible to scale so thick that the underlying plaque is totally obscured. Thickness of scale correlates directly with disease activity and is also altered by a patient's personal hygiene. When the scale is lifted from a plaque, a moist exudative surface is left, which is the epidermal layer immediately above the dermal papillae. Often this action will cause areas of pinpoint bleeding on the plaque surface from trauma to the exposed dermal capillaries. This is referred to as the Auspitz sign, and strongly supports the diagnosis (*see* Photo 26).

Distribution

Microdistribution: Rarely follicular.
Macrodistribution:

1. Classic: Scalp, pressure points over extensor surface of joints, presacral and upper gluteal clefts, glans penis. Psoriasis may occur on any skin surface (*see* Fig. 8).

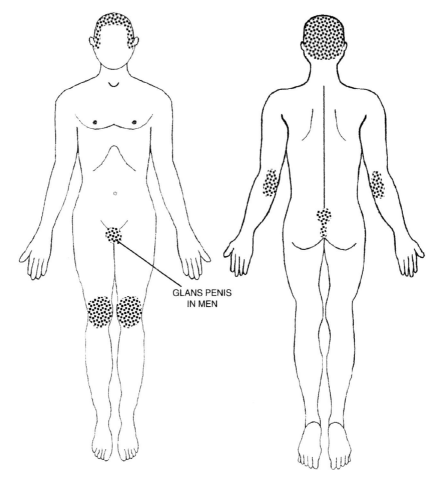

GLANS PENIS
IN MEN

Figure 8: Macrodistribution of psoriasis vulgaris.

2. Inverse: Creases and folds. An uncommon intertriginous form is referred to as inverse psoriasis.
3. Generalized erythrodermic: Generalized red skin.

Lesions tend to be symmetric from side to side and across the midline, even in extensive disease. Inverse lesions show little or no scale.

Configuration

1. Guttate (droplike) is common in eruptive exanthematic disease (*see* Photo 27).
2. Nummular (coin-sized) is common in generalized disease (*see* Photo 28).
3. Annular, gyrate, and polycyclic (*see* Photo 29). Portions of plaques may resolve or drop out, resulting in annular shapes. Gyrate and polycyclic configurations occur as these lesions merge. The solid plaque is most characteristic.

Indicated Supporting Diagnostic Data

Common patterns of PV are clinically diagnostic. A positive Auspitz sign (*see* Photo 26), Koebner phenomenon, and linear nail pitting (*see* Photo 30) provide strong clinical support. With common patterns, no supporting data are indicated.

Less common patterns of PV may simulate bacterial intertrigo, tinea corporis, tinea pedis, intertriginous monilia, seborrheic dermatitis, pityriasis rosea, subacute cutaneous lupus erythematosus, and cutaneous T-cell lymphoma (mycosis fungoides).

1. Wood's lamp examination: PV has a negative examination.
2. KOH preparation of scales: PV has a negative preparation.
3. Skin biopsy: As noted above, PV can simulate several other inflammatory dermatitides. Unfortunately, the histology of SD can also show similar changes. For this reason, biopsy of PV is not always a definitive procedure and should not be undertaken routinely. If the disease is atypical, extensive, or refractory to treatment, the patient should be referred to a dermatologist to decide whether this expense is cost-effective. Biopsy readily distinguishes psoriasis from subacute lupus erythematosus. However, distinguishing PV from other diseases, especially cutaneous T-cell lymphoma, is tricky and requires special competence and experience. Even in the most experienced hands, this is not always possible.

Therapy

The treatment of PV involves a mixture of experience, science, and art. Response to therapy is capricious, and treatment that is effective for one patient may be ineffective or actually detrimental for others. The disease often tends to become progressively refractory to treatment modalities that were previously effective. Always try to use the simplest effective means of control for as long as is possible. This section will cover very basic topical and intralesional therapy. Treatments described will essentially be useful for limited stable plaque and limited early eruptive disease. Discussion of other theraputic modalities for PV, such as topical anthralin, topical psoralens, UVB /UVA irradiation, X-ray, or the systemic administration of psoralens, retinoids, biologicals, antimetabolites, or immunosuppressants is beyond the scope of this book and should be prescribed only by a practitioner familiar with the entire armamentarium.

Topical Therapy

Topical steroids: These are available in an extensive array of vehicles and potencies (*see* Chapter 4). Side effects, both local and systemic, have been well documented, and the incidence increases with potency or with use of an inappropriate compound on an area of high permeability or with prolonged usage over large surface areas. For these reasons, topical corticoids are most useful for limited, stable plaque psoriasis and on special locations such as the scalp, genitalia, or folds where the effectiveness of other modalities is limited. Children have a greater ratio of skin surface area to body weight and are more susceptible to both the local and systemic side effects.

One of the major pitfalls of topical corticoid treatment for PV is an effect known as *tachyphylaxis*. For unknown reasons, the disease becomes increasingly refractory to corticosteroids, which requires the use of more potent preparations. Sometimes this effect can be avoided by intermittent dosing with scheduled rest periods (pulse dosing). At other times it requires a switch to alternative therapy.

Carefully review the section in Chapter 4 on topical steroids, especially with regard to potency, skin permeability, vehicles, general rules for using topical steroids, and guidelines for use of superpotent corticoids.

Topical calcipotriene: This is the first major topical alternative to topical corticoids and is effective in the treatment of limited stable plaque PV. Calcipotriene is indicated at present only for topical therapy of psoriasis because of its selected effects on cell differentiation and replication. It cannot and should not be used as a general substitute for topical corticoids in other inflammatory skin conditions. Calcipotriene is a biologically active form of vitamin D_3 that has a 1- to 200-fold weaker effect on systemic calcium metabolism. It is available as a 0.005% ointment, cream, and scalp lotion and is applied BID to the affected area. Potency of the ointment appears to be about equivalent to a group III steroid cream. Calcipotriene cream is less potent and is more useful in maintaining areas already in remission. It is to early to know if tachyphylaxis will be a problem with prolonged use, as premarketing studies were limited to 8 weeks. Side effects consist mainly of irritation to the surrounding nonlesional skin. Therefore the patient must be carefully instructed to limit application to the plaque. There have been occasional cases of dermatitis at the application sites, and if this persists, calcipotriene should be discontinued. Systemic effects on calcium metabolism have not occurred in patients using 100 g or less per week. Hypercalcemia has been reported in a small number of patients above this dose; therefore, supplies should be carefully controlled and calcium levels checked if there is suspicion of abuse. The authors recommend a baseline serum Ca^{2+} when treatment is started and with prolonged dosing that approaches 100 g/week. Use of topical calcipotriene is not recommended for facial skin. Safety has not been established for children or for pregnant or nursing women. Established hypercalcemia is a contraindication. Sequential therapy combining calcipotriene with a superpotent topical steroid and then rapidly switching to pulse therapy can induce rapid remissions, minimize the risk of side effects, and minimize the phenomenon of tachyphylaxis.

Keratolytics: Salicylic acid 3 to 6% in petrolatum or 10 to 20% urea in a hydrophilic cream base can be used to remove heavy scale that otherwise impedes topical treatment and phototherapy. Systemic absorption with extensive use could lead to salicylism in children, persons who take salicylates, or persons with abnormal renal function.

Topical therapy of special regions: For scalp with heavy scale, apply a penetrating lotion of phenol in a mineral oil-glycerin base, such as P & S liquid® (Baker-Cummins, OTC), overnight beneath a plastic shower cap. Shampoo each morning with a tar- or salicylic acid-based antipsoriatic shampoo (several are available OTC). Have the patient gently comb out loose scale, taking care to avoid trauma that can activate the disease. Apply calcipotriene scalp lotion or a topical steroid lotion, matching potency to need. Lotions with a propylene glycol or an alcohol base are best suited to treating scalp psoriasis. For ear canals, start with a low potency oil-in-water lotion such as desonide and switch to a more potent product such as clobetasol lotion if needed.

Topical retinoids: Tazarotene gel 0.05 and 0.1% has been approved for topical treatment of mild to moderate plaque psoriasis. Premarketing studies show efficacy equivalent to a group II steroid. Use of tazarotene in psoriasis requires skill and carries very specific warnings about use in women with childbearing potential.

Combination topical therapy: In an attempt to maximize the effectiveness of calcipotriene and tazarotene while minimizing their side effects and the side effects of topical steroids, the concept of combining high-potency corticosteroids with one of these newer topicals has been introduced. A full discussion of this method is beyond the scope of this book.

Intralesional Steroid Therapy

Injection of dilute solutions of corticosteroids into stable plaques can result in complete clearing for months or years. This is indicated for limited disease or for resolution of stubborn areas that will not clear with other topical treatment. Triamcinolone acetonide is the drug of choice. Other preparations tend to cause more skin atrophy. Whenever possible, dilute the solution to 2.5 mg/cc with physiologic saline. Higher concentrations increase the risk of side effects. Injections should be done only with a control syringe using a 30-gage needle, withdrawing each time to prevent intravascular or lymphatic injection. Injections should be made into the high dermis, which raises a wheal. Deeper injections are less effective and increase the risk of subcutaneous atrophy. Injections into the scalp should be done with great caution because of possible embolization of this crystalline drug to the retinal artery, with resulting blindness. Another safety precaution is to limit patients to a total of 10 mg of triamcinolone acetonide in any 1-month period.

Patients with more active disease or disease so extensive that it requires more than these treatments should be referred to a dermatologist.

Conditions That May Simulate Psoriasis Vulgaris
Seborrheic Dermatitis

SD of the scalp, face, and ears may be clinically and microscopically indistinguishable from PV. Biopsy is often of no value because at this point both diseases can show similar findings. Family history and follow-up will usually separate the two. The lesions of PV develop a deeper color, are more raised, and develop a silvery rather than yellow scale. In addition, PV lesions tend to be more fixed and circumscribed than SD lesions. In the absence of other lesions, the presence of linear nail pitting points to a diagnosis of PV.

Pityriasis Rosea

Eruptive PV in its early stages can be indistinguishable from early PR. This diagnosis must always be considered in a patient with a positive family history for PV. In general, PV will progress unless treated, and as the lesions mature they develop the deeper color and loose silvery scale typical of that disease. Eruptive PV should always be considered with fixed PR. Usually PV lacks a herald plaque and the classic Christmas tree pattern. At this stage, the biopsy findings are generally inconclusive. A short period of observation will usually spare the victim the discomfort, scar, and expense of biopsy. As with SD, the presence of nail pitting favors a diagnosis of psoriasis.

Nummular Eczema

The resemblance is usually superficial. Lesions of PV tend to be more profuse and more symmetrical than those of nummular eczema. Scale of PV is also more prominent, loose, and silvery. Eczema lesions are often moist and the scale has a crackled or fissured pattern. Itching can occur in both diseases but is usually intense with nummular eczema.

Secondary Syphilis

Secondary papulosquamous syphilis can closely resemble eruptive guttate PV. Patients with syphilis usually have associated constitutional symptoms of fatigue, fever, and myalgias. In addition, there are often palmar lesions, mucous membrane lesions, and generalized lymphadenopathy. A syphilis serology with the same precautions regarding prozone effect is definitive.

Cutaneous Lupus Erythematosus

Discoid and subacute lupus erythematosus (LE) can occasionally resemble PV in onset, distribution, and lesional morphology. Lupus lesions usually have a deeper hue with telangectasias. Scarring, which is absent in psoriasis, tends to occur early in discoid LE. Arthralgias and systemic symptoms may be present, especially with subacute LE. When suspected, a skin biopsy is helpful along with an antinuclear, anti-Ro (SS-A), and anti-La (SS-B) antibodies.

ANSWERS TO CLINICAL APPLICATION QUESTIONS

History Review

A 32-year-old man comes to your office complaining of a thick crusted flaking scalp dermatitis of 6 weeks' duration. You suspect psoriasis vulgaris.

1. What history should you elicit from this patient to support your suspected diagnosis and rule out other possibilities?

Answer:
   a. Is there a family history of psoriasis vulgaris?
   b. Is the patient aware of any other past or present persistent or recurrent skin rash?

2. What are the primary lesions of psoriasis vulgaris?

Answer: Erythematous scaling papules and plaques.

3. What are the secondary lesions of psoriasis vulgaris?

Answer: Loose silvery (mica-like) scale.

4. What distribution of lesions on the head would support your suspected diagnosis of psoriasis vulgaris?

Answer: Seborrheic dermatitis and atopic dermatitis of the scalp tend to remain limited to the hair-bearing scalp. Psoriasis frequently extends off the scalp onto adjacent skin such as forehead and postauricular areas.

5. Where else on the patient's body should you look for evidence of psoriasis vulgaris?

Answer:
   a. Pressure points such as knees and elbows.
   b. Presacral skin.
   c. Glans penis.
   d. Fingernails (fine linear nail pitting).

10 Lichen Planus

Lichen planus (LP) is a disease that has great variation in onset, appearance, and course. This section will present only the common features and usual course.

CLINICAL APPLICATION QUESTIONS

A 41-year-old woman presents with a slowly evolving intensely pruritic papular skin eruption over both volar forearms and pretibial areas. This is of 3 months' duration. She also complains of a painful erosion on the right buccal mucosa, a chronic pruritic scaling eruption on the soles of both feet, and intermittent irritated erosions on the outer vulva that interfere with intercourse.

1. Which, if any, of the above lesions may be lichen planus?
2. If any of these lesions are not lichen planus, what are they?
3. If you are uncertain of the diagnosis of lichen planus on clinical findings alone, how can you confirm the diagnosis?
4. What are the causes of lichen planus?
5. How should this patient be treated?
6. What is the prognosis for lichen planus?

APPLICATION GUIDELINES

Specific History

Onset

LP is very uncommon in children and occurs most often in adults in their fourth, fifth, and sixth decades. Family clusters are occasionally seen. Most cases begin insidiously with the onset of intensely pruritic red to deeply violet-colored papules that gradually increase in number and extent until the patient is sufficiently symptomatic to seek relief. A small number of cases present with a dramatic generalized exanthematic onset. These patients are immensely uncomfortable and socially devastated. Occasionally, painful oral lesions predominate. Uncommon nail, follicular, and ulcerating variants will not be discussed in this chapter.

Evolution of Disease Process

A small number of cases will resolve spontaneously within a few weeks. Ninety percent of cases will resolve by 24 months. About 10% of patients will develop chronic LP, usually in the form of oral mucous membrane lesions or hypertrophic lesions on the lower limbs. Occasionally, patients present with recurrent episodes that are separated by

From: *Current Clinical Practice: Dermatology Skills for Primary Care: An Illustrated Guide*
D.J. Trozak, D.J. Tennenhouse, and J.J. Russell © Humana Press, Totowa, NJ

symptom-free periods. Some patients have only a small number of lesions in a very limited area, while others have hundreds of lesions over much of the body surface. Almost all complain of intense itch that is disproportionate to the visible rash.

Evolution of Skin Lesions

LP begins with tiny papules that retain the skin marking lines and are therefore geometric or polygonal in shape. When first seen they are usually 3 to 5 mm in size and are palpably raised. Individual lesions can enlarge up to 1 cm. When lesions are grouped, they can merge to form tight aggregates of considerable size. They may then evolve into plaques or their papular origin may remain evident.

Provoking Factors

Some cases of LP are precipitated by a chronic tinea pedis and will resolve and recur with the activity of the fungal infection. Like psoriasis, LP will activate at sites of trauma and therefore shows a true Koebner phenomenon. In this disease, however, trauma induction is an incidental sign that supports the diagnosis but does not contribute in any significant way to the extent of the disease. A wide range of medications produce LP-like drug eruptions; however, it is uncertain at present whether these represent a separate entity or unmasking of idiopathic LP.

Self-Medication

Self-treatment is not a problem in LP, except where a covert medication might cause an LP-like drug eruption.

Supplemental Review From General History

A careful medication history is essential, and any medication reported to cause an LP-like eruption should be discontinued. The features of these drug eruptions are sometimes strikingly similar to the idiopathic disease both clinically and microscopically, and offending drugs will be uncovered only by careful history. The list of medications that cause these reactions continues to grow and any agent should be suspect. These drug-induced eruptions are slow to clear and it is not unusual for improvement to take 2 or 3 months. LP has also been associated with an increased incidence of autoimmune diseases (Sjögren's syndrome, sicca syndrome, alopecia areata, vitiligo, ulcerative colitis, myasthenia gravis, and diabetes mellitus), chronic dermatophyte infections, and chronic liver disease (primary biliary cirrhosis, alcoholic cirrhosis, chronic active hepatitis B and C). The presence of a fungal infection is usually significant: the authors have seen many cases of LP that clear and exacerbate with its activity. LP-like lesions are seen in patients with graft-versus-host reactions.

Dermatologic Physical Exam

Primary Lesions

Primary LP lesions are red to deep violet, flat-topped, angular geometric (polygonal) 1- to 3-mm papules. The papules may be separate or tightly grouped (*see* Photo 31).

Wickham's stria are a lacy network of white lines seen on the surface of the papules considered pathognomonic for LP (*see* Photo 32).

Early lesions tend to be red to dusky deep red. As the papules mature they acquire a deep violaceous hue, which is considered typical. As pigment is dropped from the basal cell layer some lesions may also have a brown cast.

Secondary Lesions

1. Scale is adherent and white, but not a prominent feature except in some hypertrophic variants (*see* Photo 33).
2. Large plaques form from coalescing papules, and the original papular morphology may be obscured. Satellite papules are frequently present at the periphery as a clue (*see* Photo 34).
3. Erosions are common with mucosal LP and occur on occasion in chronic hypertrophic lesions (*see* Photos 32,35,36).
4. Scarring and atrophy are common with LP of the hair-bearing scalp, the nail matrix, and chronic hypertrophic lesions. Permanent hair and nail loss can occur, sometimes rapidly (*see* Photo 37).
5. Although victims complain bitterly of itching, excoriations are seldom seen in LP.
6. Dense purple or deep brown hyperpigmentation can occur as lesions resolve. This pigmentary change may last for years.

Distribution

Microdistribution: Follicular distribution is encountered on rare occasions. The disease may attack any hair bearing area. Follicular LP may be seen with other typical skin and mucous membrane lesions or may occur alone. It presents as pin-head-sized conical, rough red papules pierced by a hair. Permanent hair loss may occur.

Macrodistribution: The oral cavity shows a lacy white reticulated or arborizing pattern, most commonly on the posterior buccal mucosa opposite the molars. It will not rub off with a tongue blade. Oral lesions occur in 30 to 70% of cases depending on the series. Rare cases occur with oral, genital, and anal involvement only.

Classic papular lesions have a predilection for flexural surfaces of joints and forearms. Other frequent sites are the dorsal hands, extensor shins, lateral neck, buttocks, sacrum, glans penis, and ankles (*see* Fig. 9). The face, scalp, palms, and soles are only rarely involved.

In the exanthematic form, lesions can be distributed uniformly over much of the body surface and the characteristic distribution pattern is lost. The morphology of the primary lesions is usually diagnostic and oral lesions are found in a high proportion of cases as a supporting feature.

Configuration

1. Grouped papules are the most common pattern. If the grouping is follicular rather than random, the papules are small and evenly spaced following the anatomic spacing of the follicles.
2. Annular (ring) lesions with central clearing or central atrophy may occur but are uncommon. These are most often located on the glans penis.
3. Linear (long narrow band) lesions occur very rarely.
4. Reticulated (net-like or arborizing) configuration may occur with oral lesions.

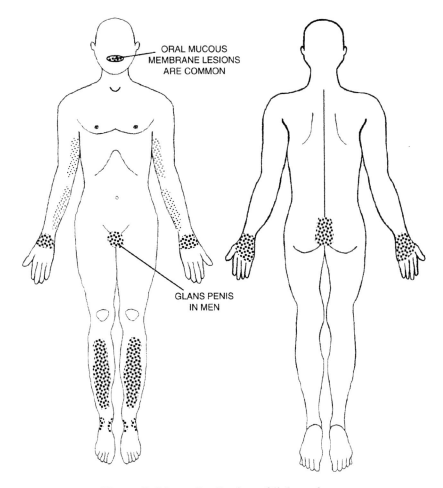

Figure 9: Macrodistribution of lichen planus.

Indicated Supporting Diagnostic Data

In many instances, oral and cutaneous lichen planus are clinically diagnostic and no specific laboratory testing is indicated.

Skin Biopsy

This test is indicated when the disease is strongly suspected but the diagnosis is clinically uncertain. Although LP and LP-like drug eruptions may show identical histology, subtle differences can sometimes point toward the latter diagnosis. Biopsy is particularly helpful for differentiating lichen planus and lupus erythematosus.

Direct Immunofluorescence

Although rarely needed, this test can be helpful in supporting a diagnosis of LP where other parameters are confusing. The pattern is quite different from that of lupus erythematosus; however, it is identical in an LP-like drug eruption.

General Laboratory Testing

The strong association of LP with chronic liver disease and hepatitis in some European series has led some authors to recommend routine screening. This association has not been confirmed in North America, and at present it would seem prudent to coordinate additional testing with information revealed in the review from the general history.

Therapy

Because LP is generally a self-limiting disorder, the aim should be to provide the patient with as much comfort as is possible with minimal risk. It must be kept in mind that the pruritus of limited disease can be very distressing, and eruptive LP is socially humiliating. Whenever possible, try to limit treatment to topical or intralesional regimens. When disease is extensive, this is not always possible and there is a point where systemic therapy is needed.

Topical Therapy

Limited LP will respond to topical steroids but effective treatment usually requires the most potent topical that is safe in a given skin region (carefully review the section in Chapter 4 on topical steroids). Resistant areas will often respond to a combination of a steroid cream alternated with topical tretinoin cream in the highest concentration tolerated. The prescribing practitioner should pay careful attention to surface area and total amount of topical steroid in use. If either of these is excessive, systemic treatment should be considered rather than trying to accomplish the same effect with an uncontrolled topical treatment.

Hypertrophic LP may respond to topical corticoids, but is less steroid-sensitive than other inflammatory skin conditions and often requires a group I steroid in an optimized vehicle. An alternative is to use a weaker product with plastic wrap occlusion. This method, which was developed prior to the arrival of the superpotent steroids, has a higher incidence of side effects and often leads to patient compliance problems.

Oral LP often responds well to a regimen of topical 0.05% fluocinonide ointment administered three to four times during the day. This agent is poorly absorbed from the bowel and systemic absorption has not been a problem. At bedtime, topical tretinoin cream is applied starting with the highest strength tolerated. Consider starting with the 0.05% cream and switching to the 0.1% concentration as the membrane responds. Tacrolimus ointment 0.1% has also proved quite effective in the treatment of oral LP. This immune modulator avoids the cutaneous atrophy associated with topical steroids but is fairly new and unique side effects may not yet be fully appreciated. Keep in mind that persisting ulceration of oral LP may signal a rare conversion to squamous cell carcinoma and a timely referral to a dermatologic consultant may be life-saving.

Intralesional Therapy

Intralesional therapy is useful for resistant localized LP and hypertrophic LP. Consider starting at a concentration of 2.5 mg/cc of triamcinolone acetonide diluted in physiologic saline. Often 5- or even 10-mg/cc concentrations are needed with thick hypertrophic areas. More concentrated solutions limit the area that can be safely treated without risk of systemic effects. The total monthly dose should always be recorded and monitored. On occasion, this technique may be useful with resistant oral lesions.

Systemic Therapy

Generalized disease that is too extensive for safe or effective topical treatment, and nail or scalp involvement that can leave disfiguring scarring, are indications for systemic therapy. If the practitioner is unsure of the situation, prompt referral to a dermatologist is then indicated. Among the multitude of systemic agents which have been reported effective, the following drugs are worth consideration.

Griseofulvin: Several years ago, this antifungal agent was reported in a controlled study to clear a high proportion of cases. Although subsequent studies have been conflicting, it is an agent with a very reasonable side-effect profile and is well worth consideration in the treatment of widespread nonscarring LP or LP with a concomitant dermatophyte infection. In the latter situation, it is the initial drug of choice. When griseofulvin is effective, some improvement is seen within 30 days. This is usually evident as decreased pruritus, flattening of the papules, and a cessation of new lesions. Because of its slow onset and spotty efficacy, it should not be used for rapidly advancing exanthematic LP or where significant scarring can occur. With adults, consider starting with a dose of 1 g/day of ultramicronized griseofulvin divided into four equal doses. Administration at the start of a meal, or with milk enhances absorption and minimizes GI side effects. A baseline CBC should be obtained, as well as liver chemistries if there is any suggestion of prior liver disease. The drug is continued until clearing is complete. With prolonged use, a CBC and liver panel are recommended on a 3-month schedule. Much has been said about griseofulvin causing LP-like drug eruptions. This has been a rare event but should be kept in mind in the face of worsening disease.

Systemic steroids: In cases of rapidly advancing exanthematic LP, or when scarring scalp or nail lesions are present, systemic steroids are justified. In adult cases, prednisone in a single morning dose of 30 to 40 mg/day should be initiated then rapidly tapered once control is achieved. Often small areas of resistant disease persist that require topical treatment while the systemic agent is withdrawn. A practitioner using systemic corticoids must be fully aware of the side effects, contraindications, and monitoring required for safe usage.

Other agents: Systemic retinoid therapy, dapsone, and antimalarial agents have each been reported helpful in treating special problem types of LP. As these treatments are outside of standard therapy, such cases should be referred to a dermatological consultant.

Conditions That May Simulate Lichen Planus

LP-Like Drug Eruptions

These have been reported with a large number of medications. Thiazide diuretics, gold, antimalarials, β-blocking agents, vitamins, and NSAIDs are among those most commonly cited. This differential must be carefully evaluated in every case of LP. Some reactions are clinically identical to idiopathic LP; however, subtle findings on routine biopsy may help to distinguish them. Immunopathology is not helpful. LP-like drug reactions resolve slowly and require a good deal of support and confidence on the part of the treating practitioner. Clinical features that help to distinguish the two include a photodistribution and a psoriasis-like appearance common with the drug-induced form.

Lupus Erythematosus

Rarely cases are encountered where these two disorders seem to merge. In most instances, a biopsy combined with direct immunofluorescence will distinguish between them. Most cases turn out to be chronic discoid lupus. Rare overlap cases do occur.

Secondary Syphilis

Exanthematic LP without pruritus may be difficult to separate from a generalized papulosquamous syphilid. The latter is associated with lymphadenopathy and constitutional symptoms. A syphilis serology with precautions regarding prozone effect is definitive.

ANSWERS TO CLINICAL APPLICATION QUESTIONS

History Review

A 41-year-old woman presents with a slowly evolving intensely pruritic papular skin eruption over both volar forearms and pretibial areas. This is of 3 months' duration. She also complains of a painful erosion on the right buccal mucosa, a chronic pruritic scaling eruption on the soles of both feet, and intermittent irritated erosions on the outer vulva that interfere with intercourse.

1. Which, if any, of the above lesions may be lichen planus?

Answer: The papular skin eruption over both volar forearms and pretibial areas is a classic distribution of lichen planus. Erosive mucous membrane lesions are also a common feature of lichen planus

2. If any of these lesions are not lichen planus, what are they?

Answer: The chronic pruritic scaling eruption on the soles of both feet is not lichen planus but is typical of tinea pedis, which can be linked etiologically to lichen planus.

3. If you are uncertain of the diagnosis of lichen planus on clinical findings alone, how can you confirm the diagnosis?

Answer: Lichen planus has a characteristic histology on biopsy.

4. What are the causes of lichen planus?

Answer: Most cases of lichen planus are idiopathic. A significant number are drug-induced (thiazide diuretics, NSAIDs, β-blocking agents, etc.) or linked to chronic dermatophyte infections. Linkage to autoimmune disease and chronic liver disease is established but uncommon.

5. How should this patient be treated?

Answer: After the presence of an active tinea pedis is confirmed by KOH preparation, initial treatment should consist of systemic treatment for the tinea pedis. In many instances, the lichen planus will remit when the fungal infection is eradicated. If drug-induced lichen planus is suspected, elimination of the suspect medication is the first measure. In idiopathic lichen planus, treatment may range from topical steroids to systemic retinoids, depending on the stage and extent of the disease.

6. What is the prognosis for lichen planus?

Answer: Idiopathic lichen planus usually remits spontaneously in 12 to 24 months. Recurrences are common and chronic persistent cases do occur. Mucous membrane lichen planus has a much greater tendency to be chronic and unremitting. Drug-induced lichen planus and dermatophyte-associated cases usually remain clear once the offending drug is withdrawn or the dermatophyte infection is adequately treated.

11 Miliaria Rubra *(Prickly Heat)*

CLINICAL APPLICATION QUESTIONS

A distraught 22-year-old mother presents her 9-month-old infant with a generalized papular eruption over the neck and upper torso. The child is irritable but otherwise alert and active. There are no other constitutional or systemic signs. You suspect miliaria.

1. What questions should you ask the mother to help you distinguish miliaria from a viral exanthem?
2. What physical examination features help you distinguish miliaria from a viral exanthem?
3. If you decide this infant has miliaria, what treatment measures can be taken?
4. If you decide this infant has miliaria, what should you tell the mother?

APPLICATION GUIDELINES

Specific History

Onset

Three forms of miliaria occur, but only the common form will be discussed here. Under favorable conditions, anyone can develop miliaria. Infants and young children, however, seem particularly prone to this eruption caused by sweat-duct occlusion. The onset may be gradual or sudden and usually suggests an acute viral exanthem. Infants become cranky and irritable, while those able to verbalize complain of an intense pricking discomfort rather than pruritus.

Evolution of Disease Process

Sheets of tightly grouped geometrically distributed irritable red papules develop; these wax and wane in intensity depending on the ambient temperature and degree of activity. Because the sweat duct is temporarily blocked and the gland will continue to secrete, any sweat stimulus will cause a sudden apparent exacerbation. This can happen even after clinical resolution while the ducts are still recovering patency. In infants, crying, emotional distress, and exertion associated with feeding frequently cause short-lived flares.

Evolution of Skin Lesions

Individual lesions may wax and wane but usually regress once the precipitating factors are removed. An exception is when secondary infection supervenes. Then the lesions may become pustular or develop into a frank impetigo.

From: *Current Clinical Practice: Dermatology Skills for Primary Care: An Illustrated Guide*
D.J. Trozak, D.J. Tennenhouse, and J.J. Russell © Humana Press, Totowa, NJ

Provoking Factors

An immature sweat gland apparatus in infants and individual genetic susceptibility play a role. Rapid change in ambient temperature, high humidity, occlusive clothing, friction from garments, and any factor that favors skin surface bacterial colonization predisposes to miliaria. A recent study implicates certain strains of *S. epidermidis* as the source of the polysaccharide plug that can be demonstrated microscopically in the eccrine duct orifice. Once occlusion has occurred, any stimulus that initiates sweating will cause a short-lived exacerbation.

Self-Medication

Self-treatment is not a problem in miliaria.

Supplemental Review From General History

Time of onset in relation to weather changes, heat stress, febrile illness, and other provoking factors will usually identify the reason for occurrence.

Dermatologic Physical Exam

Primary Lesions

The earliest primary histologic lesion of miliaria is a crystalline intraepidermal vesicle (*see* Photo 38), which evolves into a small erythematous papule (*see* Photo 39). With prolonged occlusion, pustules may occur (*see* Photo 40).

Secondary Lesions

Secondary infection may lead to frank impetiginization.

Distribution

Microdistribution: Periporal (surrounds sweat duct orifices). Examination with a magnifier will demonstrate that the interspersed hair follicle openings are spared (*see* Fig. 10).

Macrodistribution: Large numbers of geometrically spaced tiny periporal papules arise symmetrically on covered areas of the trunk and in intertriginous regions. The face, arms, palms, and soles are spared.

Configuration

Grouped (tiny grouped geometrically spaced papules).

Indicated Supporting Diagnostic Data

None.

Therapy

General Measures

Victims should avoid any circumstance that provokes sweating, as this will exacerbate symptoms and reactivate the eruption. High ambient temperatures, especially with high humidity or while in tight occlusive clothing, will prolong the glandular plugging. Clothing should be light, loose, and absorbent to wick moisture away from the skin surface.

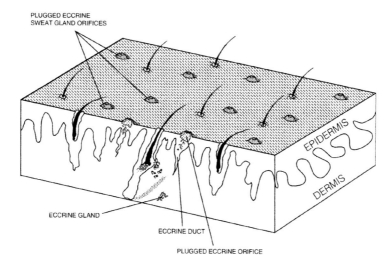

Figure 10: Microdistribution of miliaria.

Topical Therapy

The only measure ever shown to speed resolution of miliaria is epidermal lubrication. Consider using a bland OTC lubricant that contains a modest concentration of urea and an α-hydroxy acid. Topically applied anhydrous lanolin has also been reported as beneficial. Recent data suggest that use of an antibacterial bath soap might be beneficial, and in refractory cases, intermittent use of a benzoyl peroxide wash or lotion may be helpful.

Systemic Therapy

Systemic antibiotics should be used where there is clear evidence of secondary infection. They should be chosen on the basis of culture and sensitivity studies. These agents have no apparent effect on the primary process and are usually not required to treat pure miliaria. In the rare instance in which such therapy is considered for miliaria without secondary infection, culture for sensitivity should be obtained from several duct orifice lesions. Initial therapy should be directed at the spectrum of sensitivity of *S. epidermidis* and the antibiotic should preferably be one that is readily delivered to both the sweat gland and skin surface.

Conditions That May Simulate Miliaria

Viral Exanthems

Spring and summer viral illnesses may be confused with miliaria. These are usually of shorter duration and are associated with constitutional symptoms such as coryza, sore throat, fatigue, fever, or malaise. Cervical adenopathy is also common and is not seen with pure miliaria. Remember that miliaria can be a sequela of viral illness and both can have eruptions that may occur simultaneously or in sequence.

ANSWERS TO CLINICAL APPLICATION QUESTIONS

History Review

A distraught 22-year-old mother presents her 9-month-old infant with a generalized papular eruption over the neck and upper torso. The child is irritable but otherwise alert and active. There are no other constitutional or systemic signs. You suspect miliaria.

1. What questions should you ask the mother to help you distinguish miliaria from a viral exanthem?

Answer:
   a. Has there been any recent heat stress (exposure to high ambient temperature, high humidity, or tight or occlusive clothing)?
   b. Has the child been exposed to anyone else with a known viral exanthem or illness?
   c. Has the child been febrile or lethargic?
   d. Is there a history of recent sore throat or upper respiratory symptoms?
   e. Does the rash exacerbate with exposure to heat or with exertion (such as crying).

2. What physical examination features help you distinguish miliaria from a viral exanthem?

Answer: Oral findings such as an enanthem (mucous membrane rash) on the palate or mucous membranes is common with viral exanthems, but absent with miliaria. Regional adenopathy is common with viral exanthems, but absent with miliaria. Miliaria lesions are tiny red papules evenly spaced between hair follicles. Viral exanthem papules are less evenly spaced.

3. If you decide this infant has miliaria, what treatment measures can be taken?

Answer: Keep the child's environment cool and clothing light, and reduce exertion. Apply bland lubrication. On rare occasions, systemic antibiotics may be indicated for secondary infection.

4. If you decide this infant has miliaria, what should you tell the mother?

Answer: Miliaria is a benign self-limited condition that will eventually resolve. Resolution of the sweat gland blockage may take several weeks, and during that time, any heat stress or exercise will cause an immediate and apparent flare of the eruption.

12 Scabies

This discussion will be limited to human scabies.

CLINICAL APPLICATION QUESTIONS

A 16-year-old female comes to your office complaining of a pruritic generalized eruption of gradually increasing intensity over the prior 4 months. The pruritus now frequently awakens her during the night. You suspect a scabies infestation.

1. What pertinent history should you seek from this patient?
2. What primary lesions should you look for on physical examination that support a diagnosis of scabies?
3. What is the typical distribution of scabies in an adolescent female?
4. How should you establish the diagnosis of scabies?
5. What is the appropriate treatment for this patient?

APPLICATION GUIDELINES

Specific History

Onset

Human scabies is an infestation caused by an organism named *Sarcoptes scabiei var. hominis*, an obligate human parasite. The disease is most common in schoolchildren and young adults, but may be seen in all age groups and is also common in nursing home settings. Within family units, it is not unusual for the presenting case to be quite removed from the index case that brought the disease into the family. History of overnight house guests, school contacts, or close friends with symptoms is important, especially when one cannot obtain firm laboratory confirmation. Cases seen from skilled care facilities should trigger an investigation into other patients or staff with pruritus or dermatitis. When seeking this history, remember that the exposure occurred at least 1 month prior to the time the patient became symptomatic. Initial symptoms consist of discrete lesions, often on the wrists and hands, but these are frequently overlooked. Progressive pruritus, which interrupts sleep and normal activity, is what usually prompts the victim to seek help. The presence of the primary lesions is often elicited only by direct questioning. Some patients present late with extensive secondary changes. These consist of widespread dermatitis, secondary bacterial infection, and self-induced dermatitis caused by inappropriate attempts at treatment. It is estimated that the average victim has the infection for at least a month before generalized discomfort begins. Scabies should be considered in the differential of any generalized pruritic disorder. A special form called "crusted" or "Norwegian" scabies can present with minimal or no itching.

From: *Current Clinical Practice: Dermatology Skills for Primary Care: An Illustrated Guide*
D.J. Trozak, D.J. Tennenhouse, and J.J. Russell © Humana Press, Totowa, NJ

Evolution of Disease Process

Scabies begins insidiously with small comma-shaped burrows or tracks that, when viewed with magnification, have a scale at one end and a tiny papule or vesicle at the other end. The vesicle end is where the female mite is located. These lesions are initially asymptomatic and gradually increase in number. In adults, the wrists, finger webs, and lateral fingers are the most common areas. Adult men often show characteristic lesions on the genitalia, probably from autoinoculation. Adult women sometimes show characteristic lesions on the areolae or palms. Preschool children often have tracks on the palms, soles, and the lateral margins of the feet. About 4 to 6 weeks after infestation, the average patient begins to develop an immune response to the organism and the lesions become increasingly pruritic. Scratching destroys many burrows and limits but does not eradicate the infection. With persisting infestation, most victims develop an immune response that produces generalized itching, widespread papular dermatitis, and dermographism. Later, chronic generalized eczematous dermatitis and secondary impetiginization can occur. Even after successful treatment, persons with these intense immune reactions may take several weeks to become asymptomatic and inflammatory lesions may persist for weeks or months even though the organisms are no longer viable.

Persons who are immunosuppressed, physically unable to scratch, or have neurologic deficits that abolish itching, develop crusted (Norwegian) scabies. Itching may be minimal or absent and they present with thick keratotic crusted lesions of the hands, nails, elbows, knees, and ankles which may gradually progress to an erythroderma. These patients teem with organisms, are highly contagious, and may show generalized lymphadenopathy.

Evolution of Skin Lesions

The typical track lesions remain discrete and may become more erythematous or inflammatory as the immune response intensifies. This is particularly true with lesions in the genital regions. With established scabies, resolving tracks and new active tracks will be found interspersed in the same areas.

Provoking Factors

Overcrowding, poor hygiene, and close physical contact such as handholding or shared sleeping arrangements foster spread. Nursing facilities are also prone to outbreaks because of crowding and the presence of a population of patients more likely to develop the highly contagious crusted variety.

Self-Medication

Self-treatment is a significant problem in scabies cases both before and after the diagnosis is established. Because of the intense itching, victims often will try OTC remedies such as steroid creams or harsh remedies that give short-term relief by counterirritant effects. This misguided treatment either spreads the infestation or causes severe drying, which in turn worsens the pruritus. It is essential to take control of general skin care and help the patient understand that inappropriate treatment is making matters worse. After diagnosis, patients with established scabies will continue to experience symptoms for a few weeks to a month as the immune reaction winds down. It is important at the time of diagnosis and treatment to advise patients in this regard or they will often overapply irritating medications or persist in self-treatments that aggravate and prolong the discomfort.

Supplemental Review From General History

In cases of crusted (Norwegian) scabies, a general review should be undertaken seeking a reason for diminished immune response if the reason for this more severe form of the disease is not readily apparent.

Dermatologic Physical Exam

Primary Lesions

Primary lesions are comma-shaped or irregular burrows or tracks about 3 to 4 mm in length with a scale at the entrance point and a papulovesicle at the distal point where the mite is located (*see* Photos 41–43).

Secondary Lesions

1. Generalized small urticarial papules that are intensely pruritic. These occur about a month after infestation and are part of the immune reaction. Scraping these papular lesions in search of organisms is a worthless exercise (*see* Photo 44).
2. Excoriations are frequent and widespread (*see* Photo 44).
3. Impetiginization is frequent from secondary infection of excoriations (*see* Photo 44).
4. Lichenification and eczematous change may arise from persistent and repeated scratching (*see* Photo 44).
5. Warty, thick gray scaling crusts occur in crusted (Norwegian) scabies.

As the immune response becomes active during the second month, the primary burrows begin to show inflammation and become pruritic. General itching, especially bothersome at bedtime, increases and small intensely uncomfortable urticarial papules are present. Many cases show prominent immediate dermographism, which only adds to their discomfort. Persistent scratching causes excoriation, secondary infection, lichenification, and eczematous change. These patients often are simply unable to sit still during the examination process.

Distribution

Microdistribution: None.

Macrodistribution: Primary lesions in adults are found on the finger webs, finger margins, flexor surface of the wrists, elbows, axillary folds, ankles, and insteps. Adult men show a predilection for burrows on the genitalia. Adult women favor burrows on the palms and areolae of the breasts. Infants often show tracks on the palms, soles, and scalp (*see* Figs. 11–13).

Configuration

None.

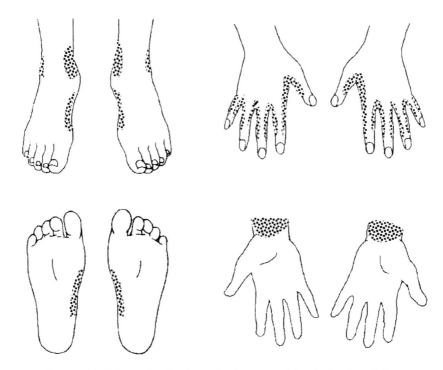

Figure 11: Macrodistribution of primary scabies lesion in adults.

Indicated Supporting Diagnostic Data

The definitive lab test for scabies is an ectoparasite examination. This is performed by identifying and scraping the distal vesicular end of one or several burrows, smearing the material on a microscope slide, and examining the specimen after adding a drop of 10% KOH or mineral oil. A positive smear will show an adult mite or mite ova, both of which are definitive (*see* Photo 45). Sometimes only the scybala or mite fecal balls are seen; these also support the diagnosis.

Therapy

General Measures

On the day of treatment, fresh clothing should be donned and bed linens should be changed. Furniture that is used frequently for lounging should be thoroughly vacuumed. Any clothing that has been worn and is launderable should be washed in the hot cycle. Any clothing that has been worn and is not launderable should be dry-cleaned. An alternative to dry-cleaning, for persons of limited financial resources, is to seal the exposed garments in a plastic bag for one week before reuse. Fastidious victims will tend to go overboard and it is important to set boundaries.

Topical Therapy

Permethrin in the form of a 5% cream formulation is currently the agent of choice in the treatment of scabies. For a typical case, it is applied from the neck down to all exter-

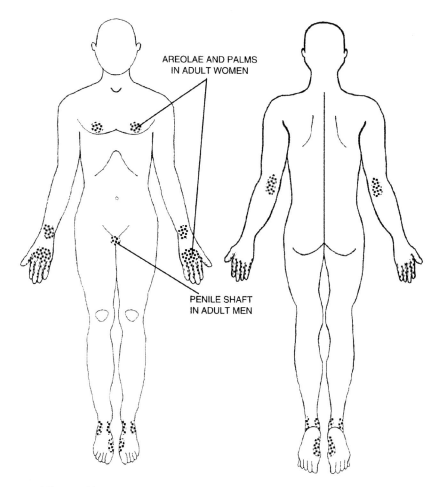

AREOLAE AND PALMS
IN ADULT WOMEN

PENILE SHAFT
IN ADULT MEN

Figure 12: Macrodistribution of primary scabies lesions in adults.

nal surfaces. You may have patients leave it on overnight and then shower it off. The application should be repeated one time only on the fourth to seventh day. This product is more effective, less irritating, and has less potential for toxicity than those previously available. Infants may on occasion require treatment of the head and neck areas, and patients with crusted scabies may require several treatments for cure. In elderly patients and in crusted scabies, special attention should be paid to the fingernails, which may be heavily infested. Subungual spaces should be manicured and medication should be applied.

Because symptoms persist for several days after effective therapy, patients must be cautioned not to continue treatment needlessly. For persisting symptoms, a topical steroid cream or a bland antipruritic ointment with 0.25% menthol and 0.5% camphor may be used. Other effective scabicides include gamma benzene hexachloride, benzyl benzoate, and 10% sulfur in yellow soft paraffin. These are inherently irritating to an already reactive skin surface. Gamma benzene hexachloride (lindane), if used to excess in children, has potential for substantial neurologic toxicity. It is no longer available in California.

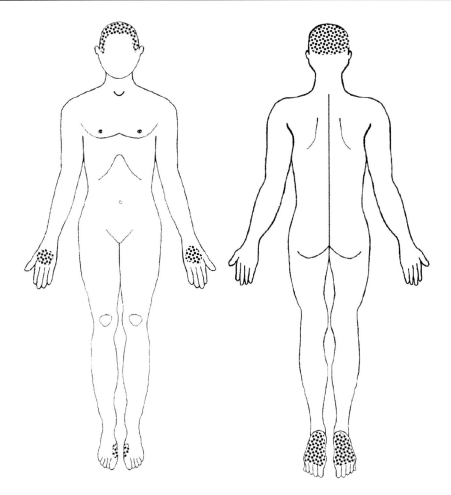

Figure 13: Macrodistribution of primary scabies lesions in infants.

Systemic Therapy

In patients with crusted (Norweigian) scabies, for resistant cases, or for patients who cannot comply with topical regimens, an oral alternative is 200 µg/kg ivermectinin two doses administered 1 week apart. Manicuring and hygiene procedures must still be observed. When combined with topical permethrin, this drug is even more effective.

Conditions That May Simulate Scabies

Scabies must be considered in the differential diagnosis of any generalized pruritic skin disorder especially with a history of nocturnal itching that interrupts sleep. Atopic dermatitis, generalized drug reactions, and widespread impetigo all show common features. A high index of suspicion that leads to a search for primary lesions is important to maintain. Crusted scabies can simulate eczema, psoriasis, or on rare occasions, an erythroderma.

ANSWERS TO CLINICAL APPLICATION QUESTIONS

History Review

A 16-year-old female comes to your office complaining of a pruritic generalized eruption of gradually increasing intensity over the prior 4 months. The pruritus now frequently awakens her during the night. You suspect a scabies infestation.

1. What pertinent history should you seek from this patient?

Answer:
  a. Are there any family members with similar symptoms?
  b. Are there any close friends or schoolmates with similar symptoms?
  c. Had any relatives or friends visited or stayed overnight prior to onset of the symptoms?
  d. Had the patient visited someone else and slept in their bed?
  e. Does the patient have any work exposure to scabies, such as direct patient care in a physician's office or nursing home facility?

2. What primary lesions should you look for on physical examination that support a diagnosis of scabies?

Answer: Comma-shaped burrows or tracks with a tiny vesicle at one end.

3. What is the typical distribution of scabies in an adolescent female?

Answer: Wrists, finger webs, finger margins, axillary folds, and the areola of the breast.

4. How should you establish the diagnosis of scabies?

Answer: Ectoparasite examination (scabies preparation) should be performed.

5. What is the appropriate treatment for this patient?

Answer:
  a. 5% permethrin cream applied from the neck down and left on overnight. This should be repeated one time only on the fourth to seventh day. Immediate household members and close contacts who are symptomatic should be similarly treated, while those without symptoms should receive a single application.
  b. Take general measures to decontaminate clothing, bed linens, and other personal items.
  c. Avoid reexposure to active cases.

REFERENCES for Part II

1. Champion RH, Burton JL, Ebling FJG. Textbook of Dermatology. 5th. ed. Oxford: Blackwell Scientific Publications, 1992, pp. 876–878, 897–911, 948–951, 1391–1457, 1675–1695, 1758–1759, 1300–1307.
2. Braun-Falco O, Plewig G, Wolff HH, Winkelmann RK. Dermatology. Berlin-Heidelberg: Springer-Verlag, 1991, pp. 21–22, 13–21, 416–417, 417–437, 447–452, 752–754, 255-258.
3. Leider M, Rosenblum M. A Dictionary of Dermatological Words, Terms and Phrases. New York-Toronto-London-Sydney: McGraw-Hill, 1968.
4. Drug Facts and Comparisons. St. Louis: Wolters-Kluwer Co., 2003 ed.
5. Cockrell CJ. Cutaneous manifestations of HIV infection other than Kaposi's sarcoma. Clinical and histologic aspects. J Amer Acad Dermatol 1990;22:1260–1269.
6. Massing AM, Epstein WL. Natural history of warts: a two-year study. Arch Dermatol 1963;87: 306–310.
7. Farthing C. HIV Disease and the Dermatologist: Who Should be tested? Fitzpatrick's J Clin Dermatol: 47–51, Nov/Dec 1993.
8. Warner LC, Fisher BK. Cutaneous Manifestations of the Acquired Immunodeficiency Syndrome. Internat J Dermatol 25: 337–350, 1986.
9. Drago F, et al. Human herpesvirus 7 in pityriasis rosea. Lancet 349: 1367-1368, 1997
10. Trozak DJ: Topical Corticosteroid Therapy in Psoriasis. Cutis 46: 341–350, 1990.
11. Gupta AC, Sauder DN, Shear NH. Antifungal agents. Part II. J Amer Acad Dermatol 1994;30: 911–933.
12. Parsons JM. Pityriasis rosea update: 1986. J Amer Acad Dermatol 1986;15:159–167.
13. Abel EA, DiCicco LM, Orenberg EK et al. Drugs in exacerbation of psoriasis. J Amer Acad Dermatol 1986;15:1007–1022.
14. Sadick NS, McNutt NS, Kaplan MH. Papulosquamous dermatoses of AIDS. J Amer Acad Dermatol 1990;22:1270–1277.
15. Dubertret L, Wallach D, Souteyrand P, et al. Efficacy and safety of calcipotriol (MC 903) ointment in psoriasis vulgaris. J Amer Acad Dermatol 1992;27:983–988.
16. Calcipotriene For Psoriasis. The Medical Letter 1994;36:70–71.
17. Kragballe K. Treatment of psoriasis with calcipotriol and other vitamin D analogues. J Amer Acad Dermatol 1992;27:1001–1008.
18. Trozak DJ. Topical Corticosteroid Therapy in Psoriasis Vulgaris: Update and New Strategies. Cutis 1999;64:315-318.
19. Boyd AS, Neldner KH. Lichen Planus. J Amer Acad Dermatol 25: 593–619, 1991.
20. Jubert C, Pawlotsky JM, Pouget F, et al. Lichen Planus and Hepatitis C Virus-Related Chronic Active Hepatitis. Arch Dermatol 1994;130:73–76.
21. Bleicher PA, Dover JS, Arndt KA. Lichenoid dermatoses and related disorders. I. Lichen planus and lichenoid drug-induced eruptions. J Amer Acad Dermatol 1990;22:288–292.
22. Sehgal VN, Abraham GJS, Malik GB. Griseofulvin therapy in lichen planus: a double blind controlled trial. Br J Dermatol 1972;87:383–385.
23. Arndt KA. Lichen Planus-like Eruptions. Cutis 1971;8:353–357.
24. Mowad CM, McGinley KJ, Foglia A, et al. The role of extracellular polysaccharide substance produced by Staphlococcus epidermidis in miliaria. J Amer Acad Dermatol 1995;33:729–733.
25. Dobson RL. Lobitz WC. Some histochemical observations on the human eccrine sweat glands. Arch Dermatol 1957;75:653–666.

From: *Current Clinical Practice: Dermatology Skills for Primary Care: An Illustrated Guide*
D.J. Trozak, D.J. Tennenhouse, and J.J. Russell © Humana Press, Totowa, NJ

26. Bellman B, Reddy R, Falanga V. Generalized lichen planus associated with hepatitis C virus immunoreactivity. J Amer Acad Dermatol 1996;35:770–772.
27. Kirk JF, Wilson BB, Chun W, et al. Miliaria Profunda. J Amer Acad Dermatol 1996;35: 854–856.
28. Wolverton SE. Comprehensive Dermatologic Therapy. W B Saunders Company, 2001.

Part III: Epidermal, Dermal, and Epidermal/Dermal Lesions

IMPORTANT ABBREVIATIONS USED IN THIS PART:

TCa	Tinea of the scalp = Tinea capitis
TB	Tinea of the beard = Tinea barbae
TF	Tinea of the face excluding the Beard = Tinea faciale
TC	Tinea of the general body surface = Tinea corporis
TCr	Tinea of the intertriginous groin = Tinea cruris
TM	Tinea of the hands = Tinea manuum
TP	Tinea of the feet = Tinea pedis
TU	Tinea of the nails (Onychomycosis) = Tinea unguium
OTC	Over-the-counter medications
NSAIDs	Nonsteroidal anti-inflammatory drugs
FDE	Fixed drug eruption
EM	Erythema multiforme

13 Erythrasma

CLINICAL APPLICATION QUESTIONS

An 80-year-old sedentary man is admitted on your hospital service for repair of a ventral hernia. During the physical examination, you note a symmetrical eruption along both inguinal creases. The patient says the eruption has been present for several months but is nonpruritic. You suspect erythrasma.

1. List the factors that can provoke erythrasma.
2. What are the primary and secondary lesions you may find with erythrasma?
3. What other common conditions may be confused with erythrasma on physical examination?
4. How would you establish the diagnosis of erythrasma?
5. What treatment could be offered to this patient?

APPLICATION GUIDELINES

Specific History

Onset

This mild superficial infectious disease usually has an insidious onset and most often is so minimally symptomatic that an observer other than the victim brings it to the practitioner's attention. Onset is common in adults, rare in children, and frequency escalates gradually with increasing age. The cause is infection of the stratum corneum by a group of aerobic corynebacteria referred to singularly as *Corynebacterium minutissimum*. Living layers of the skin are not affected.

Evolution of Disease Process

Untreated, this disease usually progresses to a maximal limit, then stabilizes, producing minimal or no symptoms. Occasional itching may be reported with inflammatory episodes.

Evolution of Skin Lesions

Macules of brown and red discoloration form and gradually coalesce to form large patches that usually stabilize at a maximal size in each affected region. Mature lesions have a dry, velvety surface.

Provoking Factors

Warm humid climate conditions, diabetes, hyperhidrosis, obesity, poor personal hygiene, occlusive clothing, increasing age, and anatomic features such as tight toe webs predispose patients to this dermatitis.

Self-Medication

Self-treatment is not a problem in erythrasma.

From: *Current Clinical Practice: Dermatology Skills for Primary Care: An Illustrated Guide*
D.J. Trozak, D.J. Tennenhouse, and J.J. Russell © Humana Press, Totowa, NJ

Supplemental Review From General History

Review of social history may reveal reasons for lack of personal skin care.

Dermatologic Physical Exam

Primary Lesions

Primary lesions are sharply marginated red or tan to brown macules (*see* Photo 1).

Secondary Lesions

1. Fine branny gray-white or brown scale gives a dry, velvety appearance (*see* Photo 1).
2. Lichenification in rare pruritic lesions.
3. Postinflammatory hyperpigmentation.

Distribution

Microdistribution: None.

Macrodistribution: Toe webs, groin, axillae, inframammary creases, vulva, and glans penis in decreasing order of frequency (*see* Fig. 1). A rare generalized form can occur on trunk and extremities.

Configuration

None.

Indicated Supporting Diagnostic Data

Wood's lamp examination will produce a distinct pink or coral-red fluorescence, which is diagnostic when combined with the clinical findings and history.

Therapy

Topical Antibacterials

Several azole-group antifungal agents have sufficient antimicrobial activity to treat most cases of erythrasma. Clotrimazole, econazole, miconazole, oxiconazole, and tioconazole have all been demonstrated effective and each is available in cream base, which is the appropriate vehicle. Ointments cause maceration in intertriginous regions and gel or aerosol vehicles are inherently irritating in these tender areas. Medication should be applied in a thin layer BID for 10 to 14 days. Erythrasma often clears with residual hyperpigmentation, which may take months to fade. One must be careful not to continue to treat this secondary phenomenon. Topical broad-spectrum antibiotics are also effective. Erythromycin, tetracycline, and clindamycin can be easily and inexpensively compounded in cream or lotions in 2 to 3% concentration for this purpose. Systemic use of azoles is ineffective.

Systemic Therapy

On rare occasions, extensive or inflammatory erythrasma may justify systemic treatment. A short course of oral erythromycin is the agent of choice. Tetracycline is an effective alternative.

Posttreatment Prophylaxis

Relapse is a problem, especially in obese, bedridden, inactive, and institutionalized patients. A regular program of cleansing with an antibacterial soap, proper aeration of

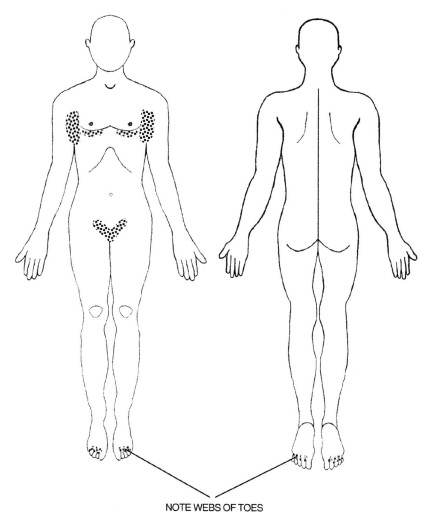

NOTE WEBS OF TOES

Figure 1: Macrodistribution of erythrasma.

intertriginous skin, loose clothing, and use of a 2% miconazole dusting power should prevent relapses.

Conditions That May Simulate Erythrasma

Pityriasis (Tinea) Versicolor

Although individual lesions may be similar in appearance, pityriasis versicolor has a distinctly different distribution.

Erythrasma is intertriginous while P. versicolor affects central regions. Generalized erythrasma can confuse the examiner; however, it still involves creases, which P. versicolor spares. Differentiation can be accomplished by KOH prep and a Wood's lamp examination. KOH exam is positive in P. versicolor. Coral-red fluorescence on Wood's lamp examination occurs only with erythrasma.

Intertriginous Dermatophytosis (Tinea)

Intertriginous fungal infections have a similar distribution but are usually more inflammatory and more symptomatic than erythrasma. They also often show a raised advancing border with loose scale. The difference can be best established by KOH prep, which is positive in dermatophytosis. Coral-red fluorescence on Wood's lamp examination occurs only with erythrasma. Intertriginous dermatophytosis does not fluoresce.

Intertriginous Monilia (Candida)

Intertriginous monilia also has a distribution similar to erythrasma. Monilia is usually very inflammatory and has a moist erosive surface with satellite lesions. Again, KOH or Wood's lamp examination should separate them. Monilia does not fluoresce.

ANSWERS TO CLINICAL APPLICATION QUESTIONS

History Review

An 80-year-old sedentary man is admitted on your hospital service for repair of a ventral hernia. During the physical examination, you note a symmetrical eruption along both inguinal creases. The patient says the eruption has been present for several months but is nonpruritic. You suspect erythrasma.

1. List the factors that can provoke erythrasma.

Answer:
   a. Inactivity.
   b. Warm humid conditions.
   c. Obesity.
   d. Diabetes.
   e. Poor personal hygiene.
   f. Occlusive clothing.
   g. Advanced age.

2. What are the primary and secondary lesions you may find with erythrasma?

Answer: Primary lesions include sharply marginated red, tan, or brown macules or patches. Secondary lesions include lichenification and branny, gray, white, or brown scale.

3. What other common conditions may be confused with erythrasma on physical examination?

Answer: Tinea cruris and intertriginous monilia.

4. How would you establish the diagnosis of erythrasma?

Answer: Examination with a Woods lamp will usually produce pink or coral-red fluorescence. KOH examination is negative.

5. What treatment could be offered to this patient?

Answer: Topical azole-group antifungal agents have sufficient antimicrobial activity to treat most cases. These should be combined with improved local hygiene.

14 Tinea *(Superficial Fungi, Dermatophytosis, Ringworm)*

INTRODUCTION

Entire references have been written on the subject of tinea. Because the goal of this book is to improve the reader's clinical skills, discussion will be limited as much as possible to common presentations at specific anatomic sites. Actual mycology will be kept to a minimum. These common superficial mycoses are caused by a number of related organisms and there is considerable variation in presentation depending on the interaction between the causative organisms, and the host. Only dermatologists have the mycology training and clinical experience to deal with difficult cases and should be consulted if the diagnosis is in question. Inappropriate treatment with systemic antifungal medication is expensive, and inappropriate topical therapy can worsen the condition or make a consultant's task nearly impossible. There are three important statements with which the authors would like to preface this section:

1. Mycolog® and its generic counterparts (triamcinolone/mycostatin combinations) do not treat tinea infections.
2. Topical steroids used alone may initially improve symptoms by suppressing inflammation, but will worsen the infection in the long run.
3. The combination of betamethasone diproprionate (a potent fluorinated corticoid) and clotrimazole (Lotrisone®) is, in the authors' opinion, inappropriate for use in intertriginous regions and, in the authors' experience, often exacerbates dermatophyte infections wherever it is used.

CLINICAL APPLICATION QUESTIONS

A 50-year-old male diabetic presents with an extensive eruption on the lower back and buttock areas. He complains of intermittent pruritus and occasional tender deep pimple-like lesions.

1. List the disorders that you should consider in the differential diagnosis of this patient's eruption.
2. How would you distinguish tinea corporis from the other disorders in your differential diagnosis?
3. Where else on this patient's body is fungal infection likely to be found?
4. If a diagnosis of fungal infection is established, what treatment is appropriate for this patient?
5. What is this patient's prognosis?

From: *Current Clinical Practice: Dermatology Skills for Primary Care: An Illustrated Guide*
D.J. Trozak, D.J. Tennenhouse, and J.J. Russell © Humana Press, Totowa, NJ

APPLICATION GUIDELINES

Specific History

Onset

Initial symptoms of tinea infections vary based on the host, site, and organism.

Tinea capitis: Tinea of the scalp (TCa) is most common in preschool children and pre-teens and is uncommon in adults. It should be part of the differential of any scalp condition that presents with patchy hair loss, inflammation, scaling, a localized inflammatory lesion, or follicular pustules. In children, the onset is usually abrupt and parents usually recount symptoms of redness, scaling, or hair loss of only a few weeks' duration. Discrete, demarcated, pruritic, circular areas of partial alopecia with scale and broken hairs are the most common initial signs. Adults with chronic pustular or less inflammatory infections may describe symptoms of months' or years' duration.

Tinea barbae: Tinea of the beard (TB) is seen in adult men and usually begins insidiously as a focal area of inflammatory folliculitis that gradually spreads with shaving.

Tinea faciale: Tinea of the face excluding the beard area (TF) occurs on the face, neck, and postauricular regions. It is common in preteen children but may also be seen in adults and is often acquired from snuggling with or handling small domestic pets. TF begins as a low-grade inflammatory dermatitis with moderate itching and spreads in a centrifugal fashion. It is frequently misdiagnosed.

Tinea corporis: Tinea corporis (TC) can occur anywhere on the outer skin surface but is most common between the waist and the knees. It is usually gradual in onset, spreads slowly in a centrifugal fashion, and causes mild discomfort. It is often associated with concomitant infection on the feet. TC may involve extensive areas of the skin surface.

Tinea cruris: Tinea cruris (TCr) is most common in adult men and affects the inner thighs, the base of the scrotum, and sometimes the gluteal cleft. It is usually a chronic infection that begins with itch, scale, and irritation. An associated foot infection is common.

Tinea manuum and **tinea pedis:** Tinea manuum (TM = hands) and tinea pedis (TP = feet) often occur together and usually present as a gradual progression of erythema, superficial scale, and moderate pruritus on the palmar and plantar surfaces. Confluent involvement is common; the classic presentation is involvement of both feet and the dominant hand, or so-called "two foot one hand disease" (*see* Photo 2). The authors have seen every possible variation, however. Disease on the dorsal surface of the hands and feet is similar to tinea corporis in onset and appearance. A deeper vesicular variant that presents with rings of intensely pruritic blisters is less common.

Tinea unguium: Tinea unguium (TU = nails) is usually of gradual onset. Symptoms other than the altered appearance of the nail relate to nail plate dystrophy as it interferes with the wearing of footgear. Distal separation of the nail plate and yellow or superficial white discoloration are common early signs.

Evolution of Disease Process

TCa and TB can undergo spontaneous cure or become a chronic indolent pustular or scaling condition, which, if untreated, will remain active for years.

TF, TC, and tinea on the dorsal surfaces of the hands and feet all follow a course of gradual centrifugal extension with varying degrees of central clearing. Gradual extension is the norm and spontaneous remission is uncommon.

TCr is usually a chronic process. This form of tinea is subject to acute exacerbations that vary with weather, physical activity levels, and other external factors.

TM and TP of the palmar and plantar surfaces are usually chronic with acute exacerbations triggered by heat and humidity. Both may remain active for a lifetime if untreated.

TU usually shows slow progression and is not subject to spontaneous cure.

Evolution of Skin Lesions

The course of TCa is variable. Changes may continue to consist only of broken hairs with minimal scale, erythema, and pruritus in noninflammatory cases. Some patients will develop thick scale, obscuring the underlying scalp, while in other cases deep follicular pustules occur. A common scenario in children is the development of a *kerion,* which is a deep, boggy plaque caused by intense immune response and is often secondarily infected with bacteria. This is an important event to recognize, as it can rapidly scar and cause permanent alopecia if untreated (*see* Photos 3–5). Enlarged posterior auricular and occipital nodes are common even in non-inflammatory cases. Certain clinical symptoms have a high predictive value in this condition which can be difficult to diagnose and may involve considerable delay before cultures turn positive. A study correlating 100 consecutive pediatric patients having one or more of four symptoms (postauricular/occipital adenopathy, alopecia, pruritus, scaling) of tinea capitis with culture results has been reported. When all four symptoms were present the correlation with a positive culture was 100%. When fewer than four symptoms were present, but with adenopathy, the positive predictive value was 94%. In the absence of adenopathy and alopecia, only 6% of cultures were positive and when both adenopathy and scaling were absent cultures were uniformly negative. These clinical signs should assist in deciding whether or not to procede with treatment while awaiting culture results.

TB rapidly progresses from erythema and scale to inflammatory papules, nodules, and in its worst form, undermining abcesses. Regional adenopathy may be present. Affected hairs can often be easily and painlessly epilated (*see* Photo 6). TB can also scar without prompt treatment.

As TF, TC, and tinea of the dorsum of the hands and feet extend peripherally, scaling is common in the central areas and, with careful inspection, an advancing border is usually present (*see* Photos 7–12). This border may be very subtle, especially in cases of TF. As the infection crosses hair-bearing regions, discrete follicular pustules, papules, and nodules occur (*see* Photos 11,12). New circular areas of activity may occur in the center of existing lesions, producing concentric circles (*see* Photo 10).

TCr is chronic and for long periods presents only minimal symptoms of pigmentation and scaling. During exacerbations, erythema, fissuring, severe itching, and centrifugal spread with a raised advancing border are noted (*see* Photo 13).

TM and TP of the palmar and plantar surfaces often present as a diffusely red surface with a fine white scale accentuated in the creases (*see* Photo 14). Areas of delicate superficial scale are often evident as vesicles dehydrate and reach the surface. Both surfaces may show deep-seated, intensely pruritic vesicles, but these are more common on the feet (*see* Photo 15). On rare occasions, large multiloculated bullae develop. Infection of both sites tends to be chronic with exacerbations triggered by heat and humidity.

TU usually starts insidiously at the distal nail plate. Distal separation and discoloration are followed by dystrophy of the nail plate when deep nail structures or nail matrix are infected (*see* Photo 16). Superficial white TU discolors the plate surface but does not produce distortion or lysis. This uncommon form of nail infection is characterized by small areas of intense white discoloration that migrate from the proximal nail fold to the distal edge (*see* Photo 17). The white spots can be easily scraped away and contain fungal elements. Onychomycosis may remain localized for months or years, then gradually spread from one nail to the next.

Provoking Factors

Common dermatophyte fungi can be cultured from soil samples so there is a vast persisting reservoir for infection and reinfection.

TCa is usually spread from one child to another by direct physical contact, or by sharing hats and grooming instruments. Epidemic cases have occurred in gym classes from the common use of infected tumbling mats. This type of activity history should be elicited to prevent community spread.

TB occurs primarily in male farm or ranch workers who handle infected livestock. Occasional cases occur from handling small infected domestic pets. The animals can be treated with similar medication by the veterinarian; otherwise, they pose a source of reinfection.

TF is often related to handling infected domestic pets that have been cuddled against the face or neck.

Tinea of the dorsal hands and wrists is a common site of infection in livestock handlers; infection at these locations should prompt a work exposure history.

TC can spread from infections on the feet or in the crural regions by autoinoculation or direct extension. These other sites should be examined. Fomites, such as common towels, may also serve as an initial source. Many patients with chronic TC have an inherent susceptibility to these organisms and exhibit anergy to fungal antigens. Extensive TC is also seen in patients who are on chronic systemic steroid therapy, on immunosuppressants, have certain lymphomas, are diabetic, or have Cushing's syndrome.

TCr is also often seen with associated pedal infection. Moisture, heat, and maceration cause acute exacerbations. Tight undergarments, wet bathing suits, exercise, and obesity all tend to predispose to TCr.

TP is also aggravated by warm moist conditions. Footgear that is occlusive (especially of synthetic materials), improperly dried, wet, or shared, all predispose to TP. Using common locker, shower, and pool facilities without foot protection is another source of infection. Persons with tight toe webs that aerate poorly have an anatomic predisposition to TP. Exacerbations of chronic TP are common with exercise and during warm weather.

Self-Medication

Self-treatment is common, especially in cases of inflammatory TCr and TP. There are innumerable over-the-counter (OTC) antifungal products, which is an indication of their overall success. Some of the newer agents are quite effective, provided they are used on a regular schedule for an appropriate time period. Unfortunately, the consumer may also choose some of the older OTC products, which are only marginally effective. These patients then present with a partially treated infection that can no longer be definitively diagnosed. Sometimes the practitioner can do nothing other than stop what is being used and reassess the situation in 5 to 7 days. The sale of OTC hydrocortisone preparations for "dermatitis" has also had an impact, as these topicals will exacerbate tinea after an initial period of apparent improvement. Recent application of weak antifungals can cause a false negative KOH exam and applications of creams, ointments, or even hand lotions can make interpretation of this test more difficult.

Supplemental Review From General History

Extensive TC that recurs rapidly after systemic therapy is occasionally seen in immunologically suppressed patients. Appropriate historical review should be taken. The authors have seen this association in patients with lymphoma, Cushing's syndrome, and in poorly controlled diabetics.

Proximal white subungual onychomycosis, a very rare finding, has been associated with, and reported as, a presenting sign of HIV disease. The proximal nail at the lunula acquires a white opaque appearance while the distal nail remains normal. In this presentation the color cannot be gently scraped away as it can in the superficial white variant. History for high-risk behavior should be sought.

Dermatologic Physical Exam

Primary Lesions

1. Dusky-red or hyperpigmented patches (*see* Photos 10,13).
2. Dusky-red indurated plaques (*see* Photo 12).
3. Inflammatory follicular papules and nodules (*see* Photos 11,12).
4. Follicular pustules (*see* Photo 11).
5. Small grouped intraepidermal vesicles in TM and TP (*see* Photo 15).
6. Large multiloculated bullae in TP.

Secondary Lesions

1. Scale, on the skin surface usually delicate and white, most evident at an active margin. Scale in the scalp can vary from loose white scale to dirty yellow-gray thickened crusts.
2. Fissures in intertriginous regions.
3. Hyperpigmentation and hypopigmentation (*see* Photos 7,9).
4. Impetiginization with secondary infection (*see* Photo 4).
5. Scarring may occur on the scalp with kerion formation and with severe TB (*see* Photos 5,6).

Distribution

Microdistribution: Follicular lesions in TCa, TB, TF, TC, and TCr (*see* Photos 3,6, 11,12).

Macrodistribution: As the forms of tinea are separated and named according to area of anatomic involvement, macrodistribution is self-evident.

Configuration

Annular, arciform, polycyclic, and serpiginous configurations may be encountered with TF, TC, and TCr (*see* Photos 7–11).

Indicated Supporting Diagnostic Data

Wood's Lamp Examination

Certain dermatophytes of the genus *Microsporum* produce substances that cause hairs to fluoresce brilliant green when exposed to a Wood's lamp in a darkened room. Another scalp dermatophyte, *T. schoenleinii*, produces pale-green fluorescence. When positive, this test is very helpful. Unfortunately, most infections in North America are now caused by nonfluorescing *Trichophyton* dermatophytes. Therefore, a negative exam is not helpful. Prior use of coal-tar-based shampoos can give a false-positive result.

KOH Preparation

A microscopic examination of hair or skin scrapings that have been digested with 10 to 30% potassium hydroxide and dimethyl sulfoxide (DMSO) often gives a rapid diagnosis. With gentle heating, these preps clear and can be read within a few minutes. Reading should not be delayed beyond 30 minutes or false negative results may occur. The presence of translucent branching hyphae (*see* Photo 18) confirms the diagnosis. Hairs should be collected by epilation, as distal portions of infected hairs may not show organisms. Scales should be collected with the edge of a scalpel; a layer of moist alcohol prep will help to keep the sample together. Skin scale samples are best collected from the active margin or from inverted blister roofs if vesicles are present.

Fungal Cultures

In typical disease where the KOH exam is positive, cultures are mainly of academic interest. In situations in which the true diagnosis is doubtful, they can be most useful. These cultures take days or weeks to grow and are not as reliably positive as bacterial cultures. Samples of hair, scale, and nail plate are used as specimens. When hair specimens are obtained by plucking, care must be taken to be sure the infected proximal end is inoculated. Scalp specimens are best obtained by vigorously rubbing the involved site with a cotton swab for 10 to 15 seconds as one would do while obtaining a bacterial culture. Inoculation of a standard bacterial culturette and plating for fungal culture after transport to a local laboratory has been shown to have equivalent positive results to specimens plated in the office. Scalp specimens are positive only about 50% of the time. In acute situations, treatment should be initiated while culture results are pending.

Therapy

Topical Antifungals

Topical treatment of dermatophyte infections is feasible when the infection is superficial, limited in extent, and the patient can comply with the regimen. Extensive areas of infection, scalp involvement, deep follicular lesions, and nails require systemic therapy. Topical antifungals can also be used in a cost-effective fashion to prevent relapses in susceptible patients after systemic treatment. This discussion will focus on the modern topical antifungals and will ignore historical treatments, even though many of these are still available OTC.

In general, cream vehicles are the most effective and are tolerated in all locations. Aerosols sting and injure inflamed skin, and powder products are messy and less effective. Modern topicals include the azole, allamine, benzylamine, ciclopirox, and morpholine derivatives. Only the first four are marketed in the United States. The azole, allamine (terbinafine only), benzylamine, and ciclopirox derivatives are effective against dermatophytes and *Candida* organisms. The azoles and allamines are also broad-spectrum antibacterial agents, which may have some utility for mixed infections at intertriginous sites. The allamine derivative terbinafine leaves a measurable level of drug for at least a week after applications cease. This repository dose may increase cure rates and shorten the course of application. These creams are applied QD or BID depending on the product. Patients should be instructed to apply them 1 to 2 cm beyond the area of visible activity, and for interdigital tinea, apply them carefully to each toe web and to the sulcus on the ventral toe surface.

Topical treatment of nails is effective in cases of superficial white onychomycosis and can be undertaken for deep nail infection with patients who cannot tolerate or do not wish systemic treatment. Topical treatment of deep nail infection is usually palliative rather than curative. The authors have had most success with a suspension containing 0.77% ciclopirox olamine combined with periodic debridement of the diseased nail plate. The suspension should be applied over the entire nail plate and proximal nail fold to the distal joint. Debridement should be carried out at regular intervals timed to each patient's rate of nail growth. An 8% ciclopirox nail lacquer preparation is available. Occasionally we have had success using topical terbinafine cream in a similar fashion. Although complete cures are not frequent, in most instances the nails will improve to the point at which patients are comfortable in shoes, and nails are more acceptable cosmetically. Surgical removal of the nail plate rarely has a place in the treatment of mycotic nails. If for some reason removal of a nail plate becomes necessary, most dermatologists can do it painlessly with a topical urea-based cream and debridement without risk to the nail unit.

Adjunctive topical treatment of TCa with ketoconazole shampoo 2% or selenium sulfide shampoo 2.5% applied two or three times per week reduces shedding of spores and should decrease spread to family members and playmates. It may improve the efficacy of the main systemic therapy.

Systemic Antifungals

Systemic therapy of dermatophyte infections is in a state of transition. At present, **griseofulvin** remains the drug of choice for TCa and other tinea infections in children. It is generally effective, well-tolerated, and has a long record of safety. Recommended doses depend on the particular preparation used and can be administered either BID or as a single oral dose. Micronized and ultramicronized preparations are available and absorption is improved if the drug is taken with a fatty meal. The recommended dose for micronized griseofulvin is 10 to 15 mg/kg/day. Because of gradual resistance that has developed over years of usage, many dermatologists prescribe 20 to 25 mg/kg/day. Griseofulvin has a wide therapeutic window. Ultramicronized preparations are dosed at one-third less than micronized preparations. The tablets are large but they can be crushed and administered with food. Liquid preparations are also available.

Treatment of TCa requires at least 8 to 12 weeks of continuous therapy, occasionally longer. Medication should be continued until all clinical evidence of infection is resolved and the hair is regrowing. Pulse-dosing using a single monthly dose of 1.5 g for three pulses has been reported effective but is not the standard method of administration. Hypersensitivity to griseofulvin, existing liver disease, porphyria, and organ transplantation are the major contraindications to this drug. Griseofulvin has a number of important drug interactions with which the prescribing practitioner should be familiar. Griseofulvin reduces the action of cyclosporine, oral contraceptives, and anticoagulants of the coumarin or indandione types. It also potentiates the effects of ethanol, and is itself less effective when given to patients taking barbiturates or primidone. Early fears regarding marrow suppression appear unfounded and routine blood counts are no longer recommended. With long-term dosing, liver function screens should be performed periodically.

Occasional cases of TCa do not respond to griseofulvin. Failures may be due to poor absorption from the gut or organism resistance. In addition, because griseofulvin is only fungistatic, poor responses are more common in persons with altered immune status. When griseofulvin is ineffective at maximal dosing, the newer systemic antifungals may be used.

Systemic **ketoconazole** is of historical interest only. The activity of this antifungal is unpredictable. In addition, it has a slow onset of action and is associated with potentially serious and sometimes irreversible hepatotoxicity.

Kerion formation in the scalp is a situation that requires prompt and aggressive intervention; otherwise, permanent alopecia may occur (*see* Photos 4,5). The inflammation in the kerion may make it impossible to obtain a positive KOH preparation or fungal culture and treatment should not be delayed by waiting for cultures. In children systemic griseofulvin should be started in the appropriate dosage and the patient should also be placed on oral prednisone in a single morning dose based on size and weight. Concomitant treatment with a broad-spectrum antibiotic is also recommended because secondary infection is common. Both the prednisone and the antibiotic can be stopped as soon as the inflammation resolves, usually after 1 to 2 weeks. The antifungal agent should be continued until hair regrowth is well-established.

In cases that do not respond to maximal doses of griseofulvin, treatment may be switched to an azole (itraconazole/fluconazole). *Microsporum canis*, a common organism in the United States and the usual cause of kerion formation, appears to be less sensitive to terbinafine. Therefore, the first alternative choice is itraconazole. For inflammatory TCa, an initial continuous dose of 5 mg/kg/day is recommended. A switch can be made to pulse dosing once the acute phase is controlled. For less inflammatory disease, itraconazole can be pulsed at 5 mg/kg/day for 1 week out of each month. Treatment of TCa has also been reported with fluconazole 6 mg/kg/day for 20 days or in single pulses at 8 mg/kg one dose per week for 8 to 16 weeks. The body of literature supporting use of fluconazole is not extensive. Terbinafine, despite its apparent diminished activity against *M. canis*, *M. audouini,* and *T. mentagrophytes*, is very effective against *T. tonsurans*. It can be used for noninflammatory infections in a continuous dose of 5 mg/kg/day. Itraconazole or terbinafine, in the absence of a kerion, should be given for 2 to 4 weeks continuously. Itraconazole may also be used in two to three monthly pulses. The same precautions and recommendations in regard to administration and testing should be followed in children, and the practitioner should become familiar with the large number of drug interactions associated with these newer medications.

Systemic treatment of fungal infections in adult patients is also currently changing. TB, TF, TC, and TCr can usually be eradicated with 4 weeks of treatment with oral griseofulvin. The drug is best taken at the start of a meal with some fat content. Intermediate doses (500 mg/day micronized or 250 mg/day ultramicronized griseofulvin) are usually effective. Maximal dosing may be required in obese patients or where there is slow response due to poor absorption. TM and TP infections are best treated for 6 to 8 weeks provided there is no nail involvement. The drug can be stopped when all signs of erythema, desquamation, vesicle formation, and peeling have ceased. Treatment of adult nail disease with this drug has such low efficacy; its use for this purpose should be abandoned. Griseofulvin and ketoconazole have been largely supplanted by itraconazole and terbinafine for adult infections.

Itraconazole, a triazole derivative, is fungistatic and shows broad activity against dermatophyte fungi, *Candida albicans, Pityrosporum obiculare* (the cause of tinea versicolor), and other systemic mycosis. The drug is delivered rapidly to the skin, hair, and nails. It binds strongly to keratinized structures, remaining there in therapeutic concentrations for months after administration ceases. These characteristics allow the pulse-dosing schedules that will be discussed. Absorption is markedly depressed in the presence of achlorhydria or medications that suppress acid secretion.

Approved indications for itraconazole are onychomycosis of the fingernails and toenails by continuous regimens, and pulse-dosing for fingernails only. Recommended continuous dosing in adults is 200 mg/day (6 weeks for fingernails, 12 weeks for toenails). Pulse doses for fingernails are 200 mg BID for one week each month for a total of two pulses. Although somewhat less effective than continuous dosing in some reports, pulse-dosing is also useful for toenails but requires four to six pulses. Nails will usually continue to clear and normalize even though they are not totally normal when treatment is stopped. Nail infections in children have been successfully treated with pulse-dosing at 5 mg/kg/day (two pulses for fingernails, three pulses for toenails). Regimens for treatment of the following dermatophyte infections have also been published.

1. Tinea corporis/cruris, 100 mg/day for 2 weeks or 200 mg/day for 1 week.
2. Tinea pedis/manuum, 100 mg/day for 4 weeks or 200 mg/day for 2 weeks or 200 mg BID for 1 week.

The liquid formulation contains cyclodextrin, which may cause severe diarrhea in children with prolonged administration. Because of higher drug levels with this liquid preparation, a lower daily dose of 3 mg/kg is recommended.

Itraconazole is teratogenic in animal studies and is contraindicated during pregnancy. It has a large list of potentially significant drug interactions with which the practitioner should become familiar. It has been reported to precipitate and aggravate congestive heart failure. Rare reports of liver toxicity have been published and liver function should be monitored if itraconazole is administered in the presence of preexisting liver disease. Despite it's cost, the shorter courses of treatment and improved efficacy make it a more cost-effective drug for the treatment of adult fungal infections. Pulse-dosing improves cost-effectiveness and may decrease the risk of drug interactions and side effects.

Fluconazole is a fungistatic *bis*-triazole derivative which is approved and marketed in the United States for the treatment of vaginal candidiasis. It has essentially the same broad antifungal activity as itraconazole. Despite the fact that it is hydrophilic rather than lipophilic, it rapidly reaches the skin, hair, and nails by direct diffusion and in the eccrine sweat. Unlike itraconazole, it does not bind strongly to keratinized tissue and when therapy is suspended the accumulated dose in the skin can slowly rediffuse to the systemic circulation. These characteristics allow for pulse-dosing but on a much different type of schedule. In hair and nails, accumulated measurable levels are present for several months. Unlike itraconazole, absorption is not significantly altered by food or GI acidity.

Although never marketed for dermatophyte infections, fluconazole is an effective alternative drug, and the following dosing schedules have been published:

1. Tinea corporis/cruris, 150 to 200 mg single weekly dose for 2 to 4 weeks.
2. Tinea pedis/manuum, 150 to 200 mg single weekly dose for 2 to 6 weeks.
3. Tinea unguium, 150 to 200 mg single weekly dose continued until the nails are clinically clear.

Fluconazole is teratogenic and although administration during the first trimester of pregnancy has been reported without problems, it should be prescribed only if the potential benefit justifies the risk. Like itraconazole, it has a sizable list of drug interactions. Pulse-dosing improves the cost-effectiveness of fluconazole and has been shown to reduce the risk of drug interactions and side effects.

Terbinafine is an allamine antifungal that is both fungistatic and fungicidal. It has broad-spectrum activity against dermatophyte fungi but may be less active against *Microsporum canis*, a common cause of inflammatory TCa in children. Activity against *Candida* species is also less reliable than the azoles, and against yeasts its action is fungistatic rather than fungicidal. Terbinafine is highly lipophilic, rapidly concentrates in sebum, and binds to skin, hair, and nails, where it can be detected for months. Therefore, like the azoles, it can be pulse-dosed. Food and GI acidity do not alter oral absorption.

Approved indications for terbinafine include onychomycosis of fingernails and toenails due to dermatophyte fungi. Recommended continuous dosing schedules are 5 mg/kg/day for children and 250 mg/day for adults (6 weeks for fingernails, 12 weeks for toenails). Nails will usually continue to clear after discontinuation of dosing due to the repository drug in the nail plate. The following dose regimens have also been published:

1. Tinea unguium, 250 mg BID 1 week each month for four to six pulses. Due to a much longer plasma half-life, pulse dosing with terbinafine may have minimal advantage over continuous therapy.
2. Tinea pedis/manuum, 250 mg/day for 4 to 6 weeks.
3. Tinea corporis/cruris, 250 mg/day for 2 to 4 weeks.

Terbinafine has a category B rating for pregnancy but should not be used for treating infections that can be deferred until after delivery. Interactions with other medications are limited compared with the azoles. The most common significant interactions would be enhanced toxicity to theophylline and tricyclic antidepressants. Administration to patients with established liver or renal dysfunction is not recommended. Rare instances of fatal liver toxicity and reversible marrow suppression have been reported, and baseline liver function tests are now recommended. Like the azoles, the shorter courses of treatment and availability of pulse-dosing improve cost effectiveness. Pulsing could also reduce the risk of drug interactions and toxicity.

Commonsense Prevention

Conditions that promote skin maceration, warmth, and moisture increase the risk of a superficial fungal infection. Susceptible persons should wear either leather footgear that breathes or open footgear. Tight clothing or prolonged wearing of wet garments after swimming can also predispose to fungal infection. Patients should be told to to avoid going barefoot in showers, locker rooms, and around public swimming pools. As noted earlier, dermatophyte fungi can be cultured with regularity from soil samples. Fomites such as shared towels, footgear, and items of clothing may also spread these organisms. Children with TCa should not be kept out of school as long as they avoid use of common fomites, such as tumbling mats or trampolines, which could infect others.

Conditions That May Simulate Tinea

Tinea Capitis

Tinea of the scalp may be confused with any scalp disorder that causes patchy alopecia, inflammation, or scale. The presence of hairs broken off a short distance above or right at the scalp surface should cause immediate suspicion. Occasionally TCa does not produce hair breakage.

The noninfectious dermatidities seborrhea and psoriasis can both cause inflammation and scaling of the scalp, but do not cause patchy hair shedding. Both are more diffuse than TCa. When any inflammatory scalp condition does not respond promptly to treatment, a KOH exam and fungal culture of epilated hairs are indicated.

Alopecia areata causes patchy hair loss and may show erythema of the scalp. Scale is absent, however, and the presence of exclamation-point and dystrophic anagen hairs should differentiate it. In older patients with alopecia areata, gray hairs continue to grow within the patches of alopecia.

Trichotillomania, which is frequent in children, presents with patchy areas of hairs that are broken off at differing lengths above the scalp. Inflammation and scale are usually absent. When inflammatory change is present, there is usually associated lichenification. These secondary changes are more common in adult cases.

An active impetigo of the scalp, on rare occasions, can produce enough inflammation to cause hair loss and may simulate a kerion. Hairs can be readily epilated but come out by the root rather than by breakage. Whenever there is a question, hair KOH exam and fungal culture are indicated.

Tinea Barbae

Chronic staphylococcal folliculitis and TB may be very difficult to distinguish because TB usually has a component of secondary infection that will respond to broad-spectrum antibiotics. One should always be suspicious when there is rapid relapse of a facial folliculitis after appropriate antimicrobial therapy.

Gram-negative folliculitis can also be confused with TB; however, the pustules are usually painful and not pruritic. They are dusky red and have a straw-colored surface pustule. Bacterial culture will usually distinguish between them.

Tinea Faciale

Because this form of tinea occurs on a sun-exposed area and subjective symptoms exacerbate with sun exposure, it is not infrequently confused with discoid lupus and other light eruptions that affect the face. The similarity can be striking. Look carefully for an active advancing margin and for follicular pustules. A simple KOH exam of the scale can prevent an important misdiagnosis.

Tinea Corporis

Patches of nummular eczema, early lesions of psoriasis, patches of impetigo, pityriasis alba in its early inflammatory phase, and the herald patch of pityriasis rosea can all be confused with TC. When other diagnostic features of these conditions are absent, a simple KOH exam should distinguish them.

Tinea Cruris

Erythrasma of the groin is less inflammatory and less symptomatic than TCr. In addition, it lacks the active border and gives a coral-red fluorescence when exposed to a Wood's lamp.

Intertriginous monilia is more inflammatory, and the usual complaint is soreness and itching. The area has a deep-red burnished or moist appearance. The margin is sharp but is not raised as in TCr and there are small satellite lesions and pustules beyond the edges.

Bacterial intertrigo is usually more inflammatory and associated with an offensive odor. This is almost always seen in obese persons and shows a symmetric sharp but not raised margin, which corresponds to the areas of skin opposition.

Tinea Manuum and Tinea Pedis

Bacterial intertrigo, candidiasis, erythrasma, or Gram-negative toe web infections may be difficult to distinguish from intertriginous tinea of the feet. Wood's lamp exam will show coral-red with erythrasma and green-blue with intertriginous pseudomonas. Otherwise a KOH preparation or fungal culture are indicated.

Eczema, although common on the feet, rarely affects the toe webs. Dry scaling fungal infections of the palms and soles are difficult to confuse with other conditions. A simple KOH exam should establish the diagnosis because the surface is usually teeming with hyphae.

Dyshidrosis or contact dermatitis may be easily confused with vesicular fungal infections of the palms and soles. A KOH exam of an inverted blister roof is almost always positive if it is a dermatophytosis. Remember, active TP can cause a sympathetic id reaction (*see* Photo 19) on the hands, and those vesicles are KOH negative. Both areas should be tested.

Tinea Unguium

Psoriasis, lichen planus, monilia of the nails, and other nondermatophyte fungal and yeast organisms that invade nail tissue must be distinguished from onychomycosis of the nails.

Psoriasis may be clinically very similar. Fine linear pitting of psoriasis is not a feature of TU. Another helpful sign is the oil-spot change on the nail bed seen in psoriasis.

Lichen planus usually attacks the proximal nail fold, causing scarring and nail dystrophy. Lysis of the plate occurs but is usually "clean" without the debris and buildup seen with TU.

Monilia can cause distal lysis and is usually tender with minimal scale distortion or debris. When the proximal nail fold is involved, there are pain and swelling not seen with TU. To confirm a dermatophyte infection versus other nail pathogens, obtain nail cultures.

ANSWERS TO CLINICAL APPLICATION QUESTIONS

History Review

A 50-year-old male diabetic presents with an extensive eruption on the lower back and buttock areas. He complains of intermittent pruritus and occasional tender deep pimple-like lesions.

1. List the disorders that you should consider in the differential diagnosis of this patient's eruption.

Answer:
   a. Tinea corporis.
   b. Nummular eczema.
   c. Psoriasis.
   d. Mild atopic eczema (pityriasis alba).

2. How would you distinguish tinea corporis from the other disorders in your differential diagnosis?

Answer: Only tinea corporis has a positive KOH preparation. If KOH preparation is negative but you strongly suspect tinea corporis, a fungal culture should be done.

3. Where else on this patient's body is fungal infection likely to be found?

Answer: Tinea corporis is commonly associated with tinea pedis, tinea cruris, and nail infections. These sites should be examined.

4. If a diagnosis of fungal infection is established, what treatment is appropriate for this patient?

Answer: Extensive fungal infections and those with follicular lesions should be treated with systemic antifungal medication.

5. What is this patient's prognosis?

Answer: With the newer systemic antifungal agents, prospects for cure are excellent. Because of the complicating diabetes, occasional new infections may be encountered.

15 Urticaria *(Urticaria Simplex, Common Hives)*

CLINICAL APPLICATION QUESTIONS

A 48-year-old woman is seen for intensely pruritic raised lesions on her trunk and extremities of 3 weeks' duration. Clinically her lesions look to you like hives.

1. What questions should you ask the patient about the lesions to support your suspicion?
2. Would this most likely be classified as acute urticaria, chronic urticaria, or chronic intermittent urticaria, and why?
3. Assuming this is acute urticaria, what history should be sought to establish a possible cause?
4. Assuming this is acute urticaria, what laboratory studies are indicated?
5. What is the appropriate treatment at this point?
6. What is the prognosis for acute urticaria?

APPLICATION GUIDELINES

Specific History

Onset

Commonplace urticaria is a monomorphous eruption of intensely pruritic wheals and is usually of sudden, sometimes explosive onset. Occasionally, victims will note gradual onset with increasing intensity, but this is not the typical presentation. A small number of patients during the acute phase will develop laryngeal or glottic edema, bronchospasm, and circulatory collapse, which can comprise fatal anaphylactic shock. This is a true medical emergency that requires prompt action. Acute urticaria is more frequent in young persons. Chronic hives are more frequent in middle-aged women. Urticarial lesions may also occur in other skin conditions, such as the peribullous areas of pemphigus vulgaris and bullous pemphigoid, or the wheal lesions seen as part of erythema multiforme. Here, however, the welts are associated with other lesions of more distinctive morphology. They are more fixed in duration, and the resemblance to true urticaria is superficial.

Evolution of Disease Process

At one time or another, urticaria is estimated to affect 15 to 20% of the population. In approximately 95% of these cases, the eruption resolves within a few days or months without sequelae. Urticaria is separated into acute and chronic forms on the basis of duration, with 6 weeks being the most generally accepted point at which chronicity begins. Acute urticaria is frequently the result of an immediate (type I) hypersensitivity reaction

From: *Current Clinical Practice: Dermatology Skills for Primary Care: An Illustrated Guide*
D.J. Trozak, D.J. Tennenhouse, and J.J. Russell © Humana Press, Totowa, NJ

or a drug-induced pseudoallergic reaction. Linkage between cause and exposure in acute disease can often be established. Chronic urticaria can persist for years and is a vexing problem for the patient and practitioner. Despite extensive workup and testing, the cause of chronic urticaria is seldom determined. An even less common type is chronic intermittent urticaria, in which symptoms can last for years, but are punctuated by symptom-free periods of varying duration. Causes of intermittent disease parallel acute urticaria, and careful history of periodic or cyclical exposures may reveal the cause.

Evolution of Skin Lesions

Discrete wheals develop rapidly on any body location. New hives may develop at one site while they are resolving in others. Lesions that remain fixed at one site longer than 24 to 48 hours' duration suggest another diagnosis.

Provoking Factors

History-taking for provoking factors in urticaria is tedious and complicated because of the large number of possible etiologies. The factors listed here are among the most common, but this does not represent an exhaustive listing. These will be found more frequently in acute and chronic intermittent urticaria. Despite the low yield in cases of chronic disease, a careful and repeated history must be taken. Provoking factors may cause hives by means of type I (IgE-mediated) hypersensitivity reactions, type III (immune-complex-mediated) hypersensitivity reactions, or by nonimmunologic release of histamine or other mediators. This latter mechanism is referred to as a *pseudoallergic reaction*. Existing acute, chronic intermittent, or chronic urticaria may also be directly exacerbated by a number of substances that stimulate direct histamine release from mast cells or initiate other mediator cascades. Also, certain substances and activities that promote vasodilation will worsen active hives.

1. Immunologic type I or type III reaction:

    Foods: Fish, shellfish (especially oysters and mussels), meats (especially pork and mutton), cheeses that are mold-containing, strawberries, citrus fruits, nuts, seeds, peanuts, tomatoes, chocolate, dairy products (especially milk), egg whites.

    Medications: Penicillins, cephalosporins, sulfonamides, sedatives, tranquilizers, laxatives, diuretics.

    Inhalant allergens: Pollens (would be among the more common causes of chronic intermittent urticaria and would cause seasonal exacerbations), tobacco smoke, tobacco additives such as menthol, house dust, airborne molds, and fungi (again often seasonal).

    Chronic focus of infection: Dental abscess (usually the patient has poorly maintained dentition on physical exam, with one or more sensitive teeth; however, occult abscess formation without signs or symptoms has also been reported), chronic sinusitis, chronic dermatophytosis, candidiasis, intestinal parasitosis, diverticulitis.

    Infectious disease: Hepatitis B, mononucleosis, Coxsackie infections.

    Insect bites or stings may provoke attacks of urticaria of varying duration.

2. Substances that cause pseudoallergic urticaria or may exacerbate existing urticaria by direct mediator release:

   Foods: Lobster, crayfish, scombroid fish (usually old or improperly processed), strawberries, yeast and yeast-containing cheeses, spinach, chicken livers, red wines, egg whites, tomatoes, tonic water (quinine content).

   Food additives: Salicylate derivatives, tartrazine and azo dyes (also widely used in medications, these dyes are listed with each medication in the *Physicians' Desk Reference* [PDR]), benzoates, sulfites.

   Medications: Morphine, codeine, scopolamine, atropine, salicylates, indomethacin, thiamine, quinine and quinine derivatives, polymyxin B, D-turbocurarine, succinylcholine, decamethonium, certain radiographic contrast materials, gallamine, ACTH, dextran, halothane, ACE inhibitors (may provoke angioedema by direct action on the kinin cascade).

3. Diseases reported to provoke urticaria: atopy, systemic lupus, dermatomyositis, lymphoma, dysproteinemias, hyper- and hypothyroidism. With the exception of hyperthyroidism, these are rare associations. Atopy and thyroid disease are associated with common hives while the others are usually associated with urticarial vasculitis, a disease distinct from common hives that will be covered in the differential diagnosis section.

Self-Medication

Although antihistamines are readily available over the counter, they are not a problem because they merely suppress but do not alter the disease process.

Supplemental Review From General History

At the initial visit for acute urticaria, history-taking should focus on the provoking factors previously listed. With ongoing symptoms or when investigating chronic urticaria, an exhaustive review is indicated.

Dermatologic Physical Exam

Primary Lesions

Edematous plaques: wheals or hives (*see* Photos 20–22). These raised plaques have sharp margins and the central color can vary from pink to yellow to white. A peau d'orange effect may be present in the center and there is often a peripheral dusky blotchy red border, which is the axon reflex. Individual hives may vary from a few millimeters to greater than palm-sized. Hives may remain discrete or may become confluent, forming geometric and polycyclic shapes. Pruritus is usually severe, especially at onset, and the lesions usually evolve rapidly, then resolve within a few hours.

Secondary Lesions

Although they are usually primary lesions, rarely bullae may develop as secondary lesions on the hive surface when edema is rapid and severe. Also very rarely purpura may occur in hives with marked vasodilation.

Distribution

Microdistribution: Follicular (rare).

Macrodistribution: May occur at any site.

Configuration
1. Annular.
2. Polycyclic (*see* Photo 22).
3. Serpiginous.

These configurations have no diagnostic or etiologic significance.

Indicated Supporting Diagnostic Data

Case history is critical to the discovery of a specific cause in acute, intermittent, or chronic urticaria. Testing should be guided by historical data, and extensive blind testing is seldom productive. History should be repeated periodically, as the victim may recall forgotten information or, over time, may make new associations.

Biopsy

Biopsy is seldom indicated for urticaria; when a question arises regarding common hives versus urticarial vasculitis (*see* Differential Diagnosis section), biopsy will help to distinguish them.

Avoidance Testing

This should be done in a staged fashion, eliminating first any suspect allergens and any substances known to cause pseudoallergic hives or nonspecific histamine or mediator release. With severe symptoms or with chronic disease, an avoidance diet with staged reintroduction of different food groups may be useful.

CBC

If there is a significant eosinophilia, this suggests either a type I hypersensitivity reaction or possibly intestinal parasites.

Stool Exam for Ova and Parasites

This is indicated if travel history, GI history, or CBC suggests this possibility.

Radiologic Studies

In chronic urticaria, sinus films and apical dental films have the highest yield. They may be positive even when symptoms are absent. Other X-rays should be ordered strictly by indications from a general history and physical exam.

Skin Testing

This form of testing requires special skills and may on occasion provoke a life-threatening reaction. Interpretation and a familiarity with the proper concentrations and quality of the antigens is essential. In the authors' opinion, these studies should be carried out only by a qualified allergist or a practitioner with equivalent training.

Serum IgE Determination

Although this test may support suspicion for an allergic cause, it is a very nonspecific test especially in the presence of atopic disease. It is rarely indicated.

Radioallergosorbent (RAST) Testing

These tests are expensive, controversial, difficult to interpret, and subject to false-negative results. Their use should be authorized by a qualified allergist.

Therapy

Acute Urticaria

Most cases of acute urticaria resolve within 1 or 2 weeks. For this reason, emphasis should be placed on taking a thorough history and on safe symptomatic relief. Extensive laboratory or radiologic testing is seldom indicated and should be guided by history.

At the initial interview, history-taking should concentrate on the common provoking factors, especially foodstuffs, medications, pseudoallergens, and any substances that are nonspecifically aggravating the urticaria. Travel history, dental history, and a general review of symptoms for hidden infection is indicated. This encounter will be closest in time to the exposure and offers the best single opportunity to establish an etiology.

All suspect allergens, pseudoallergens, and mediator-releasing substances should be discontinued, along with any nonessential medications.

An antihistamine (H_1-receptor blocker) should be started on a regular schedule until all symptoms have abated for at least 3 or 4 days. The choice of antihistamine depends on the patient and on the practitioner.

When it is important for the patient to remain alert, the use of second generation, minimally sedating, H_1-receptor blockers is recommended. Cetirizine, fexofenadine, loratidine, and desloratidine are all available in the United States. Of this group, cetirizine may cause some sedation at recommended doses. Loratidine and desloratidine can cause sedation at doses above those routinely recommended. Fexofenadine has not been reported to sedate, even at doses above those recommended. All these antihistamines have a rapid onset of action and all are free of the cardiotoxic side effects encountered with the earlier products terfenadine and astemizole (which have been withdrawn from the US marketplace). None of these products have any significant drug interactions and no dose adjustment is required for elderly persons. Dosage adjustments are recommended for cetirizine, loratidine, and desloratidine when impaired liver or renal function is present.

1. Cetirizine:
   Dose: Adults and children over age 6 years: 5 or 10 mg once daily. Children 2–5 years: 2.5 mg once daily, but may be increased to 5 mg per day depending on age and severity of disease.
   Preparations: 5 and 10 mg tablets; syrup 5 mg/5 mL.

2. Fexofenadine:
   Dose: Adults and children over age 12 years: 60 mg BID or 180 mg QD Children 6–11 years: 30 mg BID.
   Preparations: 30, 60, and 180 mg tablets.

3. Loratidine:
    Dose: Adults and children over age 6 years: 10 mg once daily.
                         Children 2–5 years: 5 mg once daily.
    Preparations: 10 mg tablet, 10 mg readitab, syrup 1 mg/1 mL.

4. Desloratidine:
    Dose: Adults and children over age 12 years: 5 mg once daily.
    Preparations: 5 mg tablet.

Anxious patients are better treated with a sedating preparation, particularly when pruritus is interrupting normal sleep patterns. Hydroxyzine 25 to 50 mg QID, 10 mg doxepin TID, 25 to 50 mg diphenhydramine QID, and 12.5 to 25 mg promethazine QID all have significant sedative effects. Hydroxyzine, diphenhydramine, and doxepin have particularly wide dosing schedules in adults. Because of well-established safety records, the first two are particularly appropriate for childhood cases and dosage should be adjusted on the basis of age or weight. With all the traditional H_1-blocking agents, adult patients should be cautioned about driving and also regarding the additive effects of ethanol.

When an attack does not respond to the H_1 blocker alone, occasional patients seem to improve with the addition of an H_2 blocker. In this situation, 300 mg cimetidine QID is combined with a traditional H_1 agent to augment its effect. This combined therapy is recommended only in adult patients.

On very rare occasions when the cited measures fail or with an extremely aggressive onset of hives, a short course of systemic corticosteroids may be helpful. Oral methylprednisolone in a single morning dose of 32 mg is given until symptoms improve and then is rapidly tapered. Steroids do not have to be continued until all hives are clear, but only until the situation is manageable. They should not be used for chronic treatment. If there is no improvement within 3 to 7 days, continued use will only add the risk of a steroid side effect.

Severe type I reactions can, on rare occasions, progress to anaphylaxis with oropharyngeal edema, glottic edema, bronchospasm, and vascular collapse. If you are contacted by phone, it is best to have the victim head for the nearest emergency facility where support measures are readily available. If the reaction occurs at a site where medication is available, immediate action will usually prevent progression. If possible, the patient should be given initial treatment and then transferred when stable, or released if the reaction has been terminated.

A patient with hives and evidence of syncope, upper airway obstruction, or bronchospasm should be immediately placed on vital-sign monitoring and should receive aqueous epinephrine solution 1:1000 dilution. Initial adult dose is 0.3 to 0.5 mL SC or IM and may be repeated every 20 minutes until a response is noted. In the case of vascular collapse, IV dosing may be indicated using a slow infusion of up to 3 mL of a 1:10,000 dilution.

Doses in children (excluding preterm infants and full-term newborns) are 0.01 mL/kg or 0.3 mL/m^2 of 1:1,000 aqueous epinephrine solution, SC only. This is repeated on a 20-minute basis until a response is noted.

When there is any suggestion of vascular collapse, an IV line should be established to increase vascular volume. With airway compromise, the patient should be given supplemental oxygen, and preparations should be made for emergency intubation or tracheostomy. Once the above measures have been accomplished and the victim is stable, administer 40 mg diphenhydramine IV in adult patients. In children, oral dosing is preferable. In both, a regularly scheduled H_1 oral antihistamine should be prescribed for at least a week to minimize the risk of a recurrence.

Once the attack is clearly receding, it is useful to give a final dose of longer-acting epinephrine suspension (Sus-Phrine®) 1:200 dilution to adult patients. This is given SC only and should be timed about 20 to 30 minutes after the last dose of aqueous epinephrine so that the immediate release component does not overlap. This long-acting preparation reduces the risk of a delayed exacerbation.

After the patient is stable, a dose of rapid acting hydrocortisone sodium succinate is usually given IV or IM and followed by a short course of oral glucocorticoid as recorded above. Glucocorticoids are not effective in the early progression of anaphylaxis and should not be of concern during initial treatment.

Chronic Intermittent Urticaria

The symptomatic management of this form of urticaria is essentially the same as in acute disease. Anaphylactic episodes are unlikely, however. Because of the duration of the symptoms, an exhaustive history, review of symptoms, and search for provoking factors should be done. The history should focus especially on intermittent exposures or symptoms that have a temporal relationship to the attacks. Travel history dating back to the time of onset should be discussed. Physical examination should be thorough and should focus on anything revealed in the history, any possible focus of chronic infection, and endocrine disease.

All suspect allergens, pseudoallergens, and mediator-releasing substances should be discontinued, along with any nonessential medications.

A CBC, urine with microscopic exam, and basic thyroid function screen are indicated. Additional lab testing should be based on positive historical data or physical findings.

The use of a diary is an inexpensive and often valuable aid in the diagnosis of intermittent hives. The patient keeps a daily record of food, proprietary and prescription medication, plus any unusual or cyclical exposures. Any exacerbations are recorded and compared to the journal to look for connections.

With severe or frequent recurrences in the absence of other positive findings, a set of sinus films and a set of apical dental films seeking occult infection may be justified.

Chronic Urticaria

Symptomatic therapy of chronic urticaria is essentially the same as that for acute disease. Because of the protracted course, the use of systemic steroids, other than short courses for exacerbations, is discouraged. Reports of control with addition of the leukotriene receptor antagonist montelukast have been published. Immediate (type I) hypersensitivity appears to play a minor role in chronic urticaria while a substantial number of cases are the result of pseudoallergy. In about 50% of cases, no causative agent or mechanism can be found. Roughly half the victims will go into remission within 1 year. An exhaustive history, review of systems, and physical exam should be done with special attention to seasonal exacerbations (suggesting inhalant antigens), and chronic infections (sinusitis, dental abscesses, intestinal parasites, urinary tract infections, and pelvic infections lead the list). Also consider endocrine diseases (thyroid disorders and diabetes), insulin allergy, and underlying conditions such as connective tissue diseases, lymphomas, leukemias, and dysproteinemias.

All suspect allergens, pseudoallergens, and mediator-releasing substances should be discontinued, along with any nonessential medications.

A CBC, urine with microscopic exam, basic chemistry panel, and thyroid function screen are indicated. Additional lab testing should be based on positive historical data or physical findings.

Although not quite as useful as in chronic intermittent urticaria, a daily diary may be valuable in uncovering a cause or some of the exacerbating factors. The diary is kept in the same way and the patient comments daily on the severity of symptoms. Exposures may correlate with increased severity.

With severe or prolonged disease, even in the absence of other positive findings, a set of sinus films and a set of apical dental films seeking occult infection is justified.

Also, in severe or prolonged disease where there is no clue as to etiology, an empirical attempt at elimination of antigens is justified. A 5-day course of 1 to 2 g/day oral tetracycline along with two tablets oral mycostatin TID will alter intestinal flora, and effects on the symptoms can be observed. If candidiasis in other locations is suspected, a 5-day course of 150 to 200 mg/day of fluconazole can be given.

Additional challenge testing, dietary elimination testing, and the use of specific hyposensitization should be left to practitioners with allergy training.

Conditions That May Simulate Common Urticaria

Adrenergic Urticaria

These are pruritic generalized hives that show a central wheal surrounded by a small blanched halo (halo hives). Attacks can be triggered by emotional stress and reproduced by intradermal sympathomimetics. Epinephrine and other sympathomimetics are contraindicated. Symptomatic therapy with H_1 blockers may help, but β-blocking agents such as 25 mg propanolol BID are more specific and reduce attacks. Andrenergic pruritus is a variant that produces generalized itching without visible hives. Both conditions are very rare.

Idiopathic Angioedema

Angioedema presents as massive soft tissue edema of the face, genitalia, or soft tissues around joints. It may occur with common urticaria or as an isolated symptom in the context of a type I allergic reaction, pseudoallergic reaction, or rarely on a recurring basis with chronic urticaria. Oral, pharyngeal, or laryngeal edema may lead to asphyxia. Treat as described for anaphylaxis in the section for acute common urticaria. The very rare syndromes of hereditary angioedema normally do not present as common hives and do not enter into this differential.

Aquagenic Urticaria

Urticarial lesions develop within 5 to 30 minutes of water exposure at any temperature. Lesions are confined to the skin areas in direct water contact. Pruritus is intense and often described as having a prickling or burning quality. Hives are small (1 to 3 mm) and are often surrounded by a large axon flare as in cholinergic urticaria. Partial response may be seen with traditional H_1 blockers. There are reports of improvement with addition of 50 to 200 g sodium bicarbonate (6 to 24 rounded teaspoons) to the bath water. Also reported are beneficial responses to ultraviolet B phototherapy and to transdermal scopolamine. A variant is aquagenic pruritus, in which the sites of exposure itch without visible hive formation.

Cholinergic Urticaria

Pruritic hives, 1 to 3 mm with a large red axon flare, develop after a stimulus that causes sweating. The primary lesions are papules and they may occur at any site, but are most common on the upper torso. Attacks can be triggered by severe stress, exercise, heat exposure, and even hot food. Symptoms can be readily reproduced by exercise or intradermal cholinergic agents. Cholinergic hives show partial response to standard H_1 blockers. Transdermal scopolamine or small doses of other oral anticholinergic agents may be helpful.

Cold Urticaria

Common-appearing hives occur within minutes of cold exposure or even a significant drop in ambient temperature. Two major types occur: an acquired form, which may be associated with underlying disease, and a rare familial type. Lesions develop at cold-exposed sites (contact type) or may be generalized (reflex type) following ingestion of cold food or drink. Generalized sudden cold exposure may lead to hypotension and syncope and may be responsible for some unexplained drownings. During water sports, patients should avoid sudden immersion, premedicate 1 hour before swimming, and swim with a buddy who is aware of the problem. Diagnosis can be confirmed in more than 90% of cases with an ice cube test. Traditional H_1 antihistamines are effective but must be taken on a regular basis or prior to exposure. Oral cyproheptadine has been reported as particularly effective.

Contact Urticaria

Contact urticaria occurs at the site of skin exposure to the offending contactant, and because the reaction is immediate, the cause is readily apparent. This reaction may be a true type I allergic reaction or may be nonimmunologic due to mediator release from stings, bites, or absorption of histamine-releasing chemicals. In either type, a generalized reaction may occur due to sufficient absorption.

Urticarial Dermographism

The term literally translated means the ability to write on the skin. The immediate form is quite common and any light stroking or pressure against the skin will elicit an exaggerated triple response of Lewis with a welt following the line of trauma, a large axon flare, and intense itching. Symptoms also are common at sites where clothing binds, and occur frequently when undressing. Although this phenomenon can occur in relation to common urticaria, stings, and anaphylactic reactions, most cases begin suddenly for no apparent reason. History should reveal that the attack begins as pruritus without visible lesions. The lesions arise after and at the sites of scratching. Once initiated, they result in an orgy of itching. The attacks are most frequent in the evening hours. Generally no workup is indicated. This condition responds to modest doses of H_1 antihistamines, and these should be given in 1-month courses until symptoms regress. Most cases resolve within 6 months, but rare cases last for years. There is a very rare delayed form reported.

Heat Urticaria

Localized erythema and welting develop at a site of heat application. This rare disorder is of uncertain cause and treatment is symptomatic. Traditional antihistamines should be tried first. If these are ineffective, beneficial results have been reported with a combination of indomethacin and chlorpheniramine. Variants exist.

Pressure Urticaria

This is a rare but disabling disorder that may occur in the context of common hives, but usually occurs alone and is more easily confused with urticarial vasculitis. Following sustained pressure, deep soft tissue swelling occur at the site after a 3- to 6-hour delay. Erythema or hive-like change may overlie the swellings. Lesions are usually painful rather than pruritic and persist for 1 to 2 days. The soles and buttocks are the most common sites, and constitutional symptoms are common. Most cases respond to systemic steroids; however, the condition is chronic and the steroids cannot be justified except on a short-term crisis basis. Recently, success has been reported in five cases treated with 50 mg/day dapsone. Cetirizine, a nonsedating H_1 blocker, has also been reported as effective. NSAIDs may also be helpful.

Solar Urticaria

This is a chronic, rare disorder with generalized whealing shortly after exposure to ultraviolet radiation. A wide spectrum of wavelengths act as the trigger, and vary from case to case. Hives occur on exposed skin while unexposed areas may be relatively spared. Extensive solar exposure may trigger all the symptoms of anaphylaxis. A type I hypersensitivity reaction to endogenous photoallergens is postulated. Diagnosis and therapy are complicated and these cases should be referred.

Urticarial Vasculitis

This condition is mediated by a chronic type III immune-complex reaction and the causative antigen is only occasionally evident. Although common hives may occur, the skin lesions are more typically fixed and last 24 hours or more. Pain, tenderness, and bruising are more common than itching. Constitutional symptoms, arthralgias, frank arthritis, and renal complications including glomerulonephritis can occur. Evaluate for possible underlying systemic lupus, hepatitis B, EB virus infections, and Lyme disease. Cases in which the patient is hypocomplementemic during attacks have a strong association with systemic lupus. Cryoproteins should be measured to rule out a cryopathy. Biopsy of established lesions shows a fibrinoid, necrotizing venulitis. Direct immunofluorescence of lesional skin may show deposition of immunoglobulins around vessels and at the dermoepidermal junction. Early lesions may not show characteristic findings. Therapy should start with 25 to 50 mg indomethacin TID combined with regular doses of a traditional H_1 antihistamine.

Vibratory Urticaria and Angioedema

This rare problem occurs after exposure to low-frequency vibration. Sporadic and familial cases are reported. After common activities, such as walking, jogging, hand clapping, or operating a power mower, the victim develops pruritus, redness, and swelling at varied sites within a few minutes. The trigger is usually quite evident. Fexofenadine 60 mg BID is effective.

ANSWERS TO CLINICAL APPLICATION QUESTIONS

History Review

A 48-year-old woman is seen for intensely pruritic raised lesions on her trunk and extremities of 3 weeks' duration. Clinically her lesions look to you like hives.

1. What questions should you ask the patient about the lesions to support your suspicion?

Answer:
a. Are the lesions fixed or do they change position (resolve and recur at different sites over a short time period)?
b. Is the onset of the lesions related to emotional or physical stress, exercise, heat or cold exposure, physical injury, pressure, sun exposure, vibration, or contact with certain substances such as latex rubber?

2. Would this most likely be classified as acute urticaria, chronic urticaria, or chronic intermittent urticaria, and why?

Answer: Acute urticaria. The definition of acute urticaria is symptoms of less than 6 weeks' duration.

3. Assuming this is acute urticaria, what history should be sought to establish a possible cause?

Answer: History should concentrate on food, medications, and pseudoallergens. Also obtain a travel history, dental history, and general review of systems seeking occult infection.

4. Assuming this is acute urticaria, what laboratory studies are indicated?

Answer: Laboratory studies should be ordered in response to information from the history that suggests specific causes such as localized infection.

5. What is the appropriate treatment at this point?

Answer:
a. All suspect allergens, pseudoallergens, and mediator-releasing substances should be avoided.
b. Discontinue nonessential medications.
c. Initiate therapy with an H_1-type antihistamine.

6. What is the prognosis for acute urticaria?

Answer: Most cases of acute urticaria resolve within 4 to 6 weeks. Additional investigation is indicated only if symptoms persist.

16 Fixed Drug Eruption

CLINICAL APPLICATION QUESTIONS

A 70-year-old man on multiple medications presents with dusky, asymmetric red plaque lesions first noted upon awakening. The patient complains of a deep burning itch and states he has had identical lesions at the same sites on three previous occasions over the past 2 years. You suspect a fixed drug eruption.

1. What history should be elicited from this patient pertaining to a fixed drug eruption?
2. What other variations in appearance of lesions may characterize fixed drug eruptions?
3. What treatment is appropriate for this patient's fixed drug eruption?
4. What is this patient's prognosis?

APPLICATION GUIDELINES

Specific History

Onset

Fixed drug eruptions (FDEs) occur suddenly within 30 minutes to 8 hours of ingesting the offending substance. Because many medications are ingested at bedtime, it is common for the patient to relate a history of retiring with clear skin and first discovering the eruption upon arising.

Evolution of Disease Process

Initially, there is usually a single lesion at one site. With continued exposure, additional lesions develop and other anatomic areas may also become active. Although new sites may develop, the original site will reactivate with each episode of exposure, and the limitation of the reaction to that site is a striking feature. These attacks occur on a cyclical basis with the frequency determined by the usage pattern of the offending agent.

Evolution of Skin Lesions

Once the lesions arise, they reach their maximum activity within a few hours. The acute lesions consist of red or violet-brown dermal macules and, on occasion, palpable plaques with vesicles or bullae. Patients complain of a burning discomfort or a deep-seated itch that cannot be relieved by rubbing or scratching. The acute inflammatory phase lasts 7 to 10 days, then gradually resolves. FDE typically causes a long lasting gray-brown hyperpigmentation, which increases with subsequent episodes.

From: *Current Clinical Practice: Dermatology Skills for Primary Care: An Illustrated Guide*
D.J. Trozak, D.J. Tennenhouse, and J.J. Russell © Humana Press, Totowa, NJ

Provoking Factors

The only provoking factors are ingested foreign substances, which are almost exclusively prescription or proprietary medications. On rare occasions foods are implicated, producing a "fixed food reaction." The list of offending agents is extensive. The following list includes the more common offenders, but is not all-inclusive.

Medications:

- *• Acetaminophen
- • Acetylsalicylic acid
- • Atropine
- *• Barbiturates
- • Bisacodyl
- • Carbamazepine
- • Chloralhydrate
- • Chlordiazepoxide
- • Ciprofloxacin
- • Codeine
- • Cyclizine
- • Dapsone
- • Diflunisal
- • Diphenhydramine
- • Disulfiram
- • Erythromycin
- • Griseofulvin
- • Guanethidine
- • Hydralazine
- • Hydrocodone
- • Hydroxyurea
- • Ibuprofen
- • Ketoconazole

- • Mefenamic acid
- • Meprobamate
- • Methaqualone
- • Metronidazole
- • Naproxen
- • Nystatin
- *• Paracetamol
- • Penicillins
- • P. aminosalicylic acid
- *• Phenacetin
- †*• Phenolphthalein
- • Pipemidic acid
- • Piroxicam
- • Prochlorperazine
- *• Pyrazolon derivatives
- • Quinine derivatives
- • Quinidine
- *• Sulfonamides
- • Sulindac
- *• Tetracyclines
- • Tinidazole
- • Trimethoprim

Foods:

- • Red wine
- • Fresh grapes
- • Raisins

- • Strawberries
- • Cheese crisps
- • Saccharin

---

* Drugs most frequently implicated.

† Once found in most OTC laxative preparations. Banned for use in the United States.

Self-Medication

Periodic self-treatment with prescription or OTC medications is almost always the underlying cause of a fixed drug reaction.

Supplemental Review From General History

An intensive and repetitive review of all medication used must be undertaken. The questions should focus on medication taken intermittently. All prescription medications,

OTC drugs, foods, and nutritional substances should be included. Patients often do not think of some of these as medications or are embarrassed to admit to their use. When a fixed drug reaction is strongly suspected and the drug history is not productive, a general review of systems may uncover conditions that require periodic medication use. Additional history may then allow a deductive approach to the answer.

Dermatologic Physical Exam

Primary Lesions

1. A sharply demarcated macule or plaque, color initially pink but rapidly becoming dusky violet or violet-brown (*see* Photos 23,24).
2. Surface vesicles or bullae. Bullae may be so large as to obscure the underlying inflammatory macule or plaque (*see* Photo 25).

Secondary Lesions

1. Moist erosions as bullae separate.
2. Deep dusky brown or gray-brown hyperpigmentation that persists (*see* Photo 26).

Distribution

Microdistribution: None.

Macrodistribution: FDE may occur at any site on skin or mucous membranes. More common sites include periorbital and perioral regions of the face, genitalia, and perianal areas (*see* Fig. 2).

Configuration

Plaques are usually round or oval.

3. Indicated Supporting Diagnostic Data

Occasional positive patch tests have been reported with some drugs causing FDE. Positive results are supportive, but a negative test is meaningless. These tests are not routinely performed for FDE.

In very difficult cases, biopsy may be indicated and can support, but is not sufficiently characteristic to establish, the diagnosis. It is seldom indicated.

Drug challenge can be safely performed, but is rarely done due to the discomfort involved.

4. Therapy

The only definitive treatment for FDE is discovery and avoidance of the offending agent. Therapy of the acute lesions is disappointing. Neither topical nor systemic steroids seem to have any significant effect on the natural history of the lesions.

Conditions That May Simulate Fixed Drug Eruption

Early vesicular or bullous lesions on mucous membranes could be confused with a herpetic infection or an early localized stage of pemphigus vulgaris. There should be no confusion with an established FDE once the history of acute onset and cyclical recurrence is elicited.

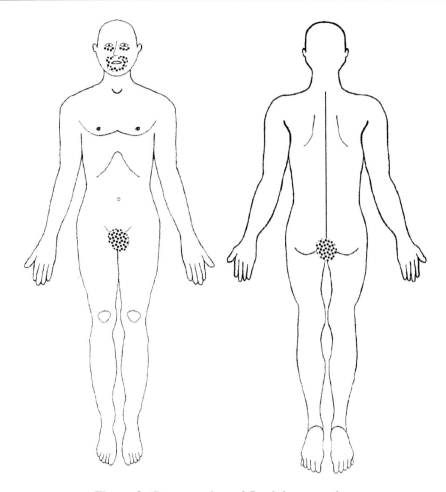

Figure 2: Common sites of fixed drug eruption.

ANSWERS TO CLINICAL APPLICATION QUESTIONS

History Review

A 70-year-old man on multiple medications presents with dusky, asymmetric red plaque lesions first noted upon awakening. The patient complains of a deep burning itch and states he has had identical lesions at the same sites on three previous occasions over the past 2 years. You suspect a fixed drug eruption.

1. What history should be elicited from this patient pertaining to a fixed drug eruption?

Answer: An exhaustive history of prescription and over-the-counter medications, food, and nutritional supplements. Be especially concerned about medications used on an intermittent basis.

2. What other variations in appearance of lesions may characterize fixed drug eruptions?

Answer: Primary lesions may include sharply demarcated pink or dusky violet macules or plaques. Vesicles or bullae may also be present. Secondary lesions may include moist erosions and dusky brown or gray-brown pigmentation that is persistent.

3. What treatment is appropriate for this patient's fixed drug eruption?

Answer: Avoidance of the offending substance is essential.

4. What is this patient's prognosis?

Answer: The prognosis is excellent if the offending substance can be found and avoided. If not, the eruption will recur and gradually extend.

17 Erysipelas/Cellulitis

INTRODUCTION

Erysipelas and cellulitis are now considered as variants of the same bacterial disease. Erysipelas is a more superficial and more acute infection of the upper subcutaneous tissue and dermis. Cellulitis affects the deeper loose subcutaneous tissue. As in any continuum of disease, some overlap can occur. Despite their common etiology, significant differences in presentation, signs, and clinical course are noted.

CLINICAL APPLICATION QUESTIONS

A 27-year-old park ranger presents at your office with a spreading erythema of the right volar forearm. He complains that the area has been sensitive to touch since he scratched the forearm while clearing brush at a campsite 3 days before.

1. What disorders should you consider in this patient?
2. What additional history should you attempt to obtain from this patient?
3. To establish a diagnosis of cellulitis, what physical findings may be present?
4. What treatment is appropriate for this patient?

APPLICATION GUIDELINES

Specific History

Onset

Erysipelas starts abruptly and can spread with impressive rapidity, often in a matter of hours. Systemic symptoms of fever, chills, and general feeling of malaise often occur, and constitutional symptoms may be quite severe. The most common site is the lower limb, where a distal portal-of-entry wound is often evident in the form of an abrasion, ulcer, interdigital fissure, or paronychia. The face is the second most frequent area to be affected. Cellulitis evolves more slowly. Usually patients indicate that symptoms developed gradually over a period of days or even a few weeks, and systemic symptoms usually occur only with longstanding disease. Cellulitis is also seen most frequently on the lower limb and face; however, involvement of skin over the perineum or abdominal wall is not uncommon.

Evolution of Disease Process

Untreated or ineffectively treated erysipelas/cellulitis will progressively spread, resulting in an ascending lymphyangiitis and sometimes septicemia. Deep extension can result in dermal necrosis, subcutaneous abscess formation, fasciitis, gangrene, and even muscle destruction. Facial involvement with erysipelas and periorbital or orbital cellulitis

From: *Current Clinical Practice: Dermatology Skills for Primary Care: An Illustrated Guide*
D.J. Trozak, D.J. Tennenhouse, and J.J. Russell © Humana Press, Totowa, NJ

can, on rare occasions, result in dread complications such as cavernous sinus thrombosis, brain abscess, meningitis, or periorbital abscess formation.

Evolution of Skin Lesions

Erysipelas begins with the classic signs of infection. Areas of bright red erythema (rubor) develop in the form of sharply demarcated palpable plaques. If the margin edge is inked, spread beyond the markings is noted within a matter of hours. The area is palpably warmer (calor) than the adjacent skin and the involved area is either tender to palpation (dolor) or at the very least is hypersensitive to touch. Sometimes skin sensitivity is the earliest sign. Superficial vesicles or bullae are common. Hemorrhage into the blisters may occur, and in older patients hemorrhage into the intact skin is not unusual. Cellulitis also shows the classic signs of infection but there are subtle differences. The erythema is more of a pink rather than a bright red color, and the affected part has a feel of deeper doughy swelling. The margin of color change is indistinct and there is no clearly defined plaque. The afflicted area is palpably warmer than adjacent skin and the area is painful to palpation; however, it is a deep discomfort and not the hyperalgesia noted in early erysipelas. Hypoalgesia or anesthesia with either of these conditions is an ominous sign signaling fascial or deeper compartment involvement. Very rare complications include chronic lymphedema of the affected skin, glomerulonephritis, or cardiovascular complications of septicemia.

Provoking Factors

A simple scratch or nick can trigger an episode. On the face and head, infection may be secondary to fissuring of chronic eczema or may complicate trauma to the auditory meatus as patients manipulate the canal while relieving the itch of a chronic dermatitis. In children, periorbital cellulitis has been associated with middle-ear infections, and orbital cellulitis has been associated with chronic sinusitis in older children and in adults. On the lower extremities, fissuring from dermatophytosis or chronic stasis ulceration is a predisposing factor. These conditions often act in concert with long-standing lymphatic injury from old trauma or chronic phlebitis. A recently defined syndrome of recurrent cellulitis of the lower extremities has been reported in cardiac bypass patients where vessel harvesting in the lower extremities has disrupted the normal venous and lymphatic return. Diabetes mellitus, neutropenia, IV drug abuse, and immunosuppression predispose patients to the more severe forms of cellulitis and a wider array of organisms.

Self-Medication

Self-treatment is not a problem in erysipelas/cellulitis.

Supplemental Review From General History

When the cause such as a local trauma is obvious, extensive review is not essential. When there is no obvious cause, then a history for possible predisposing factors should be sought. This is especially important in cases of recurrent infection.

2. Dermatologic Physical Exam

Primary Lesions

1. Sharply defined, bright red, sensitive plaques that are warmer than the adjacent or contralateral skin (erysipelas: *see* Photo 27).

2. Indistinct macular areas of pink erythema that are tender to deep palpation. They are warm, and the affected part may be visibly or palpably edematous (cellulitis: *see* Photo 28).
3. Vesicles and bullae (*see* Photo 29).

Secondary Lesions
1. Purpura secondary to dermal hemorrhage.
2. Erosions.
3. Ulceration.
4. Gangrene.

Distribution

Microdistribution: None.

Macrodistribution: The lower extremity is the most common site for both forms of infection. The next most common is the facial skin. Cellulitis is common in periorbital locations and is also fairly common on the perineal and lower abdominal skin (*see* Fig. 3).

Configuration

None

Indicated Supporting Diagnostic Data

In most cases, the diagnosis is clear and supporting laboratory data are not indicated. When there is a question regarding the diagnosis, or special circumstances prevail, the following laboratory testing may be indicated.

1. **CBC:** Elevated white count with leukocytosis.
2. **Sedimentation rate:** Elevated.
3. **Culture:** Culture may be taken if the diagnosis is in question, when there is lack of response to standard therapy, or where circumstances suggest the possibility of an unusual organism. Culture of the nasopharynx may be helpful with facial involvement, and culture of intact vesicles or bullae will sometimes reveal the offending bacteria. Cultures of entry wounds are often misleading and help only if they correlate with other cultures. If the victim is septic, blood cultures are an excellent source. In a desperate situation, aspiration of involved skin after saline infiltration or culture of minced tissue from a carefully obtained punch biopsy may identify an organism, but the yield is low.

Therapy

Group A streptococci remain the overwhelming cause of erysipelas and cellulitis. On rare occasions, Group C or G strep may be responsible, and in neonates group B strains have been reported. Occasionally, *Staphylococcus aureus* has been implicated in cellulitis. Childhood facial and periorbital cellulitis is commonly caused by *H. influenzae* type b. With the introduction of effective vaccines against *Hemophilus* bacteria in the last decade, an immunization history is critical. Facial or periorbital cellulitis in an immunized child is now likely to be some other organism. Rare causes of an erysipelas/cellulitis-like picture include *Aeromonas hydrophilia* (fresh water or soil wound contamination), *Pasturella*

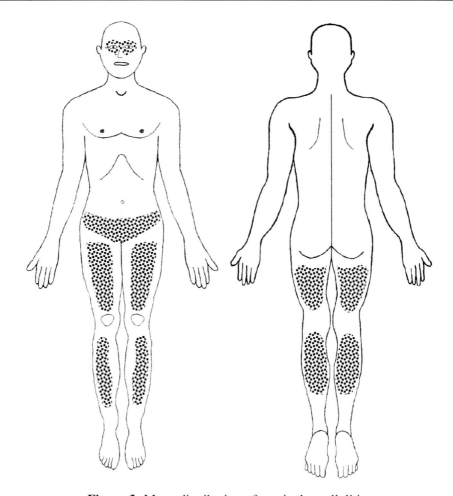

Figure 3: Macrodistribution of erysipelas cellulitis.

multocida (animal bites), or *Vibrio* species (salt or brackish water exposure or contact with raw seafood). Immunocompromised patients may be infected by a number of unusual organisms and vigorous attempts at culture are indicated.

Antimicrobial Therapy

Early or mild episodes of erysipelas can be treated with 250 to 500 mg oral penicillin V (phenoxoymethyl penicillin) QID. In penicillin-sensitive patients, 250 to 500 mg erythromycin orally QID is a reasonable alternative. Severe or advanced cases should be hospitalized and treated with 600,000 to 2 million units IV aqueous penicillin every 6 hours. Early cellulitis of suspect streptococcal origin can be treated in a similar fashion but usually requires maximal dosing and more often demands hospitalization. Rest, elevation, and immobilization of the affected part are an important part of therapy for cellulitis.

When response to therapy is slow or when staphylococcal organisms are suspected, treatment should consist of 500 to 1000 mg oral oxacillin QID, or in the case of more severe infections, 1.0 to 1.5 g iv nafcillin every 4 hours. In penicillin-sensitive patients with severe cellulitis, or cases in which the patient is neutropenic or otherwise immunologically compromised, consultation with an infectious disease specialist is recommended. Periorbital disease, especially when associated with developing proptosis, pain, loss of extraocular motion, change in pupil reaction, or visual acuity, should prompt appropriate scans and an ophthalmologic or combined ENT consult. Periocular cellulitis in children was classically due to *H. influenzae* prior to the advent of the HIB vaccine. Initial therapy now recommended for this condition is IV cefotaxime or ceftriaxone until culture and sensitivity results are available. The patient's vaccine history should also be reviewed. If the response to therapy is not prompt, a subperiosteal or orbital abscess should be suspected.

Topical Therapy

Topical medications are indicated when surface changes occur that breach the integrity of the overlying epidermis. This fragile tissue should be elevated to reduce edema and promote the delivery of the systemic antimicrobials. A foot cradle prevents additional trauma, and if the surface is moist or exudative, evaporative soaks of 0.25% acetic acid solution cleanse, dry, and inhibit secondary infection. Once the exudative phase is past, applications of an ointment containing polymyxin B sulfate and bacitracin is recommended.

Prevention

Treatment of any local skin condition that is near the site of acute infection is essential. This is particularly important with interdigital tinea and intertrigo in diabetics, or with patients who have chronic lymphatic damage to the lower extremities from trauma, phlebitis, or surgery. If recurrent erysipelas/cellulitis occurs despite these measures, prophylaxis with chronic low-dose 250 mg erythromycin BID or 250 mg cephalexin BID is usually effective and can be justified on the basis of both overall cost and prevention of progressive lymphatic destruction.

Conditions That May Simulate Erysipelas/Cellulitis

Allergic Contact Dermatitis

This may at first seem strange; however, early erysipelas and an acute contact reaction show similar degrees of erythema and induration, and both have a sharp margin with small vesicles. Contact dermatitis lacks the warmth seen in erysipelas. Although both may itch, the pruritus of erysipelas rapidly gives way to tenderness or frank pain while the itch of a contact reaction intensifies. Contact dermatitis does not have the constitutional symptoms that often accompany erysipelas.

Erysipeloid

This is an infection caused by a Gram-positive facultative anaerobic rod named *Erysipelothrix insidiosa* (former name: rhusiopathiae). It is usually acquired by occupational exposure, and is common among veterinarians, butchers, poultry handlers, and seafood handlers. The infection occurs 1 to 4 days after exposure through a minor skin breach or scratch. The dorsal fingers, hand, wrist, and distal forearm are the most common sites. A slow-moving area of dusky violaceous erythema develops, often around an obvious injury site. Central clearing with peripheral extension may occur. Throbbing and burning are prominent; however, there is no pitting edema and no increasing pain with palpation. Although erysipeloid can resolve spontaneously, symptoms may persist for a year or more and demand therapy. In addition, diffuse and septicemic forms occur as potentially fatal complications.

Angioneurotic Edema

The edema can simulate an erysipelas; however, the warmth, redness, and tenderness of an infectious process are all absent.

Other More Virulent Soft-Tissue Infections

Early stages of gangrenous and gas-forming types of cellulitis may fall into the differential diagnosisof erysipelas/cellulitis. These infections can advance with extraordinary rapidity and produce profound systemic toxicity. They usually require intensive general care and antimicrobial therapy, and almost always need surgical intervention. These disorders must always be kept in mind when treating common soft-tissue infections, and should be thought of especially when infection arises in the context of trauma, surgery, burns, malignancy, diabetes, advanced age, general debilitation, or when a foreign body is present. These infections represent clinical entities caused in some instances by a single organism, while others are caused by multiple organisms acting synergistically. This chapter will not deal with them in depth, and will only address the major clinical clues pointing to their presence. Prompt action and combined multidisciplinary care are essential because of the high morbidity and mortality rates.

Clostridial and nonclostridial crepitant cellulitis: Crepitant cellulitis is more likely to follow local trauma or surgery where wounds are contaminated by bowel flora. Extensive subcutaneous gas accumulation develops with minimal signs of cellulitis and minimal pain. Infection can progress rapidly. A nonclostridial form is common in diabetics and is often associated with a putrid odor.

Necrotizing fasciitis: This is a necrotizing process that develops at the level of the superficial fascia and subcutis. It is always more extensive than it appears clinically. Originally called hemolytic streptococcal gangrene, it is caused by several organisms. It follows minor trauma or surgery, and presents with prominent systemic toxicity. In the early stages, skin signs may be minimal. The usual picture is that of an acutely ill patient with a cellulitis that is progressing despite antimicrobial treatment. Erythema and edema are variable and may be minimal. The presence of blistering, cyanosis, and especially anesthesia point to this diagnosis. Pain is present, progression is rapid, and gas and putrid odor may occur with the mixed infection type.

Progressive bacterial synergistic gangrene: Also known as Meleney's ulcer, this gangrenous process usually occurs at an abdominal or thoracic operative site that contains wire-retention sutures. Ulceration and gangrene develop at the wound site, where a gangrenous ulcer with a border of purple cellulitis is seen. Mixed organisms are present. Despite pain and enormous tissue damage, there is little systemic toxicity.

Clostridial myonecrosis: Clostridial myonecrosis develops after penetrating trauma, bowel surgery, bowel infarction, or perforation. It progresses rapidly with localized pain and marked systemic toxicity. Crepitus may or may not be clinically evident. Skin over the site is initially blanched and tense. Later, bronze discoloration develops, followed by bullae and necrosis. True gas gangrene has a sweet or "mousy" odor.

Nonclostridial myositis: Nonclostridial myositis also follows local trauma. It is caused by various organisms, most often anaerobic strep. Onset is gradual over several days. Minimal pain and systemic signs appear early, but may become severe in late stages. Gas formation is rare and sparse when present. Skin findings consist of erythema. Odor may be foul.

Synergistic necrotizing cellulitis: Typically seen in diabetics, necrotizing cellulitis presents as an acute infection with marked systemic toxicity. It usually involves the perineum, causing patchy skin necrosis with small ulcers discharging foul "dishwater" pus. Crepitus may be present. Biopsy shows muscle necrosis without vascular occlusion. This is a mixed synergistic process with very high mortality.

ANSWERS TO CLINICAL APPLICATION QUESTIONS

History Review

A 27-year-old park ranger presents at your office with a spreading erythema of the right volar forearm. He complains that the area has been sensitive to touch since he scratched the forearm while clearing brush at a campsite 3 days before.

1. What disorders should you consider in this patient?

Answer:
   a. Cellulitis.
   b. Toxicodendron dermatitis (rhus dermatitis).

2. What additional history should you attempt to obtain from this patient?

Answer:
   a. Prior history of toxicodendron dermatitis.
   b. Exposure to suspicious plant materials.

3. To establish a diagnosis of cellulitis, what physical findings may be present?

Answer:
   a. Sharply defined bright-red warm sensitive plaques.
   b. Discrete vesicles and bullae (as distinguished from the confluent vesicles and bullae of toxicodendron dermatitis).
   c. Lymphangitic streaking.
   d. Regional adenopathy.

4. What treatment is appropriate for this patient?

Answer:
   a. Systemic antimicrobial therapy is needed if there is any possibility of an acute cellulitis.
   b. Rest and elevation of the affected part.
   c. Follow-up at 5 to 7 days, but immediate telephone call to your office if there is progression of lesions or systemic symptoms develop.

18 Erythema Multiforme

INTRODUCTION

Erythema multiforme (EM) has been divided into a minor (simplex) form and a major (bullous) form. The minor form is additionally subdivided into papular and vesiculobullous variants, and all three have been considered a continuum of the same process. Histologically, each shows varying degrees of dermal and epidermal inflammation and injury. The clinical manifestations are determined by both the intensity of the damage and the relative amount of injury to each layer. Histologic gradations show a continuum that parallels the clinical findings. The major variant is also referred to by the eponyms "Stevens-Johnson syndrome" (prominent skin and mucous membrane lesions with systemic signs) or "Fuchs syndrome" (prominent prolonged eye and oral involvement). Recent publications challenge the concept of a continuum and propose a division of erythema multiforme minor and erythema multiforme major into separate entities with different provoking causes. Overlap cases are reported, however, and until the pathogenesis of each is fully understood, the value of such a separation remains unclear. EM major shares some clinical and pathologic features with toxic epidermal necrolysis. This is a catastrophic illness with a 30 to 40% mortality rate.

CLINICAL APPLICATION QUESTIONS

A 12-year-old schoolgirl presents in your office with a 2-day history of fever, intense oral pain, crusting and blistering of the lower lip, and severe dysuria. She also has scattered skin lesions over the trunk and extremities. Some are target lesions. You suspect erythema multiforme major.

1. What history is indicated with regard to the cause of erythema multiforme major?
2. What specific areas of the body should be evaluated on physical examination?
3. What laboratory studies are indicated with regard to the cause of erythema multiforme major?
4. What treatment is appropriate for erythema multiforme major?

APPLICATION GUIDELINES

Specific History

Onset

The onset of both forms of EM is acute with lesions developing rapidly over a matter of hours. A minority of patients with EM minor complain of fever, headache, myalgias, and arthralgias; however, most have only complaints relative to the skin lesions. EM major is usually associated with prominent systemic signs of fever, weakness, myalgias, and

From: *Current Clinical Practice: Dermatology Skills for Primary Care: An Illustrated Guide*
D.J. Trozak, D.J. Tennenhouse, and J.J. Russell © Humana Press, Totowa, NJ

even prostration. Both forms may be preceded by a viral-like prodrome consisting of malaise, fever, headache, sore throat, rhinorrhea, and cough. This prodrome occurs 1 to 2 weeks prior to onset of the EM and almost always precedes the major variant. Adults in their third and fourth decades account for most cases. Up to 20% of victims are children and adolescents.

Evolution of Disease Process

EM minor is usually characterized by lesions that erupt over a 3- to 5-day period, then stabilize and resolve within 2 weeks. New lesions may occur for up to 2 weeks with complete healing in 1 month, but this long duration is unusual. Healing of vesiculobullous lesions is usually more prolonged than healing of papular lesions.

The course of EM major is more protracted. New lesions typically occur for 2 to 4 weeks, but sometimes for more than a month. Healing is usually complete at 6 weeks, but may be much longer in some cases.

EM minor may be further characterized as classic, recurrent, or persistent. Classic EM minor is sporadic, acral in distribution, and symmetrical. Except in drug-induced cases, the average duration is 2 to 3 weeks. Frank blistering is uncommon and symptoms other than the skin eruption itself are minimal. Medications, herpes simplex virus, and other infections are the most common triggers.

Recurrent EM minor occurs on a cyclical basis with long symptom-free intervals. Yearly recurrences are common. Clinically it is identical to the classic type except for the more common presence of photoaccentuation. Recurrent herpes labialis attacks that precede the EM episode by 1 to 2 weeks are the most common identifiable cause.

Persistent EM minor is a rare form in which the attack, despite fluctuations in intensity, continues without interruption. Vesicular and bullous lesions are more common and the eruption tends to be widespread. Associated symptoms, pruritus, and low-grade constitutional symptoms are common. More extensive vascular changes are reported on biopsy, and lab exam often shows hypocomplementemia and the presence of circulating immune complexes. Persistent EM minor has been linked to occult malignancy, chronic Epstein-Barr virus infection, inflammatory bowel disease, and lupus erythematosus.

Complications are rare in EM minor. On occasion, oral mucous membrane lesions may interfere with nutrition and fluid intake. In EM major, complications are the rule, and eye involvement can lead to visual impairment or damage to the lacrimal apparatus in up to 10% of cases. Esophagitis, esophageal stricture, renal necrosis, bladder injury, upper airway injury, and myocardial injury have been reported. Untreated, the mortality rate is estimated at 5 to 15%. Most deaths are attributable to pneumonia, secondary infection of denuded skin, and renal failure.

Evolution of Skin Lesions

The earliest lesions of EM are erythematous macules, which rapidly evolve into fixed papules. In some cases, these occur in successive waves or crops. Some lesions enlarge to form erythematous plaques, and partial clearing or superimposition of successive lesions may produce geometric, polycyclic, or arciform configurations. Central hemorrhage, blister formation, or superficial epidermal necrosis can cause a bruised, translucent, or gray color change. When multiple zones are present, concentric rings occur, which are termed iris or target lesions. These are pathognomonic. With greater degrees of epidermal injury, a central vesicle or small bullae may develop, and smaller vesicles may be present at the periphery. These lesions are typical of EM minor but may also be seen with the major variant. Lesions of EM major may consist of a fine maculopapular erythema or large areas or plaques of confluent erythema. Large bullae and extensive areas of epidermal separation may develop. Healing times as noted above are much longer in EM major and are also affected by nutritional status and secondary infection.

Provoking Factors

A causative factor can be identified in about 50% of cases. Extensive lists of provoking factors have been compiled. For purposes of brevity and clarity, this section will list the major categories and the most frequent specific causes.

1. Infections.
   Viral: Herpes simplex, most often type I (most common infectious cause of EM minor)
   Bacterial: Streptococcus; *Mycoplasma pneumoniae* (common infectious cause of EM major in children and young adults); **Protozoan**; **Fungal**, most often deep fungal infections.
2. Immunizations and hyposensitizations.
3. Drugs (most common cause of EM major)
   Topical medications; systemic agents: Sulfonamides, especially long-acting; carbamezapine; phenylbutazone; diphenylhydantoin; penicillins; nonsteroidal anti-inflammatory agents.
4. Neoplasms.
5. Lupus erythematosus.
6. Physical agents, especially irradiation of malignancies.

Self-Medication

Self-treatment is a problem when the medication is the provoking factor.

Supplemental Review From General History

When the provoking factor is not evident, a complete review is indicated in order to establish an etiology and to eliminate any exogenous cause or treat an endogenous one.

Dermatologic Physical Exam

Primary Lesions

1. Small and large erythematous macules.
2. Erythematous papules (*see* Photo 30).
3. Small and large erythematous plaques (*see* Photos 30,31).
4. Vesicles and bullae (*see* Photo 32).

Secondary Lesions

1. Purpura.
2. Necrosis.
3. Erosions.

4. Impetiginization.
5. Hemorrhage, vesicle formation and necrosis combine in secondary lesions in concentric rings to form the clinically pathognomonic target or iris lesions (*see* Photo 33).

Distribution

Microdistribution: None.

Macrodistribution: In EM minor, lesions are symmetrical and are typically found on the palms, dorsum of the hands, wrists, extensor forearms, dorsum of the feet, elbows, and knees (*see* Fig. 4). Lesions may occur in any location.

Mucosal lesions may occur in EM minor but are limited to one site, usually the oral cavity. Involvement of more than one mucosal site is considered evidence for EM major. In EM major, all mucous membranes, the lining of the esophagus, the upper respiratory epithelium, and the lining of the urinary bladder may be involved. The most characteristic mucosal sign is the bloody denuded vermilion of the upper and lower lips (*see* Photo 34). Since EM is a clinical spectrum, these different distributions are not mutually exclusive, and a fair degree of overlap can exist.

Configuration

1. Iris (rainbow-like).
2. Targetoid (*see* Photo 35).
3. Annular and polycyclic.

Indicated Supporting Diagnostic Data

EM minor is readily diagnosed on clinical exam, and in the absence of systemic signs, supporting diagnostic data are seldom indicated. Vesiculobullous EM and EM major may at times enter into the differential of drug eruptions, lupus erythematosus, cutaneous vasculitis, dermatitis herpetiformis, pemphigoid, toxic epidermal necrolysis, and other toxic erythemas. On these rare occasions, the following laboratory studies may be helpful. Otherwise, lab data are indicated mainly for the management of the complications of EM major.

Skin Biopsy

EM does not show clearly defining features under the microscope. The main utility of a biopsy is to establish whether or not the findings are compatible, and to rule out other entities that have more defining features.

Direct Immunofluorescence

This test should be performed primarily when there is a need to rule out other major bullous diseases. Although the patterns of fluorescence seen in EM are not specific, they can support the diagnosis and may offer a clue as to the general etiology.

Therapy

Elimination or Eradication

The initial goal in treating any form of EM should be establishing an etiology and the elimination of any offending drug or the eradication of any treatable internal cause. If an

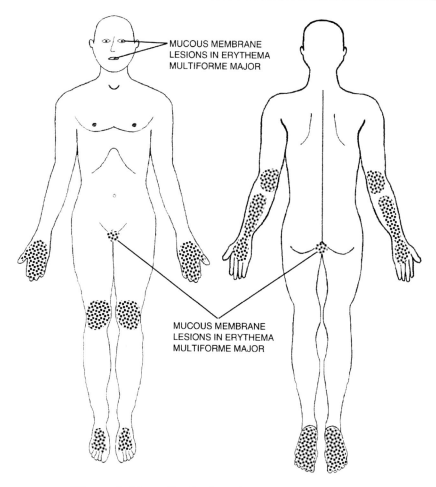

Figure 4: Macrodistribution of erythema multiforme.

obvious provoking factor is not evident from the history, all medications (prescription, OTC, and topical) become suspect. In the minor forms, one can begin by eliminating non-essential or most suspect medications. In EM major, if possible, all medications should be stopped. The list of medications associated with EM is extensive and is constantly expanding. Most cases of EM minor without an obvious cause do not recur, and laboratory investigation is not warranted. In the case of recurrent EM minor or EM major where history and physical exam are unremarkable, the following diagnostic laboratory studies are justified, and may be revealing:

1. CBC.
2. Cold agglutinin titers.
3. Throat and sputum cultures-for B-strep and mycoplasma.
4. Chest X-ray, PA and lateral.

In rare cases of persistent EM minor, once medications have been absolved as a possible source, the patient should receive a complete history and physical examination followed by any lab workup indicated from that examination. If this is not productive, then complement levels, circulating immune complex titers, a connective tissue screen, and complete serologies for Epstein-Barr virus should follow. Biopsy for direct immunofluorescence may be needed to distinguish vesiculobullous lesions from other blistering diseases. Finally, an exhaustive workup for occult neoplasm is next. The only case of this EM variant in the authors' experience had a walnut-sized adenocarcinoma of the ileocecal junction, and the eruption resolved with resection of the tumor.

EM Minor Without Mucous Membrane Involvement

Treatment in this instance is primarily symptomatic unless there are recurrent episodes with an identifiable, treatable cause. Antihistamines, in the form of a sedating H_1 blocker, help when there is intense pruritus. Hydroxyzine 25 to 50 mg QID or 10 mg doxepin TID are excellent choices. A high-potency or superpotent topical steroid can also be helpful. Myalgias, arthralgias, and deep skin tenderness will improve with aspirin or acetaminophen. Extensive EM minor or EM minor with a significant vesiculobullous component will respond to oral corticosteroids. Provided there are no contraindications, short courses are justified in patients who are uncomfortable or must maintain a busy work schedule. Adults usually clear promptly on a single morning dose of prednisone in the range of 20 to 30 mg/day administered over 10 to 14 days. Topical therapy of oral lesions in EM minor is the same as in the major form discussed below.

Recurrent EM Associated With Recurrent Herpes Simplex Virus

Attacks of EM, most often simplex type, follow both labial and genital herpes in a small but significant number of individuals. The lag time from cold sore to EM is usually 10 to 14 days. Simple measures such as avoidance of sunburns and the use of a sunscreen in a lip pomade can greatly help some; however, attacks may continue to occur at frequent intervals. Suppressive therapy with 200 mg oral acyclovir BID or TID will usually prevent both problems. Episodic acyclovir therapy at the first sign of a herpetic lesion will usually temper the viral lesion but often has no effect on the subsequent EM. Acyclovir given for an established herpetic lesion will not affect either process.

EM Major

Treatment of this problem usually requires hospitalization, intensive nursing care, and a multidisciplinary approach. Superimposed infection, particularly pulmonary, is responsible for a number of deaths. Full isolation precautions are recommended and any focus of infection should be treated promptly. Alimentation may be a major problem in the first 2 or 3 weeks and must be addressed so that the patient can respond to this significant injury. Fortunately, modern hyperalimentation can prevent much of this early debilitation. Most cases require a period of IV fluid maintenance, and in extensive cases, fluid therapy can be as complicated as that for a burn injury. Treatment of the mucous membranes and vermilion should be active but gentle, and despite their crusted appearance, debridement of the lips is contraindicated.

The oral cavity can be gently debrided with swishes of dilute saline or 1.5% (half-strength) hydrogen peroxide every 3 to 4 hours. Gentle cleansing with glycerin swabs will lubricate and freshen. Gargles of 4% lidocaine solution or viscous 2% lidocaine prior to meals will help minimize pain while eating. Urethral involvement may be so severe that catheterization is needed. Pain on micturition can be severe, especially in female patients where the outer vaginal and vulvar membranes are affected. Having the patient void in a shallow tub of lukewarm water may relieve much of this discomfort. Additional relief can be obtained with topical 5% lidocaine ointment. When the pain is primarily of urethral origin, 200 mg phenazopyridine HCl TID for adults, and 12 mg/kg/24 hours in three divided doses for children 6 to 12 years old, is indicated.

Topical treatment for intact skin lesions is similar to that discussed under EM minor. Involvement of the ocular mucous membranes can lead to blindness, and permanent scarring of the lacrimal apparatus has been documented. Because of the severe sequelae, an ophthalmologic consultant should be engaged early in the course.

Treatment of the EM major itself is controversial, and a debate over the use of systemic steroid therapy has raged in the literature for two decades. While we await more definitive prospective studies, a moderate, thoughtful approach seems most sensible. A dermatologic consultant should be engaged immediately to assist with topical therapy, and of greatest importance, to aid in a decision regarding steroid therapy or possible tertiary referral. There is evidence for both immune-complex and type IV hypersensitivity mechanisms in EM. Both show a response to systemic corticoids. If steroids are given vigorously in early EM major prior to maximal tissue injury, there is a rationale for their use. Once maximal tissue injury has developed, or where there is greater than 25% surface loss, they may contribute to mortality and morbidity by depressing tissue repair and predisposing the patient to secondary infection. If a decision is made to start steroids, they should be initiated in doses of 60 to 80 mg/day of prednisone in adults, or 1 to 2 mg/kg/day in children. Doses should be maintained until the patient is afebrile and free of new lesions for 3 days. These can then be tapered over a 2- to 3-week period.

When greater than 10 to 15% second-degree surface loss has occurred, strong consideration should be given to transferring the case to a tertiary burn unit, where fluid management and use of biological dressings can be initiated.

Conditions That May Simulate Erythema Multiforme

Hand, Foot, and Mouth Disease

This painful viral exanthem is caused by several strains of coxsackievirus. The oral lesions are usually small, and the vermilion margin injury seen with EM is not present. In addition, flat vesicles oriented along skin lines are seen on the palms and soles.

Bullous Pemphigoid

This major bullous disease may simulate EM especially when oral lesions are present. Pemphigoid usually has a gradual onset, systemic toxicity is absent, and it occurs in an older patient population. Biopsy combined with direct and indirect immunofluorescence should distinguish between them.

Dermatitis Herpetiformis

Like pemphigoid, the onset of dermatitis herpetiformis is gradual and the course is chronic. Systemic signs are absent and biopsy and direct immunofluorescence should distinguish the two.

Allergic Vasculitis

Some cases of hypersensitivity vasculitis show polymorphic lesions that may resemble EM. Usually the distribution is different and the biopsy shows a leukocytoclastic angiitis, which is absent in biopsies from EM.

ANSWERS TO CLINICAL APPLICATION QUESTIONS

History Review

A 12-year-old schoolgirl presents in your office with a 2-day history of fever, intense oral pain, crusting and blistering of the lower lip, and severe dysuria. She also has scattered skin lesions over the trunk and extremities. Some are target lesions. You suspect erythema multiforme major.

1. What history is indicated with regard to the cause of erythema multiforme major?

Answer:
   a. A careful history of prodromal upper respiratory or pulmonary symptoms.
   b. Any antecedent infections.
   c. Any systemic medications taken within 1 week of onset of symptoms.

2. What specific areas of the body should be evaluated on physical examination?

Answer: Mucous membrane sites should be evaluated for blistering and surface loss, which can cause severe pain and interfere with urination and food intake. Ocular mucous membranes must be examined, early treatment is mandatory to avoid damage to the lacrimal duct.

3. What laboratory studies are indicated with regard to the cause of erythema multiforme major?

Answer:
   a. Throat culture and sputum cultures for beta streptococcus and mycoplasma.
   b. Cold agglutinin titers for mycoplasma.
   c. ASO titer for streptococcal infection.
   d. Chest X-ray for pneumonia.
   e. Urinalysis for evidence of hematuria and casts indicating possible kidney or bladder involvement.

4. What treatment is appropriate for erythema multiforme major?

Answer: Immediate hospitalization for a complex potentially life-threatening multisystem insult requiring a multidisciplinary medical team.

REFERENCES for Part III

1. Champion RH, Burton JL, Ebling FJG. Textbook of Dermatology. 5th ed. Oxford: Blackwell Scientific Publications, 1992, pp. 996–998, 1127–1170, 1865–1880, 845–847,861–863, 992–993, 1834–1838.
2. Braun-Falco O, Plewig G, Wolff HH, Winkelmann RK.Dermatology. Berlin-Heidelberg: Springer-Verlag, 1991, pp. 181–182, 219–232, 292–315, 396, 409–412.
3. Provost TT, Farmer ER. Current Therapy in Dermatology-2. Toronto-Philadelphia: B.C. Decker Inc., 1988, pp. 212, 277.
4. Leider M, Rosenblum M. A Dictionary of Dermatological Words, Terms and Phrases. New York-Toronto-London-Sydney: Mc Graw-Hill, 1968, pp. 123.
5. Gupta AK, Sauder DN, Shear NH. Antifungal agents: An overview. Part I. J Amer Acad Dermatol 1994;30:677–698.
6. Gupta AK, Sauder DN, Shear NH. Antifungal agents: An overview. Part II. J Amer Acad Dermatol 1994;30:911–933.
7. Gupta AK, Diova N, Taborda P, et al. Once weekly fluconazole is effective in the treatment of tinea capitis: a prospective multicentre study. Br J Dermatol 2000;142:965-968.
8. Elewski BE. Clinical Pearl: Proximal white subungual onychomycosis in AIDS. J Amer Acad Dermatol 1993;29:631–632.
9. Freidlander SF, et al. Use of the cotton swab method in diagnosing tinea capitis. Pediatrics 1999;104:276-279.
10. Physicians Desk Reference. Thomson, 57th ed., 2003.
11. Drug Facts and Comparisons. St. Louis: Wolters-Kluwer Co., 2003 ed.
12. Wolverton SE. Comprehensive Dermatologic Therapy. W B Saunders Company, 2001.
13. Elewski BE. Tinea capitis: Itraconazole in Trichophyton tonsurans infection. J Amer Acad Dermatol 1994;31:65–67.
14. Freiden IJ, Howard R. Tinea capitis: Epidemiology, diagnosis, treatment and control. J Amer Acad Dermatol 1994;31:S42–S46.
15. Degreef HJ, Piet RG, DeDoncker MSc. Current therapy of dermatophytosis. J Amer Acad Dermatol 1994;31:S25–S30.
16. Dover JS, Shear NH. New systemic treatments for onychomycosis. Journal Watch 3, 1995; 154:36–37.
17. Legendre R, Escola-Macre J. Itraconazole in the treatment of tinea capitis. J. Amer Acad Dermatol 1990;23:559–560.
18. del Carmen Padilla Desgarennes M, Rubio Godoy M, Beirana Palencia A. Therapeutic efficacy of terbinafine in the treatment of three children with tinea tonsurans. J. Amer Acad Dermatol 1996;35:114–116.
19. Dragos Vlasta, Lunder Majda. Lack of efficacy of 6 week treatment with oral terbinafine for tinea capitis due to Microsporum canis in children. Ped Dermatol 1997;14:46–48.
20. Monroe EW, Jones HE. Urticaria, An Updated Review. Arch Dermatol 1977;113:80–90.
21. Kozel MM, Mekkes JR, Bossuyt PM, et al. Natural course of physical and chronic urticaria and angioedema in 220 patients. J Amer Acad Dermatol 2001;45:387-391.
22. Jacobson KW, Branch LB, Nelson HS. Laboratory Tests in Chronic Urticaria. JAMA 1980;243:1644–1646.
23. Bernstein IL, Huffman Jr. BL, Knight AK. Diagnosis and Management of Histamine Mediated Allergic Diseases. Clinician 1986;4 #3:18–21.

From: *Current Clinical Practice: Dermatology Skills for Primary Care: An Illustrated Guide*
D.J. Trozak, D.J. Tennenhouse, and J.J. Russell © Humana Press, Totowa, NJ

24. Champion RH. Urticaria: then and now. Br J Dermatol 1988;119:427–436.
25. Dobson RL, Thiers BH. Westwood Western Conference on Clinical Dermatology III. J Amer Acad Dermatol 1982;6 #4:552.
26. Kennard CD, Ellis CN. Pharmacologic therapy for urticaria. J Amer Acad Dermatol 1991;25:176–189.
27. Newer Antihistamines. The Medical Letter April 30, 2001;43:35.
28. Cetirizine—A new antihistamine. The Medical Letter March 1996;38:21–23.
29. Haustein UF. Adrenergic urticaria and adrenergic pruritus. Acta Derm Venreol (Stockh) 1990;70:82.
30. Shelly WB, Shelly ED. Adrenergic urticaria: A new form of stress induced hives. Lancet 1985; II:1031.
31. Bircher AJ, Mier-Ruge W. Aquagenic Pruritus, Water-Induced Activation of Acetyl-cholinesteraase. Arch Dermatol 1988;124:84–89.
32. Bayoumi A-HM, Highet AS. Baking soda baths for aquagenic pruritus (letter). Lancet 1986; II:464.
33. Neittaanmaki H. Cold Urticaria, Clinical findings in 220 patients. J Amer Acad Dermatol 1985;13:636–644.
34. Ryan TJ, Shim-Young N, Turk JL. Delayed Pressure Urticaria. Br J Dermatol 1968;80: 485–490.
35. Estes SA, Yung CW. Delayed Pressure Urticaria: An investigation of some parameters of lesion induction. J Amer Acad Dermatol 1992;1981;5:5–31.
36. Cosky RJ, Dermatologic therapy.J Amer Acad Dermatol 1993;29:603.
37. Kontou-Fili K, Maniatakou, Demaka P, et al. Therapeutic effects of cetirizine in delayed pressure urticaria: Clinicopathologic findings. J Amer Acad Dermatol 1991;24:1090–1093.
38. Leenutaphong V, Holzle E, Plewig G. Pathogenesis and classification of solar urticaria: a new concept. J Amer Acad Dermatol 1989;21:237–24.
39. Olson JC, Esterly NB. Urticarial vasculitis and Lyme disease.(letter) J Amer Acad Dermatol 1990;22:1114–1116.
40. Millns JL, Randle HW, Solley GO, et al. The therapeutic response of urticarial vasculitis to indomethacin. J Amer Acad Dermatol 1980;3:349–355.
41. Monroe EW. Urticarial vasculitis: An updated review. J Amer Acad Dermatol 1981;5:88–95.
42. Davis MD, Daoud MS, Kirby B, et al. Clinicopathologic correlation of hypocomplementemic and normocomplementemic urticarial vasculitis. J Amer Acad Dermatol 1998;38:899-905.
43. Vibratory angioedema: lesion induction, clinical features, laboratory and ultrastructural findings and response to therapy. Br J Dermatol 1989;120:93–99.
44. The Guide to Drug Eruptions. 5th ed. Amsterdam: Free University Amsterdam; File of Medicines, 1990, pp. 46–48.
45. The Guide to Drug Eruptions. 6th ed. Amsterdam: Free University Amsterdam; File of Medicines, 1995, pp. 21–22.
46. Mandell GL, Bennett JE, Dolin R. Principles and Practices of Infectious Diseases. 4th ed. New York, Edinburgh, London, Madrid, Melbourne, Milan, Tokyo: Churchill-Livingston, 1995, pp. 913–916, 1134.
47. Leppard BJ, Seal DV, Colman G, et al. The value of bacteriology and serology in the diagnosis of cellulitis and erysipelas. Br J Dermatol 1991;1985;112:59–567.
48. Broadhurst LE, Erickson RL, Kelly PW. Decreases in invasive Haemophilus influenzae disease in US army children, 1984 throug. JAMA 1993;269:227–231.
49. Adams WG, Deaver KA, Cochi SL, et al. Decline of childhood Haemophilus influenzae type b (Hib) in the Hib vaccine era. JAMA 1993;269:221–226.
50. Duvanel T, et al. Quantitative cultures of biopsy specimens from cutaneous cellulitis. Arch Intern Med 1989;149:293.
51. Bisno AL, Stevens DL. Streptococcal infections of skin and soft tissues. NEJM 1996; 334:240–245.

52. McCoy JA. Erysipelothrix Rhusiopathiae Infection in Animals and Man. J Assoc Mil Dermatol VIII 1982;no.1:28–30.

53. Feingold DS. Gangrenous and crepitant cellulitis. J Amer Acad Dermatol 1982;6:289–299.

54. Huff JC, Weston WL, Tonnesen MG. Erythema multiforme: A critical review of characteristics, diagnostic criteria, and causes. J Amer Acad Dermatol 1983;8:763–775.

55. Finan MC, Schroeter AL. Cutaneous immunofluorescence study of erythema multiforme: Correlation with light microscopic patterns and etiologic agents. J Amer Acad Dermatol 1984;10:497–506.

56. Rasmussen JE. Erythema multiforme in children: response to treatment with systemic corticosteroids. Br J Dermatol 1976;95:181–186.

57. Ginsburg CM. Stevens-Johnson syndrome in children. Pediatr Infec Dis 1982;1:155–158.

58. Ruiz-Maldonado R. Acute disseminated epidermal necrosis types 1, 2, and 3: Study of sixty cases. J Amer Acad Dermatol 1985;13:623–635.

59. Weston WL, Morelli JG, Rogers M. Target lesions on the lips: Childhood herpes simplex associated with erythema multiforme mimics Stevens-Johnson syndrome. J Am Acad Dermatol 1997;37:848-850.

60. Garcia-doval I, LeCleach L, Bocquet H, et al. Toxic epidermal necrolysis and Stevens-Johnson syndrome: Does early withdrawal of causative drugs decrease the risk of death? Arch Dermatol 2000;136:323-327.

61. Cote' B, Wechsler J, Bastuji-Garin S, et al. Clinicopathologic correlation in erythema multiforme and Stevens-Johnson syndrome. Arch Dermatol 1995;131:1268-1272.

62. Renfro L, Grant-Kels JM, Feder Jr. HM, et al. Controversy: Are systemic steroids indicated in the treatment of erythema multiforme? Pediatr Dermatol 6 1989;no. 1:43–50.

63. Drago F, Parodi A, Rebora A. Persistent erythema multiforme: Report of two cases and-review of literature. J Amer Acad Dermatol 1995;33:366–36.

64. Tay Y, Huff J, Weston W. Mycoplasm pneumoniae infection is associated with Steven's-Johnson syndrome, not erythema multiforme (von Hebra). J Amer Acad Dermatol 1996;35: 757–760.

65. Update on Superficial Fungal Infections, A Special Report: Postgraduate Medicine: 1-45, July 1999.

66. Elewski BE. Treatment of tinea capitis: beyond griseofulvin. J Amer Acad Dermatol 1999;40:S27-S30.

67. Hubbard TW. The Predictive Value of Symptoms in Diagnosing Childhood Tinea Capitis. Arch Pediatr Adolesc Med 1999;153:1150-1153.

Part IV: Epidermal and Dermal Lesions, Eczematous Lesions, and Atrophies

IMPORTANT ABBREVIATIONS USED IN THIS PART:

AD	Atopic dermatitis
ANA	Antinuclear antibody
DLE	Discoid lupus erythematosus
NSAID	Nonsteroidal anti-inflammatory drugs
OTC	Over-the-counter
RIF	Rapid immunofluorescence test
SCLE	Subacute cutaneous lupus erythematosus
SLE	Systemic lupus erythematosus
SPF	Sun protection

19 Lupus Erythematosus

INTRODUCTION

The purpose of this chapter is to improve the participant's skill in the clinical diagnosis of the cutaneous manifestations of lupus erythematosus (LE). Discussion will focus on characteristic disease patterns without an exhaustive review of obscure variations. Laboratory parameters that support the clinical findings will be discussed, along with a review of current therapy. The material on LE will conclude with comparisons between cutaneous LE and other common dermatitides that can be confused with both discoid and systemic LE.

Cutaneous lesions can occur in all of the major forms of LE. In classic presentation, each form is quite different from the others. However, considerable overlap can occur and a final classification of any solitary case will depend on a composite of data from history, skin examination, general examination, and laboratory tests. This chapter will emphasize the morphologic differences, but the reader must be wary that these are not mutually exclusive.

CLINICAL APPLICATION QUESTIONS

A 35-year-old woman seeks help regarding a progressive skin eruption that began on the ears and facial skin late in the previous summer. The lesions stabilized during the winter months but rapidly progressed with the return of warm, sunny weather. Physical examination reveals a scaling dermatitis with discrete and confluent plaques. Some plaques have a depressed center and scarring. Telangectasia, hypopigmentation, and hyperpigmentation are evident. The rash is asymmetric on the face and ears but is symmetrically distributed over the V of the chest, dorsal arms, and forearms with sharp limitation at the collar and short-sleeve protection line.

1. What is the most likely diagnosis: localized discoid lupus erythematosus (DLE), disseminated DLE, subacute cutaneous LE (SCLE), or systemic LE (SLE)?
2. What other findings on physical exam would be helpful in distinguishing one form of lupus from another?
3. What additional supplemental historical data would help to distinguish one form of lupus from another?
4. History reveals an unexplained episode of pleurisy 4 years ago. What supporting laboratory data are indicated?
5. If laboratory parameters are consistent with a diagnosis of SLE with discoid skin lesions, what are your treatment options?
6. If laboratory parameters are consistent with a diagnosis of disseminated DLE, what are your treatment options?

From: *Current Clinical Practice: Dermatology Skills for Primary Care: An Illustrated Guide*
D.J. Trozak, D.J. Tennenhouse, and J.J. Russell © Humana Press, Totowa, NJ

APPLICATION GUIDELINES: DISCOID LUPUS ERYTHEMATOSUS (CUTANEOUS LUPUS ERYTHEMATOSUS)

Specific History

Onset

The onset of DLE is usually rather abrupt and frequently related to solar exposure. Because the lesions have a striking appearance, patients often recall very specifically the time of onset. Sometimes it is possible to elicit a history of transient prior episodes following intense sun exposure. DLE may cause severe disfigurement and permanent scarring; it should not be approached in a cavalier fashion. Localized and disseminated forms occur. About 15% of patients with SLE show lesions indistinguishable from those of DLE at some stage of their disease.

Evolution of Disease Process

Localized DLE: This condition usually begins on the exposed skin of the face and neck, and lesions are limited to the scalp, face, and neck areas. These patients seldom have any general complaints, and the risk of conversion to systemic disease is estimated at about 1%.

Disseminated DLE: This variant of DLE usually begins on, and is more prominent on, sun-exposed skin. Widespread lesions develop above and below the neck, some of which may occur on non-sun-exposed sites. These patients have a greater incidence of systemic complaints such as arthralgias or Raynaud's phenomenon. This form of DLE has about a 20% risk of conversion to systemic lupus. Because localized DLE is more common than disseminated DLE, the overall risk of any single case of DLE converting to SLE is about 5%.

Evolution of Skin Lesions

DLE lesions usually remain fixed and tend to progress unless treated. They rarely cause any subjective symptoms such as pruritus or pain and are mainly of cosmetic concern to the patient.

Provoking Factors

Sunburn, emotional stress, and various medications have been reported to exacerbate DLE. These medications include isoniazid, penicillamine, griseofulvin, and dapsone. Sunburn and medications are the most common triggers.

Self-Medication

Self-treatment is usually not a problem in DLE. The lesions do not cause any compelling subjective symptoms and do not respond to the relatively weak over-the-counter (OTC) corticosteroids.

Supplemental Review From General History

Because of the systemic variant, a comprehensive review of systems is indicated with special emphasis on lupus-associated findings in the joints, lungs, central nervous system (CNS), and cardiovascular systems. Although the risk of SLE in a patient with DLE lesions is small, this history should target those patients at greatest risk and foster selective use of the laboratory. Only a small portion of DLE patients need extensive serologic surveys.

Dermatologic Physical Exam

Primary Lesions

The early primary lesions of DLE are raised, sharply demarcated papules and plaques. Both are smooth, dusky-red with a shiny surface and loss of skin lines (*see* Photo 1). Size varies from a few millimeters to several centimeters. As these plaques mature, secondary changes occur.

Secondary Lesions

1. White adherent scale (*see* Photos 2,3).
2. Atrophy, both epidermal and dermal.
3. Telangiectatic (dilated) blood vessels (*see* Photos 4,5).
4. Hyper- and hypopigmentation (*see* Photos 4–6).
5. Significant scarring is common (*see* Photos 5–8).

The lesions extend peripherally while a central adherent white scale develops (*see* Photo 2). The scale fills the hair follicles; this follicular pattern may be clinically evident as discrete geometrically speckled dots (*see* Photo 2). When the scale is lifted, conical projections may extend downward, giving the "carpet-tack" sign (*see* Fig. 1). Follicular accentuation and a positive "carpet-tack" sign strongly support a diagnosis of DLE. Scale may be barely evident (*see* Photo 2) or may be so thick as to simulate the scale of psoriasis (*see* Photo 3). With continued activity, damage to the epidermis and upper dermis causes central thinning, resulting in the characteristic disklike or "discoid" lesion (*see* Photo 9). In long-standing lesions, the central region evolves into a white depressed or punched-out scar. The margin shows erythema, telangectasia, and hyperpigmentation. Inactive or treated sites often show combined hyper- and hypopigmentation (*see* Photos 5,6).

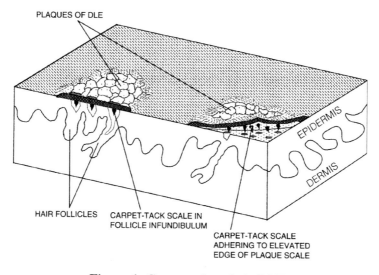

Figure 1: Carpet-tack scale in DLE.

Distribution

Microdistribution: Hair follicles. Follicular accentuation of scale produces the "carpet-tack" sign.

Macrodistribution: Most cases show accentuation on sun-exposed skin. DLE may occur as a butterfly pattern but has a greater tendency to be asymmetric than does SLE (*see* Photo 10). The localized type is limited to the head and neck. The disseminated variant shows extensive lesions over large body areas above and below the neck (*see* Photos 10,11).

Configuration

Discoid or disklike (*see* Photo 9). A late sequela of scarring DLE is the development of squamous cell carcinoma (*see* Photo 12).

Indicated Supporting Diagnostic Data

Localized DLE Without Associated Symptoms

Skin biopsy should be the first step and should be read by a dermatologist or dermatopathologist.

Direct immunofluorescence of lesional skin and nonlesional skin should be considered when routine biopsy is inconclusive. Also known as the "lupus band test," this examination is positive in about 90 to 95% of lesional biopsies of DLE and SLE. The test is generally negative on nonlesional skin in cases of DLE and positive on nonlesional skin in SLE. There can be a 25% false-positive rate on heavily sun-exposed areas, therefore a sun-protected site is recommended for the nonlesional biopsy.

ANA should be done in every case. If negative, it virtually excludes SLE. Exceptions are cases with marked photosensitivity, which may be SCLE or SLE overlap disease. In cases with prominent photosensitivity, obtain Anti-Ro and Anti-La antibodies. Fluorescent ANA titers less than two or three times the standard deviation of normal mean are considered equivocal. Positive titers of 1:160 to 1:320 should raise suspicion of SLE; however, false-positives at these levels are seen in otherwise healthy individuals. False-positives are also seen in pregnancy, older populations, and relatives of patients with connective tissue diseases. A positive ANA alone does not establish a diagnosis of connective tissue disease. When fluorescent ANA patterns are reported, peripheral and homogeneous patterns are highly suggestive of SLE.

Disseminated DLE or Localized DLE With Symptoms Suggesting Systemic Disease

1. Both a skin biopsy and direct immunofluorescence (described above) should be performed.
2. If SLE is strongly suspected, a lupus band test can be done on a biopsy from lesional skin, nonlesional sun-exposed skin and nonlesional sun-protected skin. Fluorescence is positive 90 to 95% of the time in lesional skin, 70 to 80% in nonlesional sun-exposed skin, and 50% in nonlesional sun-protected skin. A positive reaction in a nonlesional, sun-protected site strongly supports a diagnosis of SLE and portends aggressive disease and renal involvement.
3. CBC, multichemistry panel, urinalysis, ESR.
4. Lupus serology screen: ANA is positive in 35% of DLE cases, and is supportive but not specific. It does not distinguish DLE from SLE. Anti-nDNA (dsDNA) anti-

bodies, when positive, indicate SLE. Anti-single-stranded DNA (ssDNA) antibodies are not specific. They may be positive in active DLE, and are seen in several connective tissue diseases including SLE. Anti-Ro (SS-A) antibodies are positive in subacute lupus and other connective tissue syndromes. Anti-La (SS-B) antibodies have a profile similar to the Anti-Ro antibody, but are positive less often. Anti-Sm, when present, is specific for SLE. Anti-ribonucleoprotein (U_1RNP) antibodies support a diagnosis of systemic disease and are often seen in other connective-tissue diseases. Antihistone antibodies are positive in 30% of idiopathic SLE patients, and are positive in 90% of drug-induced SLE cases. When encountered with idiopathic SLE and other ANA antibodies, they are usually positive.

Be aware that these lab tests support or confirm a diagnosis of lupus only in conjunction with the history and physical exam.

4. Therapy

Photoavoidance and Photoprotection

Simple and basic as this may seem, sun avoidance and appropriate sun protection must be taught, emphasized, and reemphasized. Initial patient noncompliance should be expected. Photosensitivity can start at any point in the course of lupus and can trigger severe exacerbations with permanent sequelae of both a cosmetic and a systemic nature. Constant photoprotection is very difficult for active patients, as it means a significant alteration in lifestyle.

1. All lupus patients should avoid midday sun exposure, especially from about 10 AM to 3 PM.
2. When exposed, patients should wear protective clothing and a hat that shades the face and neck.
3. Patients should apply a sunscreen with both UVB and UVA protection with an SPF number of at least 30, containing the ingredient Parsol®.
4. Female patients should always wear makeup over the sunscreen, as the opaque materials in the makeup add protection against wavelengths where sunscreens are less effective. This simple cost-effective therapy is often overlooked.

Topical Therapy

Mild DLE can often be controlled with a combination of solar protection and a topical steroid. The mildest effective preparation is the best, and on facial skin try to use a non-fluorinated preparation whenever possible.

1. Start with a low-potency group VI product such as desonide or aclometasone diproprionate (*see* Chapter 4, Table 1).
2. If one of these steroid preparations is not effective within 1 to 2 weeks, then switch to prednicarbate cream or one of the two potency-enhanced hydrocortisone preparations in group V.
3. If these are ineffective, mometasone furoate cream, a group IV steroid, should be tried next.
4. Finally, if other measures have failed, the use of a potent fluorinated group I product such as clobetasol proprionate is warranted. This must be done very carefully,

and as lesions resolve, the steroid should be stopped or a less potent steroid should be substituted. This approach will be effective only in mild, limited disease, and with proper sun protection. Topical therapy is used as adjunctive treatment in SCLE and SLE but is generally effective only in conjunction with systemic treatment.

Systemic Therapy

This section will be limited to systemic therapy used in the treatment of the cutaneous symptoms. Treatment of the visceral lesions of SLE is complicated, individual, and beyond the scope of this book.

1. **Antimalarials:** One of the most valuable classes of medications in severe cutaneous lupus is the aminoquinolines. At this time, hydroxychloroquine sulfate is the preparation most frequently used. These drugs are very effective in treating skin lesions of severe localized DLE, and are also effective against the cutaneous and arthritic components of disseminated DLE, SCLE, and SLE. They are ineffective against other visceral manifestations, such as renal disease.

   Hydroxychloroquine is usually initiated at a dose of 200 mg BID and is then tapered to a minimum once a complete response is achieved.

   A G-6-PD level should be obtained prior to treatment. Aminoquinolines can cause severe hemolysis in patients who are deficient in this enzyme.

   Periodic monitoring of hematologic and liver indices is indicated. Monitoring of CBC, platelet count, and liver function studies should be carried out at least monthly for the first 3 months, quarterly for the remainder of the first year, then semiannually.

   All the aminoquinolines have been reported to cause severe retinal toxicity with blindness as a sequela. This side effect is related to rate of administration, total dose, and individual susceptibility. A baseline eye examination should be done when therapy is initiated, then repeated every 6 months. This very specific examination must be performed by a fully trained ophthalmologist who is aware of the reason for the examination. These examinations should be repeated immediately if any intercurrent visual symptoms occur.

   Other quinoline compounds have fallen into disfavor due to lack of availability or an unacceptable side-effect profile.

2. **Systemic corticosteroids:** Only on rare occasions are systemic steroids justified for cutaneous symptoms alone. Examples would include short-term initial treatment of extensive pruritic papulosquamous lesions, painful ulcerated lesions, or rapid control of scalp involvement where severe permanent hair loss may occur. In these instances, use of steroids should be decisive and followed by a rapid taper as other systemic agents take over.

3. **Sulfones:** Dapsone can be an effective agent in severe DLE and annular SCLE. Anyone using this drug should be familiar with its potential neurologic, bone marrow, and liver toxicity. Baseline CBC with platelet count and liver function studies should be performed prior to initiating treatment. Repeat these studies twice per month for the first month, monthly for the next 2 months, then semiannually.

   Like the antimalarials, a G-6-PD level should be done prior to therapy.

Coadministration of 400 IU of vitamin E helps to mitigate the mild hemolytic anemia that invariably accompanies the use of dapsone. This can be extremely important to patients with underlying cardiac disease.

Dosing is usually started from 25 to 50 mg daily, and then adjusted. Toxicity increases at dosing above 100 mg/day.

Note that there are rare reports of dapsone causing exacerbations of DLE. If there is any evidence that this is occurring, dapsone should be discontinued immediately.

4. **Alternative systemic agents:** Systemic retinoids, thalidomide, clofazimine, and gold have all been used in the treatment of cutaneous LE. At the present time these treatments should be considered experimental. Some are unavailable in the United States.

Common Skin Conditions That May Simulate DLE, SCLE, and SLE

See section on SLE.

APPLICATION GUIDELINES: SUBACUTE CUTANEOUS LUPUS ERYTHEMATOSUS

Specific History

Onset

SCLE often begins abruptly. Photosensitivity is very prominent and onset may immediately follow an acute sunburn. Patients almost always recall the time of onset because this striking eruption is usually quite distressing. A history of transient past eruptions associated with intense sun exposure can sometimes be obtained. The skin lesions of SCLE are most distressing during periods of activity, although they usually heal with minimal or no scarring. Differentiation of SCLE from true systemic disease may be difficult.

Evolution of Disease Process

The skin lesions spread rapidly and usually cover large areas. Photoaccentuation is a frequent feature; however, involvement of sun-protected skin is usually also present. About two-thirds of cases show extensive papulosquamous lesions (*see* Photos 13,14) that may resemble pityriasis rosea early on and later may resemble psoriasis vulgaris. The eruption is subject to exacerbations and remissions over many years. One-third develop evolving annular lesions (*see* Photo 15) that can simulate annular psoriasis and tinea corporis.

Evolution of Skin Lesions

SCLE lesions are usually numerous and multiply quickly. Patients rarely complain of pruritus or pain. Cosmetic appearance and social acceptance are what usually prompt the patients to seek medical care.

Provoking Factors

Sunlight, heat (elevated ambient temperature), and a large variety of medications have been reported to exacerbate SCLE. Sunlight is by far the most consistent aggravating factor. Among the medications most commonly implicated are terbinafine, griseofulvin, ACE inhibitors, hydrochlorthiazide, calcium-channel blockers, interferons, and the "statins."

Self-Medication

Self-medication is not a problem in SCLE for the same basic reasons as in DLE.

Supplemental Review From General History

Approximately one-half of SCLE cases have additional systemic manifestations and fulfill the criteria for SLE. Arthritis is most common. Fever, fatigue, pleuritis, CNS symptoms, carditis, and cytopenia also occur. Renal disease is noted in up to one-quarter of cases, but is usually mild. A distinct subset of patients with SCLE also have associated Sjögren's syndrome, rheumatoid arthritis, or complement deficiencies. Therefore, a comprehensive review of systems is indicated. SCLE patients require more extensive serologic surveys than do DLE patients.

Dermatologic Physical Exam

Primary Lesions

1. Sharply defined plaques (*see* Photos 13,14,16).
2. Sharply demarcated areas of erythema that can rapidly enlarge and coalesce. Size varies, but lesions are often several centimeters in diameter, and as they mature, secondary changes occur.

Secondary Lesions

1. Loose nonadherent white scale that does not carpet-tack (*see* Photo 14).
2. Telangiectatic (dilated) blood vessels (*see* Photos 14,16).
3. Central gray-white annular hypopigmentation (*see* Photo 16).
4. Epidermal atrophy.

A loose white scale develops in some cases, and the lesions may simulate a papulosquamous disease. There is no follicular accentuation as in DLE, and the "carpet-tack" sign is negative. As the lesions evolve, they exhibit telangiectatic vessels and a dusky color not seen with pityriasis rosea or psoriasis. When the lesions regress they may leave mild epidermal atrophy, telangectasia, and hypopigmentation, but they do not scar. Annular lesions usually enlarge peripherally with a border that has erythema and loose white scale. The central areas show gray-white hypopigmentation. These lesions tend to coalesce to form polycyclic and gyrate patterns (*see* Chapter 2).

Distribution

Microdistribution: None.

Macrodistribution: Extensor surfaces of extremities, face, and lateral trunk are regularly involved. Lesions are rare below the waist. Photoaccentuation is a common feature (*see* Photo 17, Fig. 2).

Configuration

Annular and polycyclic patterns (*see* Photo 15).

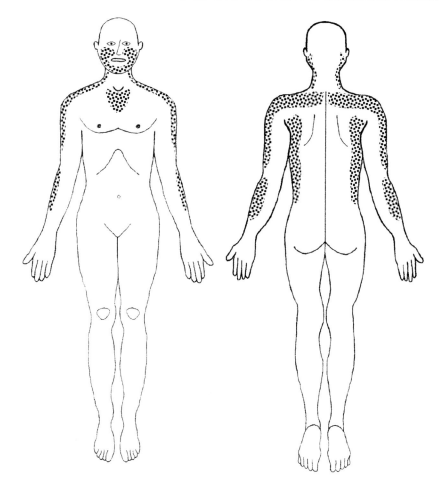

Figure 2: Macrodistribution of SCLE.

Indicated Supporting Diagnostic Data

Skin biopsy is always indicated.

Direct immunofluorescence of involved skin is always indicated.

If associated features suggest SLE, positive direct immunofluorescence of nonlesional sun-protected skin supports a diagnosis of SLE.

CBC, multichemistry panel, urinalysis, ESR, complement screen (specifically C3, C4, and CH50), lupus antibody screen, and rheumatoid factor are always indicated.

Anti-Ro (SS-A) and Anti-La (SS-B) antibodies are always indicated. Thirty percent of SCLE cases are ANA negative, but are often positive for Anti-Ro antibodies.

Therapy

See Therapy in DLE section above.

Common Skin Conditions That May Simulate DLE, SCLE, and SLE

See section on SLE below.

APPLICATION GUIDELINES: SYSTEMIC LUPUS ERYTHEMATOSUS

Specific History

Onset of Cutaneous Manifestations

If a malar rash is present at onset, it usually appears abruptly. Photosensitivity can be present but is not as prominent a feature in SLE as in cutaneous lupus erythematosus. Although skin lesions occur in 80% of SLE patients during the course of their disease, they are a presenting sign in only about 13%. Joint and other visceral symptoms predominate. Cutaneous lesions are nevertheless important because they constitute four of the 11 criteria used by the American Rheumatism Association to establish a diagnosis of SLE. The four defining cutaneous signs that can be present at onset are the following:

1. Fixed malar rash.
2. Photosensitivity.
3. Scarring discoid lesions.
4. Nasal or oropharyngeal ulcerations.

Cutaneous symptoms may occur at any point in the course of SLE. Skin manifestations in SLE are quite variable when compared to other cutaneous forms, and wax and wane with disease activity. The overall breakdown of cutaneous involvement in SLE is as follows:

1. Lesions typical of SLE: 50%.
2. Lesions more typical of SCLE: 15 to 20%.
3. Lesions more typical of DLE: 10 to 15%.
4. No cutaneous involvement: 20%.

Evolution of Disease Process

The course of SLE is so variable that there is no set pattern for the cutaneous lesions. Skin lesions of vascular origin may reflect widespread vascular injury in other organs. Onset or exacerbation of skin lesions in a patient with SLE often signals disease activity and should initiate a reassessment of lab parameters and current therapy.

Evolution of Skin Lesions

There are no consistent history findings characterizing the cutaneous manifestations of SLE.

Provoking Factors

Solar exposure is a common exacerbating factor for SLE and is reported in 30 to 75% of cases. The true incidence appears to be about 60%. A substantial number of patients seem to flare with extrinsic emotional or physical stress. There is a very extensive list of medications that have been reported to trigger SLE, exacerbate established SLE, or cause an SLE-like syndrome. Whenever possible, these should be avoided in patients with any form of LE.

Self-Medication

Self-medication is a problem in SLE mainly if patients indulge in the use of medications not specifically prescribed for them that exacerbate their disease.

Supplemental Review From General History

1. Patients with skin lesions that could be cutaneous manifestations of suspected SLE should have a comprehensive review of systems directed at symptoms of SLE.
2. Patients with established SLE who develop cutaneous manifestations consistent with LE should have a comprehensive re-evaluation of their SLE to determine if an exacerbation is occurring.

Dermatologic Physical Exam

Primary Lesions

1. Sharply defined malar erythema.
2. Sharply defined papules that may coalesce.
3. Widespread indurated erythema of the face, neck, upper chest, shoulders, extensor arms, and back of hands.
4. Urticarial lesions (rare).

Approximately 40% of patients in one large series developed a fixed malar eruption considered by many to be a hallmark of SLE (*see* Photo 18, Fig. 3). The malar eruption begins as a telangiectatic blush or a discrete maculopapular eruption with fine scale in the facial area. Although highly suggestive of SLE, this can occur in DLE, SCLE, and occasionally with dermatomyositis. Also, other common skin conditions such as rosacea, severe seborrhea, and on rare occasions tinea faciale, will simulate this finding. Prominent edema may suggest the facial eruption of dermatomyositis.

Extensive, pruritic, papular eruption of the extensor surfaces of the fingers, hands, and forearms occurs (*see* Photos 19,20).

Secondary Lesions

1. Telangiectatic (dilated) blood vessels (*see* Photo 21).
2. Scarring, necrosis, and gangrene with vascular lesions (*see* Photo 22).
3. SLE with discoid lesions may show all the changes seen in DLE (*see* Photo 23).
4. Sclerosis (rare).
5. Calcinosis (rare).
6. Proximal nail fold capillary changes (*see* Photo 21).
7. Opaque nail bed with ragged cuticles (*see* Photo 21).
8. Dermal vascular occlusion or infarcts may present as chronic ulcers or peripheral gangrene (*see* Photo 22).

Generally, skin involvement in SLE shows fewer tendencies toward scarring. Exceptions are scalp lesions, DLE-like lesions, and ulcerative lesions of vascular origin.

Distribution

Microdistribution: None.

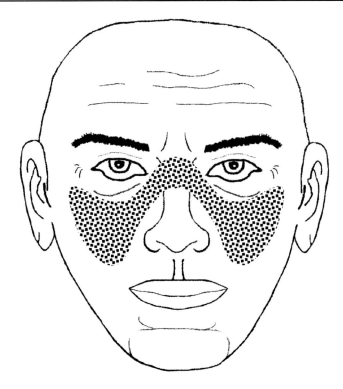

Figure 3: Butterfly rash of SLE.

Macrodistribution:

1. Malar (butterfly) in some cases (*see* Photo 18, Fig. 3).
2. Photoaccentuation in some cases, less pronounced than in other forms of LE.

Configuration

    Discoid in a small number of cases.

Indicated Supporting Diagnostic Data

    Skin biopsy is indicated when it assists in establishing a diagnosis of SLE or is needed to identify the skin lesion as part of an already established diagnosis of SLE. If the patient has established SLE and has cutaneous manifestations characteristic of LE, biopsy is unnecessary.

    Direct immunofluorescence of lesional skin is indicated under the same circumstances as skin biopsy.

    If associated features suggest SLE, and other serologic tests are inconclusive, positive direct immunofluorescence of nonlesional sun-protected skin supports a diagnosis of SLE.

    CBC, multichemistry panel, urinalysis, ESR, complement screen (specifically C3, C4, and CH50), lupus antibody screen, and rheumatoid factor are always indicated.

With active vascular lesions (infarcts and ulcerations) or with CNS involvement, screen for lupus anticoagulant and antiphospholipid antibodies.

Therapy

See Therapy in DLE section above.

Common Skin Conditions That May Simulate DLE, SCLE, and SLE

Seborrhea can simulate DLE, SCLE: Onset of seborrhea is gradual, and tends to wax and wane. Diffuse erythema occurs with very loose white or greasy yellow scale. Atrophy, scarring, telangectasia, and pigment change are absent. "Carpet-tack" sign is negative. The macrodistribution may overlap and cause confusion. No photosensitivity is present.

Rosacea can simulate DLE, SLE: Erythematous telangiectatic rosacea can simulate the facial erythema of early DLE and SLE. Onset is usually gradual with a long history of ease of flushing. Scale is absent, as are atrophy, scarring, and pigment change. The macrodistribution and prominent telangectasia can cause confusion. Dusky papules and pustules help with the differential diagnosis. Photosensitivity is common.

Psoriasis vulgaris can simulate DLE, SCLE: The onset, lesions, and distribution can be strikingly similar to DLE and SCLE. Only a biopsy and serologic tests will distinguish them. Generally, the lesions of LE have a deeper more violaceous hue, and telangectasia is not a feature of psoriasis. Although uncommon, sun sensitivity can occur in psoriasis vulgaris.

Pityriasis rosea (PR) can simulate early SCLE: Early papulosquamous lesions of SCLE can simulate PR. The persistence of SCLE, the telangectasia, and eventually the differences in macrodistribution should separate the two. In addition, PR improves rather than flaring with light therapy.

Tinea faciale can simulate DLE: Early DLE on the facial area can be clinically indistinguishable from tinea. When present, indolent follicular pustules should suggest the diagnosis of tinea faciale. A KOH preparation can prevent an embarrassing mistake.

Annular tinea corporis can simulate SCLE: Annular SCLE can simulate an active inflammatory annular tinea. Telangectasia and dark violaceous color help to distinguish them. A KOH prep is usually definitive.

Parvovirus B-19 can simulate SLE: Parvovirus B-19 infection, a cause of the common childhood exanthem called "fifth" disease, has been reported to exacerbate established SLE and to produce temporary symptoms in some patients that meet the criteria for SLE. Malar rash, arthralgias, fatigue, and low-titer positive ANAs are reported. History of exposure to affected children, or occurrence during epidemics of parvovirus B-19 infection, should lead to suspicion. Symptoms and serologies usually revert to normal within 1 to 3 months in patients who do not have SLE. Parvovirus arthritis may last beyond 3 months. Discoid lesions, alopecia, renal lesions, and cardiac lesions are not reported. Neurologic findings and serositis are uncommon with parvovirus B-19 infection. The anemia seen with the infection is usually associated with low reticulocyte counts, whereas reticulocytes are usually elevated in the hemolytic anemia of SLE. Parvovirus B-19 antibody titers may be helpful.

ANSWERS TO CLINICAL APPLICATION QUESTIONS

History Review

A 35-year-old woman seeks help regarding a progressive skin eruption that began on the ears and facial skin late in the previous summer. The lesions stabilized during the winter months but rapidly progressed with the return of warm, sunny weather. Physical examination reveals a scaling dermatitis with discrete and confluent plaques. Some plaques have a depressed center and scarring. Telangectasia, hypopigmentation, and hyperpigmentation are evident. The rash is asymmetric on the face and ears but is symmetrically distributed over the V of the chest, dorsal arms, and forearms with sharp limitation at the collar and short-sleeve protection line.

1. What is the most likely diagnosis: localized DLE, disseminated DLE, SCLE, or SLE?

Answer: The skin lesions described are most consistent with disseminated DLE. Scarring plaques in a photosensitive distribution above and below the neck are typical. Skin lesions of SCLE are also photodistributed but show little tendency toward scarring and have a tendency to spill over onto areas of sun-protected skin. SLE with disseminated DLE-like skin lesions will have to be ruled in or out.

2. What other findings on physical exam would be helpful in distinguishing one form of lupus from another?

Answer: An examination of the underside of the elevated scale will help to distinguish DLE from SCLE. Both forms of LE have scale but DLE lesions, when elevated, show conical follicular projections, a feature referred to as "carpet-tacking."

Examination of fingernails may help to distinguish disseminated DLE from SLE with discoid skin lesions. The presence of coarse dilated capillary loops on the proximal nail folds supports a diagnosis of SLE.

3. What additional supplemental historical data would help to distinguish one form of lupus from another?

Answer: A comprehensive review of systems should be carried out with special attention to any CNS, cardiovascular, pulmonary, renal, or joint symptoms, or to Raynaud's phenomenon. A positive history in this regard would raise suspicion of SLE with discoid skin lesions or disseminated DLE with a high probability of later conversion to SLE.

4. History reveals an unexplained episode of pleurisy 4 years ago. What supporting laboratory data are indicated?

Answer: This patient clearly has disseminated DLE skin lesions with historical data that raises the possibility of systemic disease. Therefore a full laboratory screen is indicated, including the following:

    a. A lesional skin biopsy.

    b. Direct immunofluorescence of a lesional skin biopsy.

    c. Direct immunofluorescence of a non-sun-exposed nonlesional skin biopsy.

    d. CBC.

    e. Multichemistry panel.

    f. Urinalysis with microscopic exam.

    g. ESR.

    h. A complete lupus serology screen.

5. If laboratory parameters are consistent with a diagnosis of SLE with discoid skin lesions, what are your treatment options?

Answer: DLE-like skin lesions in a patient with SLE may respond to topical steroids; however, this is not practical with widespread activity. Antimalarials and dapsone may be effective for the skin lesions but are not useful against visceral manifestations such as renal disease. Systemic corticosteroids should control both problems.

6. If laboratory parameters are consistent with a diagnosis of disseminated DLE, what are your treatment options?

Answer: Disseminated DLE lesions usually respond well to a regimen of systemic antimalarials or dapsone therapy. Topical steroids can be used to treat resistant focal lesions. Careful photoavoidance and photoprotection are of critical importance.

20 Toxicodendron Dermatitis *(Poison Oak, Poison Ivy, Poison Sumac; Also Known as Rhus Dermatitis)*

INTRODUCTION

Plants of the genus *Toxicodendron* are found throughout East Asia, North America, and South America. Five species common to North America cause more cases of allergic contact dermatitis than all other contact antigens combined. These species are known best by their common designations:

1. Poison ivy (two varieties).
2. Poison oak (two varieties).
3. Poison sumac.

When these plants are bruised or injured, they emit a sap called urushiol, which contains a mixture of highly allergenic, cross-reacting catechols. Contact with this sap in sufficient quantity can induce immune recognition (sensitizing dose), and with subsequent exposure (eliciting dose), a delayed hypersensitivity reaction will occur. Once allergic, an immunologically competent person will continue to react with any threshold reexposure to the offending antigen.

Some portion of the plant must be damaged for exposure to occur. Smoke from wood that contains part of a toxicodendron plant can contain enough antigen to cause severe exposure. The plant resin dries rapidly under fingernails and on skin, clothing, tools, and sporting equipment. It will retain antigenicity indefinitely unless removed. Toxicodendron dermatitis is important not only because of its frequency, but also because it serves as a model for understanding other types of allergic contact dermatitis.

CLINICAL APPLICATION QUESTIONS

A young mother seeks help for an uncooperative 5-year-old with a 7-day history of dermatitis of the right posterior thigh, right buttock, and right foot. Examination reveals patches of secondarily infected (impetiginized) dermatitis. Some areas are urticarial, while others are clearly vesicular. Excoriations are present, and the mother states that the eruption has gradually spread over several days. The vesicular eczematous areas and excoriations lead you to suspect toxicodendron exposure.

1. What additional pertinent history should you obtain?
2. The history reveals that 2 days prior to onset the 5-year-old went fishing with the father down by the river. What physical features of the rash would offer additional support for the diagnosis?

From: *Current Clinical Practice: Dermatology Skills for Primary Care: An Illustrated Guide*
D.J. Trozak, D.J. Tennenhouse, and J.J. Russell © Humana Press, Totowa, NJ

3. What laboratory data are indicated in this case?
4. Should hyposensitization with urushiol extract be considered in this patient?
5. What is the appropriate treatment for this patient?

APPLICATION GUIDELINES

Specific History

Onset

Toxicodendron dermatitis occurs most often in teenagers and young adults after recreational outings, and in young and middle-aged adult patients following both occupational and recreational exposure. Forestry, utility maintenance, timber, landscape, and agricultural workers are among those most frequently affected. The symptoms typically start with erythema and pruritus about 48 hours after the exposure. Exquisitely sensitive victims may react in as little as 6 hours, whereas persons with low levels of sensitization or minimal antigen exposure may take up to a week to react. Different body regions have varied reaction times and some sites may require several days to respond.

When new sites continue to develop late in an episode (7 to 10 days or more), it is necessary to look for continuing exposure from fomites such as contaminated clothing, tools, or sporting equipment.

Evolution of Disease Process

The duration and severity of an individual reaction will be determined by the patient's level of sensitivity, the degree of exposure to the antigen, and the skin areas involved. In average cases, the rash and pruritus worsen for the first week. During this period, new areas of involvement may develop. These are caused by variations in skin reactivity and the uneven distribution of the antigen. Blister fluid from active lesions does not spread the dermatitis. An average episode lasts 14 to 18 days. Without treatment, severe episodes may last as long as 1 month.

Evolution of Skin Lesions

Early lesions consist of pruritic patches of erythema that evolve within a few hours into raised erythematous plaques. Within 12 hours some areas will progress to a coarse orange-peel appearance composed of tiny vesicles. If the reaction is severe, 1- to 5-mm vesicles will follow. As noted above, new areas of dermatitis may occur for at least a week while the initial lesions intensify.

Because of the marked itching, the blisters are usually excoriated and ruptured so that secondary infection is a common complication. The presence or absence of secondary impetiginization should always be assessed when treating any acute contact dermatitis.

Extensive facial or genital involvement may be accompanied by massive local edema that interferes with vision or micturition, respectively. When extensive lesions are present in these locations, prompt systemic therapy should be considered.

As the reaction wanes, the pruritus diminishes, the plaques of erythema regress, the vesicles deflate, then the vesicles dry and desquamate. The duration and intensity can be dramatically altered by early treatment.

Provoking Factors

In addition to the obvious cause, there are several hidden sources for this type of acute contact reaction. Several related plant and plant products contain identical or related cross-reacting antigens. Persons who are sensitive to toxicodendrons will also react to mango rind, lacquer produced from the sap of the lacquer tree (Japanese, Burmese, and black varieties), cashew nut oil (found in the cashew shell), ink produced from the resin of the India marking nut tree, and the fruit of the ginkgo tree.

Self-Medication

Self-treatment with myriad OTC medications for poison oak and poison ivy is common. Many of these proprietary products are themselves potent sensitizers and should not be applied to dermatitic skin. Products that should be avoided in particular are those that contain "caine" anesthetics and diphenhydramine. OTC steroid creams that contain 0.5 to 1.0% hydrocortisone are readily available but are not potent enough to alter the course of this reaction, and the cream base may be irritating enough to contribute to the problem.

Supplemental Review From General History

None.

Dermatologic Physical Exam

Primary Lesions

1. Linear patches of erythema (*see* Photo 24).
2. Linear plaques of erythema (*see* Photo 24).
3. Vesicles, from pinpoint to 5 mm (*see* Photo 25).

Secondary Lesions

1. Excoriations.
2. Crusting (*see* Photo 26).
3. Impetiginization (*see* Photo 26).
4. Scale, late in the course (*see* Photo 26).

Distribution

Microdistribution: None.

Macrodistribution: Exposed skin will be heavily involved, while covered areas are protected or minimally affected. Doubly covered skin areas are spared except in instances where the antigen is transferred from the hand to the anogenital region. The palmar and plantar skin seldom reacts despite heavy exposure. Airborne exposure from burning toxicodendron leaves and stems frequently affects the face and neck (*see* Photo 27).

Configuration

1. Streaks and linear plaques of vesicles on an erythematous plaque are characteristic (*see* Photos 24,25).

2. Large irregular plaques are sometimes present due to spread from contaminated palms to other skin areas. Occasionally, recognizable handprints can be seen.
3. Confluent lesions are common with airborne exposure (*see* Photo 27).

Indicated Supporting Diagnostic Data

Toxicodendron dermatitis is a clinical diagnosis. Laboratory testing is not indicated except in rare instances as mentioned under Conditions That May Simulate Toxicodendron Dermatitis section.

Therapy

Prevention

Avoidance: Practitioners should become familiar with the species of toxicodendron found in their geographic area and instruct patients with handouts and photographs showing the appearance of the plant and the most likely exposure sites. With the exception of poison sumac, the saying "Leaves of three, let them be!" conveys the basic message. An excellent article by Guin et al. (*see* ref. 27) contains superb color photographs and comprehensive information about the characteristics and regional distribution of each major species.

Barriers: Several effective barrier products are available OTC: Ivy Block® (EnviroDerm), Stocko Gard® (Stockhausen Inc.), Hollister Moisture Barrier® (Hollister Inc.), Hydropel® (C&M Pharmacal), Poison Oak-N-Ivy Armor® (Tec Labs) and Tecnu Poison Oak-N-Ivy Armor® (Tec Labs). When applied prior to exposure and according to the package instructions, up to 90% of a reaction can be prevented if exposure occurs.

Removal of the antigen: If exposure to an offending toxicodendron is recognized, immediate washing with mild soap and water may totally prevent the reaction. The antigen penetrates the epidermis rapidly and after 10 minutes some penetration may occur. There is agreement that washing within the first hour of exposure will mitigate the severity of the reaction, and any exposed person should cleanse thoroughly at the first opportunity to limit transfer of the resin to other skin areas. Exposure to this type of contact antigen can occur indirectly from the fur of pets wandering through the brush or from camping equipment that has come in contact with the resin. This may be the surreptitious cause of unexplained or persistent cases. Pets should be shampooed; camping equipment should be washed with detergent.

Hyposensitization: Two extracts of urushiol are commercially available for the purpose of hyposensitization. Successful treatment will result in milder and shorter reactions; however, the results are transient and do not afford complete prevention. This procedure should be undertaken only by a dermatologist or allergist familiar with the process. Because of the limited results, subjects should be carefully chosen and should be fully aware of the limited results and potential side effects.

Topical Therapy

Proprietary lotions: An array of OTC products is available at any pharmacy. These contain different combinations of ingredients that relieve the itching, dry the exudate from the vesicles, and prevent secondary infection. They may, in fact, be modestly effective in mild cases. As noted earlier, several products contain benzocaine and diphenhydramine, which are both highly sensitizing when applied to dermatitic skin. These products are not effective in cases of severe or widespread exposure except for the local drying and antimicrobial effect. A prescription cream containing 5% doxepin HCl is an effective antipruritic, but caution must be taken to avoid systemic side effects and drug interactions.

Topical steroids: Despite some claims to the contrary, topical steroid creams are of considerable value provided they are used appropriately. These products are effective in mild to moderate cases applied to the sites of active dermatitis that are not overtly blistered. In some cases, they are sufficient as monotherapy. In more severe cases, they can be used in conjunction with systemic medication on the areas of acute erythema. Once an area is overtly blistered, these medications cannot penetrate and are ineffective. Potency should be a group IV steroid or stronger.

Antihistamines: An antihistamine may be occasionally useful in an agitated patient with intense itching. In adult patients, 25 to 50 mg hydroxyzine QID or 10 mg doxepin QID can be used. In children, hydroxyzine or cyproheptadine in appropriate dosage for weight or age is recommended.

Systemic steroids: Severe reactions can be incapacitating and result in time lost from work or vacation. If a reaction is progressing rapidly, and especially if there is extensive facial or genital involvement with edema, systemic steroids should be considered. Treatment for adults should start with 30 to 40 mg prednisone STAT dose, then 30 to 40 mg in a single morning dose for the next 14 days. The prednisone can then be rapidly tapered over the ensuing week. This 3-week regimen will usually avoid late flare-ups.

Conditions That May Simulate Toxicodendron Dermatitis

Delayed Contact Allergy to Other Plants

Many other plants, reaction including house plants, trees, and ornamental garden covers, can cause a delayed hypersensitivity. Depending on the plant and mode of contact, the pattern may show streaks of acute vesicular eczema indistinguishable from toxicodendron dermatitis. The source must be sought from the history and confirmed with a patch test.

Phytophotodermatitis

Certain wild plants, some varieties of meadow grass, and some common garden plants contain a photosensitizing furocoumarin in their sap that, if deposited on the skin and exposed to sun or long-wave ultraviolet light, will produce an accelerated sunburn reaction. The pattern is often one of prominent linear streaks. These reactions are usually bullous rather than vesicular, and are accompanied by sting or pain rather than itching. The acute lesions are usually replaced by dark pigmentation, which resolves very slowly.

Other Contact Allergens

When toxicodendron dermatitis shows a patchy rather than linear pattern, it must be distinguished from other causes of delayed hypersensitivity. Careful historical data and indicated patch testing for suspect substances will need to be carried out if the problem persists. Dermatologists are specifically trained in this area.

Herpes Zoster

Peculiar as it may seem, early acute zoster can be very similar to early toxicodendron dermatitis. Both eruptions can show a linear "dermatomal" pattern. Zoster with minimal acute neuritis may be pruritic rather than painful. Early toxicodendron dermatitis may exhibit only modest itching. Both conditions may have an orange-peel surface and similar-sized vesicles (*see* Photo 28). History of recreational exposure helps. Dysesthesia rather than itching, unilateral distribution, and umbilication of the vesicles suggest zoster. Intense pruritus, widespread satellites, and extension over the midline favors toxicodendron dermatitis. When in doubt, a Tzanck smear or rapid immunofluorescence (RIF) test for herpesvirus will help distinguish between them.

Bedbug Bites

The bedbug (*C. lenticularis*) can cause linear, vesicular bite patterns in a sensitized victim. Hemorrhagic puncta from the bite helps to distinguish it from toxicodendron dermatitis.

ANSWERS TO CLINICAL APPLICATION QUESTIONS

History Review

A young mother seeks help for an uncooperative 5-year-old with a 7-day history of dermatitis of the right posterior thigh, right buttock, and right foot. Examination reveals patches of secondarily infected (impetiginized) dermatitis. Some areas are urticarial, while others are clearly vesicular. Excoriations are present, and the mother states that the eruption has gradually spread over several days. The vesicular eczematous areas and excoriations lead you to suspect toxicodendron exposure.

1. **What additional pertinent history should you obtain?**
Answer:
    a. History of prior toxicodendron sensitivity or other history of allergic contact dermatitis.
    b. History of possible toxicodendron exposure especially in the 48-hour period preceding the onset of symptoms.
    c. History of self-treatment that may have modified or worsened the problems.
In the absence of toxicodendron exposure, obtain a history of any other plant exposure, gardening, or exposure to other cross-reacting products such as mango rind.

2. **The history reveals that 2 days prior to onset, the 5-year-old went fishing with the father down by the river. What physical features of the rash would offer additional support for the diagnosis?**
Answer: A configuration with streaks and linear plaques is characteristic of plant-acquired contact allergy. This configuration is particularly typical of toxicodendron dermatitis.

3. **What laboratory data are indicated in this case?**
Answer: In this case no laboratory data are indicated.

4. Should hyposensitization with urushiol extract be considered in this patient?

Answer: No. Urushiol hyposensitization should be reserved for cases of extreme sensitivity or individuals with repeated episodes. Even in these cases, the efficacy of hyposensitization is questionable.

5. What is the appropriate treatment for this patient?

Answer:

    a. Instruct the parent as to how to recognize local toxicodendron species.

    b. Instruct the parent or victim to use an effective barrier product before anticipated exposure.

    c. Instruct the parent or victim regarding prompt antigen removal when exposure does occur.

    d. Give a broad-spectrum antibiotic such as a first-generation cephalosporin if there is significant secondary infection.

    e. Give a group IV topical steroid BID and as needed for itching to the active lesions.

    f. Give a sedating antihistamine at least at bedtime for sleep.

    g. The degree of involvement described here does not warrant the use of systemic steroids.

21 Atopic Dermatitis *(Atopic Eczema, Disseminated Neurodermatitis, Besnier's Prurigo)*

INTRODUCTION

Atopic dermatitis is the cutaneous component of a complex hereditary predisposition that also includes a tendency toward bronchial asthma and immediate type I allergy to a range of environmental antigens manifest by allergic conjunctivitis. The linkage among the three is poorly understood but with careful history taking, 75 to 80% of patients are found to have a positive family history.

Atopic dermatitis is a multifaceted problem and exhibits diverse physiological defects, which continue to lead investigators in many different directions. Among the more prominent features, there is evidence of a functioning, but disordered, immune system that overreacts through humoral mechanisms to common environmental antigens (pollen, danders, foods, house dust), while responses of the delayed or cellular immune system to certain antigens (toxicodendron, candida, tuberculin, and some viruses) are depressed. This defect of immune modulation is clinically manifest by abnormal handling of certain otherwise minor infections. Other features include inherently dry skin, altered vasomotor responses, and disturbed sweating with sweat retention.

It is beyond the scope of this book to discuss the complex interactions in atopic dermatitis, but the practitioner must be aware of their existence, as they can be important in the recognition and treatment of certain cases.

CLINICAL APPLICATION QUESTIONS

A 68-year-old retired bank executive seeks your help regarding a progressively disabling and intensely pruritic rash that has generalized over the past 6 months. Examination reveals a widespread inflammatory dermatitis with excoriations and impetiginization. Heavily involved areas include the face, neck, upper back, scalp, and the dorsum of the hands. The margins of the eruption are indistinct and the neck and flexures are more heavily involved with secondary changes of lichenification. You consider a diagnosis of late-onset atopic dermatitis.

1. What historical information might help to support the diagnosis?
2. Are there any ancillary physical findings that support your diagnosis?
3. What is the most important consideration in the differential diagnosis of late-onset atopic dermatitis?
4. What supporting laboratory data are indicated?
5. Assuming a diagnosis of adult-onset atopic dermatitis, how would you approach treatment?

From: *Current Clinical Practice: Dermatology Skills for Primary Care: An Illustrated Guide*
D.J. Trozak, D.J. Tennenhouse, and J.J. Russell © Humana Press, Totowa, NJ

APPLICATION GUIDELINES

Specific History

Onset

Atopic dermatitis can begin at any age, but onset early in life is the rule. Approximately 10% of infants are affected and 75% of cases begin within the first 6 months. The vast majority of cases are manifest by puberty, and those that begin in middle life or beyond are so unusual that the diagnosis must be carefully established to rule out other entities such as cutaneous T-cell lymphoma.

Evolution of Disease Process

This is a chronic disorder that is subject to exacerbations and remissions. Although there are exceptions, most cases tend to gradually remit with advancing age. The disorder is divided into three clinical phases, and the last two show considerable overlap.

Infantile atopic dermatitis: This usually starts during the second to sixth month on the cheeks and spreads to involve the scalp and then other regions. As the infant begins to crawl, it is common for the lesions to localize to areas of friction on the knees, elbows, and the extensor surfaces of the limbs. The diaper area is almost always spared. Mild cases are often completely controlled with modest amounts of topical medication while more severe cases are subject to periodic flares. Between the second and third years, about half the cases go into remission, while the rest evolve into the childhood phase.

Childhood atopic dermatitis: Some of these cases occur without an antecedent infantile phase. The skin lesions remain intensely pruritic but assume the more characteristic lichenified appearance considered to be the hallmark of the disease. The distribution also changes so that the flexures of the limbs, the neck, and the wrists and ankles are prominently involved.

Adult atopic dermatitis: Prominent involvement of the face, neck, upper chest, flexures, and hands occurs with lesions that are similar to those of the childhood type. Typically the disease becomes more localized during adulthood, so that only very focal lesions may remain active. Local atopic dermatitis may develop in an adult for the first time or the disorder may recur in this form following years of remission after infancy.

Sites of local predilection include the scalp, hands, vermilion of the lips and immediate perioral skin, upper and lower lids, nipples and areolae, and the vulva. These limited sites will remain active for years, but are responsive to topical therapy. With treatment, long-term or permanent remission is not unusual. Photosensitivity occurs in a small number of adult atopics, but is not encountered in the infantile or childhood phases.

Complications include the following:

1. Kaposi's varicelliform eruption. Originally two variants were described.
    *   Eczema vaccinatum has not been seen since the discontinuation of smallpox vaccinations. This dread complication may return again unless a safer killed vaccine is developed for prevention of terrorist attacks.
    *   Eczema herpeticum is a generalized cutaneous infection with herpes simplex virus often accompanied by high fever and systemic toxicity. Deaths have

occurred in the past when there was no effective treatment. Papulovesicular lesions are widely superimposed upon the eczema, which promptly worsens. A Tzanck smear or RIF test for herpesvirus should rapidly confirm the diagnosis so that systemic antiviral therapy for herpes can be initiated. There is at present no proven antiviral agent for vaccinia virus.

2. Anterior and posterior subcapsular cataracts have been reported. These were documented prior to the advent of corticosteroid therapy. Symptomatic lesions are uncommon.

Evolution of Skin Lesions

The lesions of the infantile phase are less defined than those seen later on. Poorly demarcated erythema develops with intensely pruritic papules and papulovesicles. The itching is so intense that the papular lesions are rapidly excoriated and are seldom seen intact. Usually the surface is moist and exudative from excoriations when the infant first presents. Scalp involvement in infants presents with diffuse, loose white scale over a base of erythema.

As the infant enters the childhood and adult phases, the involved areas become drier and lichenified with the skin markings characteristically accentuated. Excoriated papules, however, are often still evident. In general, lesional sites become more focal but margins of lesions remain indistinct.

Special sites of involvement include the following:

Lips. Vermilion and perioral eczema with persistent lip licking is almost always a manifestation of atopy. An acute contact allergy must be considered, and appropriate history should be taken regarding cosmetics (lipsticks, pomades, etc.) and foods (mango, cashews, etc.). In the atopic patient, wrinkling and lichenification are prominent features, while true contact reactions, in the authors' experience, are more acute and vesicular (*see* Photo 29).

Hands: Chronic dermatitis on the dorsum of the hands and digits is common in adult atopics. The palms are seldom involved. Rings and small plaques of intensely itching vesicles occur, which become tender and exudative once they are excoriated. Fissures over the extensor surface of the fingers are common and painful (*see* Photo 30).

Nails: Swelling and erythema with pruritus affects the proximal nail folds. The cuticles may be disrupted and an acute bacterial or chronic monilia paronychia may then develop. Swelling in the proximal nail fold causes cyclical rippling of the nail plate, and disease activity in the nail matrix produces irregular coarse pitting (*see* Photos 30,31).

Finger pads and soles: This variation is seen most often in preschool and school-aged children and may be the lone manifestation. The distal fingerpads acquire a burnished red appearance and the fingerprint markings are diminished or disrupted. The affected pads can be indented with light pressure and will temporarily retain the impression ("ping-pong ball sign"). Symptoms are minimal and usually consist of tenderness and sensitivity. On the distal soles and toe pads, similar changes occur and are often accompanied by itching and superficial scaling which simulates a tinea pedis. Unlike tinea pedis, however, the toe creases are usually spared. KOH prep is negative.

Scalp: Isolated scalp involvement without other activity is common. Changes consist of prominent loose, fine, white scale that covers a base of dusky-pink erythema. Excoriations and moist open areas are the rule, often with secondary impetiginization (*see* Photo 32).

Classic atopic dermatitis is relatively easy to diagnose. In more challenging cases, there are several ancillary physical findings that support the diagnosis. These include the following:

Allergic shiners: Prominent hyperpigmentation of the lower eyelid, which imparts a fatigued look (*see* Photo 33).

Morgan-Dennie lines: Prominent epicanthic line of the lower lid present at birth, most evident during childhood (*see* Photo 34).

Pityriasis alba: Diminutive patches of scaling erythema seen on the face and upper body that resolve to leave areas of temporary hypopigmentation (*see* Photos 35,36).

Atopic palms: Accentuated palmar markings that impart an aged appearance (*see* Photo 37).

Delayed white dermographism: This is common in patients with very active disease. Firm stroking of an area of erythema produces a delayed prolonged white blanching (*see* Photo 38).

Ichthyosis: Mild to moderate changes similar to ichthyosis vulgaris are seen in about 50% of cases (*see* Photo 39).

Keratosis pilaris: Spiny perifollicular papules on the posterior arms and outer thighs impart a dull, dry appearance to the affected skin (*see* Photo 40).

Buffed nails: from rubbing and scratching (*see* Photo 41).

Provoking Factors

Low humidity, airborne allergens deposited on excoriated skin, defatting chemicals such as solvents, emotional stress, environmental antigens (house dust, animal danders, dust mite antigens, skin bacterial, and yeast flora), and food allergens have all been reported to provoke atopic dermatitis.

Self-Medication

Atopic dermatitis shows little response to OTC medications. Self-treatment is seldom a problem.

Supplemental Review From General History

Seventy-five to 80% of atopics have a positive family history of other blood relatives with asthma, hay fever, or eczema. Many patients with adult-onset atopic dermatitis can recall infantile or childhood eczema that went into remission. A lifelong history of dry, irritable, sensitive skin also supports the diagnosis.

Dermatologic Physical Exam

Primary Lesions

1. Patches of poorly marginated erythema with scattered papules and papulovesicles. This is the infantile phase (*see* Photo 42).
2. Patches of poorly marginated lichenified skin with papules and excoriations. This is the childhood and adult phase (*see* Photo 43).
3. Intraepidermal vesicles often in groups or small rings in dorsal hand lesions.
4. Generalized erythema (rare). This is the erythrodermic phase.

Secondary Lesions

1. Lichenification (*see* Photos 29–32,43).
2. Excoriations; prominent in all phases (*see* Photos 30–32).
3. Fissures; common with dorsal hand involvement (*see* Photos 30,31).
4. Crusting from excoriation and secondary infection (*see* Photos 30,31).
5. White loose scale; very common with scalp lesions (*see* Photo 32).

Distribution

Microdistribution: None.

Macrodistribution:
1. Infantile—Facial area, cheeks, then the scalp may become generalized (*see* Fig. 4).
2. Childhood—Flexures of the limbs, neck, wrists, and ankles (*see* Fig. 5).
3. Adult—Face, neck, upper torso, flexures, and the dorsum of the hands (*see* Fig. 6).

Configuration

None.

Indicated Supporting Diagnostic Data

Laboratory data are not routinely required for the diagnosis of atopic dermatitis.

Biopsy may be needed on rare occasions when atypical onset or clinical features suggest another diagnosis.

Bacterial cultures may be needed when there is evidence of resistant secondary infection.

Viral cultures are appropriate in suspect eczema herpeticum.

Therapy

Support and Explanation

The chronic and cyclical character of this condition requires a careful explanation and support from the treating practitioner. A majority of patients and/or parents can deal with continuing care if they are given a sympathetic insight into what is required and a modicum of hope that the situation is not hopeless and can be improved. Few things are more frustrating to patients with chronic skin disorders than to experience relapse simply because no one told them that the disorder needed ongoing care. Frequently, after an explanation to a discouraged patient, the patient says, "Why didn't someone tell me? Now I can deal with it!"

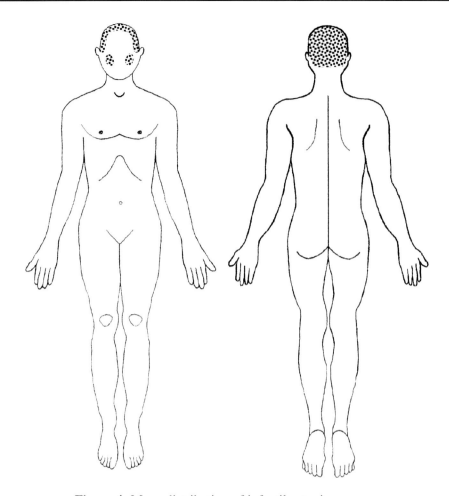

Figure 4: Macrodistribution of infantile atopic eczema.

Environmental Allergen Management

Intradermal skin tests and RAST tests in atopic dermatitis patients are mainly of negative predictive value; hyposensitization or antigen exclusion therapy based on panels of positive tests has limited value in managing the disease. This is in contradistinction to the benefits that may be seen in the treatment of allergic conjunctivitis and extrinsic asthma. A rational approach is the elimination of antigens that clearly and repeatedly cause clinical flares. Also, patients must be made aware of those things that would be best kept out of the environment. For example, they should not acquire house pets, such as cats, that may shed dander. It is important, however, especially with introspective parents, to temper their zeal so they may retain for the child surroundings that are as normal as possible.

In regard to foods, advise parents to restrict any foodstuffs that repeatedly trigger an exacerbation. Periodically review this situation to be sure that adequate nutritional balance is maintained. Food allergy appears to play a role in about 25 to 30% of a selected group

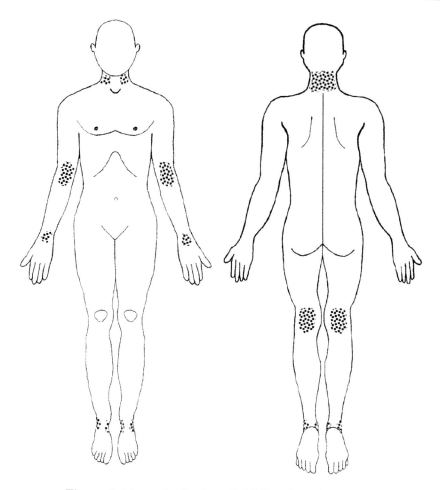

Figure 5: Macrodistribution of childhood atopic eczema.

of refractory, severe atopic dermatitis cases. The actual incidence of significant food allergy in all atopic dermatitis appears to be less than 20% and is uncommon in patients with mild or moderate disease. Food-associated flares of dermatitis typically consist of an immediate and late phase reaction and are reproducible with repeated ingestion. The immediate flare consists of a pruritic morbilliform eruption with an onset 30 minutes to 2 hours after ingestion, and lasts for 30 minutes to 2 hours. The late phase response starts 6 to 8 hours later and is more edematous and prolonged, lasting several hours. GI symptoms (nausea, cramping, vomiting, diarrhea) and respiratory symptoms (stridor, wheezing, rhinorrhea, sneezing) may occur simultaneously. Management of cases where there is a strong suspicion of food allergy should be coordinated with an allergist familiar with the technique of placebo-controlled food challenge and the negative predictive value of intradermal skin and RAST testing.

Airborne allergens such as pollens can occasionally cause acute exacerbations when they are deposited on excoriated open skin. This causes the equivalent of a positive

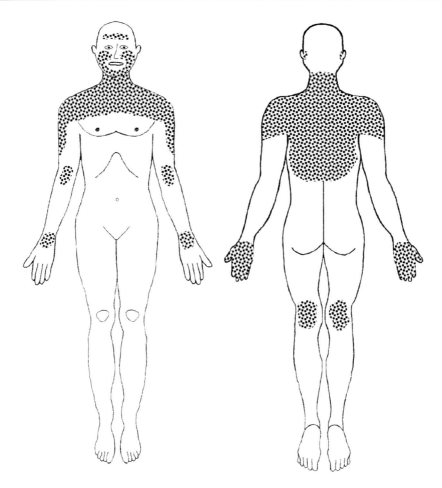

Figure 6: Macrodistribution of atopic eczema in adults.

immediate-type intradermal skin test and the onset can be very abrupt and severe. Patients with history of this type of flare should avoid exposure whenever possible, or at the very least wear protective garments. Dust-mite antigens and house dust have been implicated in some cases. Careful dust control should be encouraged, and if there is a specific history of flaring with dust exposure, specific measures such as mattress covers, hardwood floors, and the like may be indicated. A recent study demonstrates the efficacy of Goretex® mattress and pillow covers in dust control. The simple act of daily vacuuming of carpets, and quarterly spraying them with water (50 mL/m^2), markedly reduced carpet dust and the concentration of house-dust mite antigen. Atopic dermatitis patients showed a substantial improvement overall during the 6-month trial. Occasional patients react strongly to cat and dog danders. It is important to discuss this subject, as patients may not be aware of the relationship. We would not recommend orphaning a beloved pet unless there is unquestioned evidence of a reaction.

Elimination of Irritants

"Picky" or rough fabrics such as wool, sandal straps, and garments that abrade the skin can trigger nonspecific local flares. Clothing should consist of soft fabrics, such as cottons, and irritating clothing or accessories should be eliminated.

Fabric softeners added to the clothing during drying seem to irritate many atopics. We have a number of patients who have achieved much better control simply by eliminating these dryer products. Fabric softeners added to the wash cycle do not seem to be a problem.

Topical Therapy

Cleansing and general measures: Cleansing has been a controversial issue in the treatment of this disease. Many practitioners markedly restrict general bathing because it can deplete the water-holding capacity of the epidermis. While excessive dryness is a major provoking factor, so is secondary bacterial infection. We have found that these patients are immensely more comfortable and very appreciative if they are allowed to bathe daily. Advise them that they should shower rather than tub-bathe. The shower should be warm but not hot, and sufficient to cleanse but no longer than that. Cleansing should be done with a neutral pH (nonalkaline) beauty bar, superfatted soap, or lipid-free cleanser (Cetaphil Cleansing Lotion®). Immediately after the shower, they should pat dry, and before the epidermis really dries out, apply their medication to the active dermatitis, followed immediately by a general coating of the chosen emollient. This regimen allows the shower to work to their advantage.

For small children, a brief tub bath can be substituted. Bubble bath salts are irritating and should be avoided.

Fingernails should be trimmed on a regular basis to minimze excoriations and secondary infection.

Emollients: The role of emollients in the treatment and maintenance of atopic dermatitis patients cannot be overemphasized. Proper use of these hydrating agents will maintain comfort, improve appearance, control itching, and reduce the overall need for topical steroids. The emollient must have enough occlusive base to help the skin surface retain water content. At the same time, they must be cosmetically acceptable. Two products we prefer for general use in atopics are Original Formula Eucerin Cream® and Cetaphil Moisturizing Cream®. Both are also available in lotion form. Initially, patients should start on the more lubricating cream. Later when hydrated, lighter lotions can be introduced for daytime use. These should be applied in a general fashion and over any topical steroids after the shower and once or twice more during the day.

Topical antibiotics: Treatment of secondary infection is often crucial. Emollients and topical steroid therapy are ineffective if significant secondary infection is present. For focal impetiginized areas, topical 2% mupirocin ointment is effective and may reduce the need for prolonged systemic treatment. If however there are widespread open and weeping lesions, a systemic antimicrobial is more efficacious and cost-effective.

Topical steroids: Topical corticoids have become a mainstay of treatment for atopic dermatitis. They reverse inflammation, reduce pruritus, limit rubbing and scratching, and provide comfort that is not afforded by any other modality. Despite extensive use and occasional abuse, they have an unparalleled safety record. Nevertheless, caution must be exercised when treating an extensive area. Hypothalamic–pituitary axis suppression can occur, especially in children.

In the infantile cases, 1 or 2% hydrocortisone in a base of Original Formula Eucerin Cream may be used. Because infants are more susceptible to percutaneous absorption, always use the weakest steroid that is effective. The base is important, and this preparation allows the parent to apply the medication and emollient simultaneously. Emphasize to the parent that the steroid cream should be respected and not used simply as a lubricant. As areas of skin clear, then plain Eucerin is substituted for the steroid. For small resistant lesions, limited use of prednicarbate or 0.1% mometasone furoate cream is acceptable.

Childhood and adolescent disease responds to a similar regimen. However, for those patients we usually use a group IV corticosteroid cream (*see* Chapter 4, Table 1) as the main active agent. Pubescent teens are more susceptible to topical steroid complications such as striae distensae. Prednicarbate cream 0.1% or mometasone furoate cream 0.1% may be safer. Emollients are used as in the infantile cases and act in a similar fashion.

Most adult cases can be treated with a group IV preparation in an identical fashion to childhood cases. If limited areas of thick resistant eczema are present, short-term use of more potent preparations is acceptable.

Scalp involvement is best treated with a steroid lotion in a propylene glycol or foam base.

Finger fissures and paronychial lesions respond to applications of flurandrenolide tape applied over the lesions at bedtime followed by morning applications of a group I to III steroid cream with an emollient.

Topical macrolactams: Topical macrolactams are a new class of topical agents approved for the treatment of atopic dermatitis. Two products are currently available: 0.1 and 0.03% tacrolimus ointment, and 1% pimecrolimus cream. Both act by inhibiting the action of calcineurin, thus blocking the release of proinflammatory cytokines from thymic lymphocytes. Pimecrolimus also blocks the release of mediators from skin mast cells and basophils. Comparative studies have shown effectiveness in moderate to severe atopic dermatitis to be somewhat less effective than that of betamethasone-17-valerate cream (a group V corticosteroid). Both macrolactams have systemic toxicity. Toxicity, however, has not been problem with current topical formulations of tacrolimus. Pimecrolimus is so minimally absorbed that blood levels cannot be detected. These agents appear to be free of the side effects of cutaneous atrophy, telangectasia, and stria formation seen with topical corticosteroids. Furthermore, the current formulations used appropriately have not been associated with hypothalamic–pituitary–adrenal (HPA) axis suppression or any systemic suppression of the immune system. The main side effect of both products has been application site stinging, burning, and irritation, which does not appear to be vehicle-related. Neither agent has current approval for use in children under 2 years of age.

Based on their modest potency and irritant side effects, the macrolactams appear to be most valuable when used in conjunction with, rather than as replacements for, topical corticoids. They are too irritating for use on acute, open areas of eczema, but are valuable substitutes once the acute phase is controlled. A large study of children with atopic dermatitis where ad lib use of pimecrolimus cream was allowed once their disease was controlled showed a dramatic reduction in disease flares and virtually no ongoing topical steroid usage. The utility of these current agents appears to be as adjuvants to topical corticoids in the acute phase of the dermatitis, and once control is achieved, prevention of flares.

Finally, a word of caution: The macrolactams are being marketed aggressively as the safe alternative to topical steroids. Considering their extensive use and abuse, topical steroids have been uniquely safe medications. It took about 20 years of experience before we were aware of most steroid side effects. The macrolactams have had only limited use and testing and there may be adverse effects that have yet to surface. In addition, studies in lower animals have raised a theoretical concern regarding carcinogenicity, which will be resolved in humans only with use over time.

Systemic Therapy

Antihistamines: H_1-blocking agents have been widely used in the past to treat atopic dermatitis. Their effect is mainly to provide sedation and allow the patient to rest rather than having any direct therapeutic effect on the disease process. For these reasons, prescribe them primarily at bedtime. In adults, 25 to 50 mg hydroxyzine, 10 mg doxepin, 25 to 50 mg diphenhydramine, or 12.5 to 25 mg promethazine 30 minutes before retiring are usually quite effective.

In children, hydroxyzine, diphenhydramine, or cyproheptadine in appropriately adjusted doses are used in a similar fashion. Be aware, however, that children can occasionally have paradoxical reactions and become agitated rather than sedated.

Systemic antibiotics: Superficial secondary infection is common in atopic dermatitis because of the chronic excoriation, and once established, it will spread and drive the dermatitis. The normal responsiveness of the rash to topical medication may remain blunted until the secondary infection is controlled. The organisms involved are usually staphylococci of low pathogenicity. Short, 7- to 10-day courses of 250 mg oral erythromycin BID or a first-generation cephalosporin are usually effective. When there is no apparent response, obtain bacterial culture and sensitivities.

Systemic steroids: Systemic steroid use is a sign of defeat in the management of this disease. Systemic steroids offer only temporary improvement, which may be followed by a significant rebound. In addition, they discourage patient compliance with more time-consuming, but safer, topical regimens. An atopic dermatitis patient who cannot be handled with topical treatment should be promptly referred to a dermatologic consultant. Resist the temptation to place such patients on oral or repository steroids. It can place a colleague in a very difficult situation.

Conditions That May Simulate Atopic Dermatitis

Seborrheic Dermatitis of Infancy

This eruption is partially eczematous and partially papulosquamous. Onset and distribution are similar to those for infantile atopic dermatitis. Differentiation is particularly difficult when the eczema component is predominant. Both conditions may exhibit heavy scale. While the scale of seborrhea is yellow and greasy, that of atopy is white and dry. The distinction is not always easy to make. Seborrhea lesions tend to have sharp margins, while those of atopic dermatitis are indistinct. In addition, involvement of the facial creases, crural folds, and diaper area favors seborrhea.

Scabies

Infantile or childhood atopic dermatitis with widespread papular morphology and excoriations is very similar in appearance to the papules and vesicular lesions of advanced scabies. In addition, the two diseases may coexist. It is fairly common for an atopic patient to acutely deteriorate during a concomitant scabies and/or bacterial infection. The practitioner must maintain a high index of suspicion. Family and contact history are helpful, and a scraping for ectoparasites should be obtained from several sites if there is any question.

Nonbullous Impetigo

Widespread nonbullous impetigo with excoriations can enter into this differential diagnosis. Crusting is more extensive and the lesions are usually more circumscribed with a minor degree of erythema.

Nummular Eczema

Lesions of nummular or discoid eczema are usually more discrete, coin-shaped, and have a moist exudative surface. Intervening skin areas are usually normal and the general dryness and other supporting signs of atopy are absent.

Lichen Simplex Chronicus (LSC)

This condition is also known as localized neurodermatitis, and because of the striking clinical similarity to atopic dermatitis, a linkage was postulated. Lesions of LSC are marked by intense pruritus and prominent lichenification. Unlike lesions of atopic dermatitis, they tend to be solitary or symmetrical. In addition, there are specific sites of predilection, which include the nuchal area, mid-shins, ankles, scalp, vulva, and posterior scrotum. A relationship to family or job-related stress is common.

Contact Dermatitis

Delayed contact dermatitis enters into the differential diagnosis of atopic dermatitis, and the two may coexist. An airborne contact allergy can simulate photosensitive atopic dermatitis. Shoe material allergy can simulate atopic dermatitis localized to that site. Both allergic and irritant contact reactions can simulate adult atopic hand dermatitis. Differentiation requires a high index of suspicion, careful history taking, and delayed patch testing when appropriate.

Tinea Corporis

Again the two diseases may coexist. With concomitant tinea, the course of the eczema usually deteriorates. In addition, the fungal infection is driven by the application of topical steroids. Unexplained deterioration of an atopic patient, especially with annular lesions or focal follicular pustules, should raise this question. KOH exam should be done from several sites.

Cutaneous T-Cell Lymphoma

This condition, also known as mycosis fungoides, can be very difficult to distinguish in its early stages from adult-onset atopic dermatitis. Unfortunately, even biopsy at times is not helpful. Nevertheless, any atypical features such as induration, areas of poikiloderma, sharp margins with islands of spared normal skin, or persistent adenopathy should prompt a skin biopsy.

Other Conditions

The following diseases are associated with a skin eruption that resembles atopic dermatitis:

1. Sex-linked agammaglobulinemia.
2. Selective IgA deficiency.
3. Anhidrotic ectodermal dysplasia.
4. Ataxia telangectasia.
5. Celiac disease.
6. Heterozygous cystic fibrosis.
7. Hurler's syndrome.
8. Jung's disease.
9. Nephrotic syndrome.
10. Netherton's syndrome.
11. Phenylkeytonuria.
12. Wiskott-Aldrich syndrome.
13. HTLV type-1 associated infective dermatitis.

ANSWERS TO CLINICAL APPLICATION QUESTIONS

History Review

A 68-year-old retired bank executive seeks your help regarding a progressively disabling and intensely pruritic rash that has generalized over the past 6 months. Examination reveals a widespread inflammatory dermatitis with excoriations and impetiginization. Heavily involved areas include the face, neck, upper back, scalp, and the dorsum of the hands. The margins of the eruption are indistinct and the neck and flexures are more heavily involved with secondary changes of lichenification. You consider a diagnosis of late-onset atopic dermatitis.

1. **What historical information might help to support the diagnosis?**

Answer:
   a. Family history of other blood relatives with asthma, hay fever (seasonal conjunctivitis), or chronic eczema.
   b. Personal history of asthma, hay fever, or infantile/childhood eczema that went into remission.
   c. Personal history of dry, irritable, sensitive skin.

2. **Are there any ancillary physical findings that support your diagnosis?**

Answer: The following physical findings support a diagnosis of atopic dermatitis. Starred items are most helpful in adult cases.
   * a. Allergic shiners.
   b. Morgan-Dennie lines.
   * c. Pityriasis alba.

  * d. Atopic palms.
     e. Delayed white dermographism.
  * f. Ichthyosis.
  * g. Keratosis pilaris.
     h. Buffed nails.

3. What is the most important consideration in the differential diagnosis of late-onset atopic dermatitis?

Answer: Cutaneous T-cell lymphoma (mycosis fungoides).

4. What supporting laboratory data are indicated?

Answer: In most instances, atopic dermatitis is a clinical diagnosis and no laboratory data are required. If there are atypical features, especially in an adult case with a negative family and personal history of atopic disease, a skin biopsy is indicated. Cultures may be of value in cases with resistant secondary bacterial infection or where viral infection is suspected.

5. Assuming a diagnosis of adult-onset atopic dermatitis, how would you approach treatment?

Answer:

All eczema patients show better compliance with an explanation of their disease and positive support. Review bathing practices, local irritants, and environmental factors.

In this case, there is clinical evidence of secondary bacterial infection. A 7- to 10-day course of low-dose antimicrobial therapy is indicated. Erythromycin or cephalexin at 250 mg BID are usually effective.

Regular applications of a medium-potency group IV topical steroid to the active lesions and general application of an emollient cream over the steroid and to any areas of dry skin are recommended.

22 Asteatotic Eczema *(Xerosis, Xerotic Eczema, Eczema Craquelé, Eczema Cannalé, Eczema Hiemalis, Winter Itch)*

INTRODUCTION

This common dermatitis is often misdiagnosed and usually overtreated. Familiarity with the physical findings will allow an accurate assessment of the underlying cause, and symptoms can usually be corrected with simple measures. The condition occurs for a number of reasons, especially the following:

1. With age, skin sebum secretion diminishes, as does the water-holding capacity of the epidermis. These changes are particularly marked on the lower extremities.
2. Bathing further depletes the epidermis of its water-retaining constituents.
3. Climate has a major effect, and most patients experience symptoms for the first time during a winter season as their skin dries from exposure to the low indoor humidity produced as buildings are heated against inclement weather. Incidence will vary from place to place, depending on the severity of the season and the overall regional weather.

CLINICAL APPLICATION QUESTIONS

In the early spring, a 75-five-year-old woman visits your office with a complaint of generalized itching. The symptoms began in late December on local skin areas, and have progressed throughout the winter. You suspect an asteatotic eczema.

1. What information from her history may help support your suspicions?
2. What are the primary lesions in areas of asteatotic eczema?
3. What are the secondary lesions seen in asteatotic eczema?
4. What typical configurations strongly support your suspicions?
5. This woman has minimal physical findings, and some provoking factors are evident in her history, but she fails to improve with treatment. What should be done next?

APPLICATION GUIDELINES

Specific History

Onset

Symptoms usually are noted in the fifth and sixth decades of life for the first time. The incidence and severity of symptoms gradually increase with advancing age. Persons with

From: *Current Clinical Practice: Dermatology Skills for Primary Care: An Illustrated Guide*
D.J. Trozak, D.J. Tennenhouse, and J.J. Russell © Humana Press, Totowa, NJ

inherently dry skin will experience problems at a younger age and earlier in a given season than those without this constitutional predisposition. The first victims usually present about midwinter, and new cases will continue to present until the spring weather pattern is established and indoor heating is curtailed. Onset can be quite abrupt in elderly patients during hospital stays. Hospitals are often kept uncomfortably warm, and because of the large central heating plant, have a low ambient humidity.

Early symptoms consist of intense itching of the extremities and axillary folds, and patients will often remark that their skin feels dry. A generalized gray or white powdery sheen is evident, and the skin surface has a dull, lifeless appearance. The itching from dry skin can be as severe as that from the worst drug reaction.

Evolution of Disease Process

If the early signs and symptoms of asteatosis are not recognized, the symptoms will generalize and the patient will complain of discomfort that may seem to exceed the physical findings. These symptoms are often mistaken for hypersensitivity reactions leading to the discontinuation of important medications.

Evolution of Skin Lesions

Without treatment, the condition of the epidermis will deteriorate from a dry sheen to a stage where it can no longer maintain its surface integrity. At this point, plates of epidermal cells lift up, producing a coarse white scale. Later fissures develop into a canal-like (cannalé) or crazy-paving (craquelé) pattern. These changes most often start as discrete patches on the lower extremities, but with time or in severe cases, may be generalized. Persistent fissures will become inflamed and erythematous, or even frankly eczematous, with changes of edema and serous exudate. Scratching may introduce an element of superficial secondary infection (impetiginization), which further excites the inflammatory reaction and promotes spread of the lesions.

Provoking Factors

1. Constitutionally dry skin.
2. Arid climate conditions.
3. Long inclement spells of wet or cold weather, which increase indoor heating demands.
4. Heating systems that deplete indoor humidity (fireplaces, wood stoves, and gas logs).
5. Excessive bathing.
6. Malnutrition (rare).
7. Medications including allopurinol, cimetidine, dixyrazine, lithium, nicotinic acid, clofibrate, and other cholesterol-lowering agents.

Self-Medication

Self-treatment can be a significant problem. Many patients will use OTC itch creams that contain highly sensitizing substances such as benzocaine or diphenhydramine. This can lead to a superimposed allergic contact dermatitis. It is sometimes difficult to convince patients that their severe pruritus is due simply to dry skin. Find out what they are using and take control of the situation. Some OTC hydrocortisone creams, for instance, have cream bases that are more irritating than the anti-inflammatory effect of the active ingredient, and would contribute to rather than resolve this problem.

Supplemental Review From General History

If changes and symptoms of asteatosis respond promptly to treatment, no additional investigation is indicated. Generalized pruritus without changes of asteatosis, and acquired ichthyosis can be signs of underlying systemic disease. If either are present without signs of asteatosis, or if an asteatotic patient continues to have severe pruritus once the dryness is corrected, then a complete history and general physical examination should be done along with a basic CBC, chemistry panel, and a thyroid function panel. Further investigation should be based on findings from that examination.

Dermatologic Physical Exam

Primary Lesions

1. Patches of skin that appear dull, fissured, scaly, erythematous, or impetiginized (*see* Photos 44,45).
2. Intervening skin that shows an accentuated dull crisscross pattern of skin markings (*see* Photo 44).

Secondary Lesions

1. Fine white scale (early).
2. Coarse white scale (later).
3. Fissures may be dry or exudative and eczematous. Color of the fissures varies from pink to a deep dusky red. They may contain small amounts of hemorrhage or exudate. The fissures often produce a canal-like (*see* Photo 46) or crazy-pavement (*see* Photo 47) pattern. This craquelé pattern has also been described as resembling the surface fractures on an old piece of Chinese pottery.
4. Impetiginization.

Distribution

Microdistribution: None.

Macrodistribution: The lower extremities, thighs, and hips are the most common sites. Axillary folds and proximal arms are next. Distribution may be generalized in severe cases (*see* Fig. 7).

Configuration

The canal-like and crazy-paving patterns are virtually diagnostic (*see* Photos 46,47).

Indicated Supporting Diagnostic Data

None.

Therapy

Prevention

Unless you explain to the patient and relatives the underlying etiology of the disorder, the problem will recur. Bathing habits should be reviewed; the patient should be using a

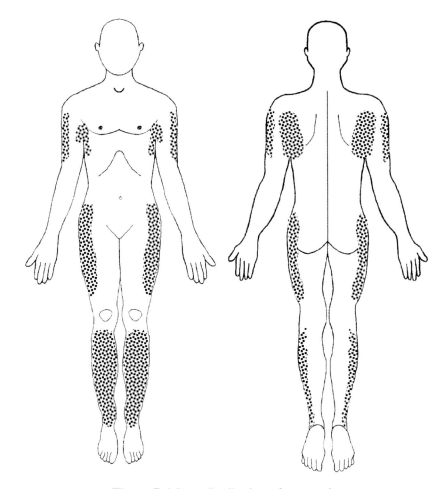

Figure 7: Macrodistribution of asteatosis.

mild bath bar with moisturizing ingredients. Showers are less drying than tub bathing. Spas and hot tubs should be discouraged. Emollients and medications must be applied immediately after toweling before the skin really dries if they are to be maximally effective. Explain the effect of dry heating sources, and encourage the use of a humidifier. Cold-water vaporizers are an inexpensive means of raising humidity, and they are portable and safe. A central humidifier attached to the furnace is ideal, but is a substantial expense. Small room humidifiers work well, but again they are expensive and have ongoing upkeep costs.

Topical Steroids

Corticoids will suppress inflammation but will not correct the underlying dryness. They should be reserved strictly for the inflamed or frankly eczematous lesions. You may use group VI or VII steroid creams for this purpose, and try to choose those with an emollient base. These products have enough potency to correct the inflammatory changes, and virtually no risk of secondary atrophy. They should be applied to the inflammatory lesions only, and should be followed immediately with a general application of moisturizer.

Moisturizers

Lubricants are the real therapeutic mainstay for correcting dry skin. Two factors must be considered when recommending a lubricant: (1) it must correct the dryness, and (2) it must have enough patient acceptance that it will be used regularly. Two effective emollients are Original Formula Eucerin® cream and Cetaphil Moisturizing Cream®. These should be applied initially TID over any dermatitic sites that have just been treated with the topical corticoid. As areas of asteatosis improve, the topical steroid is gradually discontinued. Moisturizers must initially be applied in a general fashion two or three times daily and immediately after toweling. Once asteatosis is corrected, nightly application may be sufficient.

Several products are available OTC that contain either an α-hydroxy acid or urea as active ingredients. Both ingredients improve the water-holding capacity of the epidermis. These active agents have a definite long-term beneficial effect on the appearance and function of the epidermal surface.

Products are available OTC containing 5 to 10% lactic acid, and there is a cream preparation available by prescription with a 12% concentration. Because these products produce some burning or stinging when applied to open lesions, they are not well tolerated initially. They are best added as a single daily application under the general emollient after epidermal integrity has been restored.

Urea products are available OTC in 10 to 20% concentrations. These should be used with caution in the early stages of treatment, as their concomitant use can greatly enhance the percutaneous absorption of some topical steroids. They can be used in a fashion similar to the α-hydroxy acid preparations.

Conditions That May Simulate Asteatosis

Nummular Eczema

This common condition produces coin-like circular lesions, and in elderly patients may begin initially in an area of asteatosis. Lesions are discrete and much more inflammatory than those of asteatosis. Excoriation of the lesions is prominent, the surface is moist and eczematous, and the surface lacks the canal-like or craquelé pattern. Initially, itching is confined to individual lesions.

Acquired Ichthyosis

This scaling condition in its fully developed form resembles dominantly inherited ichthyosis vulgaris. Thick dirty-brown scales occur over the trunk and extremities and encroach on the skin over the flexural aspects of the large joints. Acquired ichthyosis is usually intensely pruritic and in the early stage may suggest changes of asteatosis. It is a paraneoplastic dermatitis that may precede, follow, or coincide with an underlying malignancy. Hodgkin's disease, mycosis fungoides, other lymphomas, and visceral cancers are most commonly associated. It has also been reported with HIV infection, and does not respond to the simple measures that control asteatosis. Biopsy shows changes of ichthyosis vulgaris and may be helpful in distinguishing difficult cases.

ANSWERS TO CLINICAL APPLICATION QUESTIONS

History Review

In the early spring, a 75-five-year-old woman visits your office with a complaint of generalized itching. The symptoms began in late December on local skin areas, and have progressed throughout the winter. You suspect an asteatotic eczema.

1. What information from her history may help support your suspicions?

Answer:

    a. Similar midwinter episodes in the past with spontaneous improvement during the spring and summer.

    b. Frequent use of fireplaces or wood stove heaters, which lower ambient humidity in the home.

    c. A lifelong or prolonged personal history of dry skin.

    d. A history of excessive bathing or use of medication that alters skin texture.

    e. Unusual dietary practices (malnutrition).

    f. A severe winter season with a prolonged need for indoor heating.

2. What are the primary lesions in areas of asteatotic eczema?

Answer: Patches of skin that appear dull with an accentuated crisscross pattern of skin marking.

3. What are the secondary lesions seen in asteatotic eczema?

Answer:

    a. Fine white scale (early).

    b. Coarse white scale (later).

    c. Fissures.

4. What typical configurations strongly support your suspicions?

Answer:

    a. Canal-like fissures (eczema cannalé).

    b. Crazy-paving fissures (eczema craquelé).

5. This woman has minimal physical findings, and some provoking factors are evident in her history, but she fails to improve with treatment. What should be done next?

Answer: A complete history and physical exam, CBC, chemistry panel, thyroid function panel, and any additional laboratory or imaging studies suggested by the history and physical.

23 Senile Purpura *(Bateman's Purpura)*

CLINICAL APPLICATION QUESTIONS

A 65-year-old active sailor presents with a history of progressive bruising of the arms over the past 3 to 4 years. Bruises now occur with such frequency and following such minor trauma that his wife is concerned about some underlying medical problem. Exam reveals large bruises limited to the sun-exposed extensor surfaces of the arms, forearms, and hands. The history and physical findings suggest senile (Bateman's) purpura.

1. What additional history will support your diagnosis?
2. What are the primary lesions of senile purpura?
3. What are the secondary lesions of senile purpura?
4. What is the typical configuration of senile purpura?
5. What is the characteristic distribution of senile purpura?
6. What is the most important treatment for this problem?

APPLICATION GUIDELINES

Specific History

Onset

Recurrent, but otherwise asymptomatic patches of bruising occur over the sun-exposed surfaces of the arms, forearms, and hands in persons who have reached their sixth decade of life. The incidence increases with age, and men are more frequently affected. Involvement of the sun exposed extensor surfaces of the legs occurs occasionally in women.

Evolution of Disease Process

Once established, the condition is usually chronic, unless some provoking cofactor that can be altered is operative.

Evolution of Skin Lesions

Localization is secondary to chronic sun-induced degenerative change in the dermal connective tissues superimposed on the natural loss of connective tissue support for the small dermal vessels (a normal characteristic of aging). Skin in the involved areas is thin and wrinkled, and usually shows chronic solar exposure. Even minor degrees of shear stress will rupture small dermal vessels causing irregular areas of deep-purple purpura, which will gradually resolve over a period of several days. Skin fragility and easy tearing also occur.

From: *Current Clinical Practice: Dermatology Skills for Primary Care: An Illustrated Guide*
D.J. Trozak, D.J. Tennenhouse, and J.J. Russell © Humana Press, Totowa, NJ

Initially the lesions resolve completely; however, in some patients chronic activity results in permanent hyperpigmentation. In patients with marked fragility, white stellate scarring may develop even at sites where no overt open tear has occurred.

Provoking Factors

Anticoagulant, aspirin, and nonsteroidal anti-inflammatory drug (NSAID) therapy can precipitate symptoms and exacerbate existing activity. Chronic systemic steroid therapy can also aggravate senile purpura but will eventually affect the entire skin surface. Potent topical steroids used on the affected areas will also locally increase atrophy and activity.

Self-Medication

Self-treatment is not a problem.

Supplemental review from general history

If findings are typical, no general review or investigation is indicated.

Dermatologic Physical Exam

Primary Lesions

Irregular patches of deep-purple purpura that do not blanch with pressure. Lesions vary from coin-sized to larger (*see* Photo 48).

Secondary Lesions

1. Hyperpigmentation (*see* Photos 48,49).
2. Epidermal atrophy manifested by fine wrinkles (*see* Photo 48).
3. Stellate scars in severe cases (*see* Photo 49).

Distribution

Microdistribution: None.

Macrodistribution: Sun-exposed dorsal surfaces of the arms, forearms, hands, and the extensor surface of the legs. There is usually a sharp cutoff at the short-sleeve line on the arms (*see* Fig. 8).

Configuration

None.

Indicated Supporting Diagnostic Data

None.

Therapy

Elimination of offending medications that suppress clotting and platelet function will reduce or temporarily eliminate symptoms. Reversal of corticosteroid-induced fragility will also occur, but more slowly and not as completely.

Theoretically, topical 0.1% tretinoin cream applied over a prolonged period and combined with complete solar avoidance could partially reverse the process. This treatment is a decision between patient and practitioner after a full discussion of the costs and effort involved.

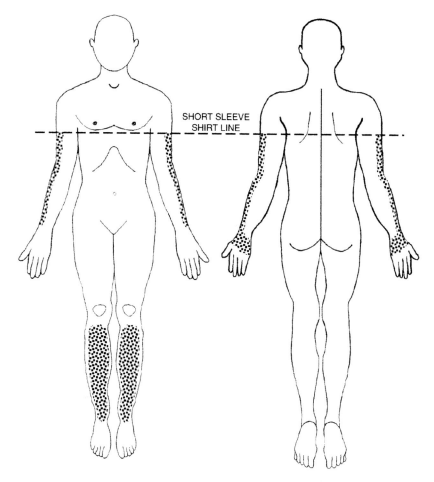

Figure 8: Macrodistribution of senile purpura.

Conditions That May Simulate Senile Purpura

Steroid Purpura

Similar findings and symptoms occur in the skin with chronic administration of systemic steroids, and in forms of adrenal cortex hyperactivity. Skin alterations are generalized, not focal, and other signs of hypercorticism are present. Local applications of potent topical steroids can simulate findings of senile purpura, and the cause is distinguishable only by history.

ANSWERS TO CLINICAL APPLICATION QUESTIONS

History Review

A 65-year-old active sailor presents with a history of progressive bruising of the arms over the past 3 to 4 years. Bruises now occur with such frequency and following such minor trauma that his wife is concerned about some underlying medical problem. Exam reveals large bruises limited to the sun-exposed extensor surfaces of the arms, forearms, and hands. The history and physical findings suggest senile (Bateman's) purpura.

1. What additional history will support your diagnosis?

Answer:
 a. Document the relative amount of lifelong solar exposure at work and recreation. The location where exposure was obtained can also be important, as latitude and elevation alter the extent of damage.
 b. Ask about associated skin fragility that is commonly present.
 c. Review provoking factors such as anticoagulant therapy, systemic steroid therapy, or use of aspirin or NSAIDs.

2. What are the primary lesions of senile purpura?

Answer: Irregular patches of nonblanching purpura, coin-sized to larger.

3. What are the secondary lesions of senile purpura?

Answer:
 a. Hyperpigmentation.
 b. Epidermal atrophy.
 c. Stellate scars.

4. What is the typical configuration of senile purpura?

Answer: Senile purpura has no specific configuration.

5. What is the characteristic distribution of senile purpura?

Answer:
 a. Dorsal sun-exposed surfaces of the upper extremities with sharp cutoff at the short-sleeve line.
 b. Extensor surface of the legs.

6. What is the most important treatment for this problem?

Answer: Elimination and avoidance of any provoking medications will have the most immediate effect on this problem.

24 Striae Distensae *(Striae Atrophicans, Striae Gravidarum, Stretch Marks)*

INTRODUCTION

Atrophic striae occur under several circumstances. They are so common as to be considered physiologic during adolescence. The microscopic features reveal a combination of findings showing epidermal atrophy and dermal scar formation. The cause of the lesions is usually apparent from the patient's age or by obtaining a pertinent history. On rare occasions, they can be an indication of underlying adrenal cortex dysfunction.

CLINICAL APPLICATION QUESTIONS

An obese, middle-aged, diabetic woman presents with a complaint of worsening stretch marks over the past year. She gives a history of marginal blood pressure readings in the past, but has never been on medication for hypertension. Exam reveals numerous wide purple-red stria beneath the breasts, in the folds of her panniculus, and on the proximal thighs just distal to the inguinal creases.

1. What underlying causes should be of concern regarding her stria?
2. History reveals stable weight for 5 years, no recent pregnancy, no history of systemic steroid therapy, and normal wound healing. The patient was diagnosed with intertriginous monilia 12 months ago by another practitioner, and was given a refillable prescription for a potent anti-yeast/steroid cream, which she has continued to use. What is the most likely cause of her stria?
3. What laboratory data are indicated?
4. What is the appropriate treatment?
5. What should the patient be told regarding the appearance of her stria?

APPLICATION GUIDELINES

Specific History

Onset

Striae occur in 35 to 40% of pubescent boys and 70% of pubescent girls, with a peak incidence about age 16 years. They occur more readily in patients with a history of rapid weight gain, and adolescents seem more prone to develop lesions associated with physical exercise and corticosteroid exposure.

From: *Current Clinical Practice: Dermatology Skills for Primary Care: An Illustrated Guide*
D.J. Trozak, D.J. Tennenhouse, and J.J. Russell © Humana Press, Totowa, NJ

Striae gravidarum develop to some extent in up to 90% of pregnant women during mid and late gestation, and are considered physiologic.

Striae associated with topical steroid usage usually occur at application sites, and may occur within weeks of initiation in susceptible persons. These may occur at any age.

Striae associated with adrenal cortical hyperactivity occur at whatever age the process becomes clinically active.

Evolution of Disease Process

The lesions themselves are minimally symptomatic and chronic.

Evolution of Skin Lesions

Early lesions may be edematous and irritable, but the central area quickly becomes depressed and is initially pink, bright red, or red-blue in color. Striae develop in parallel rows perpendicular to the direction of stretch or stress. Most lesions are 1 cm or less in width and, as they mature, the depressed central portion turns whiter than the intervening epidermis and they become less conspicuous.

Striae secondary to endocrinopathy, such as Cushing's syndrome, are wider, centrally more atrophic, more extensively distributed, and tend to retain their central discoloration. Herniation of adipose tissue into the base is common.

These are chronic lesions that leave varying degrees of chronic disfigurement once they mature.

Provoking Factors

1. Puberty.
2. Sustained and violent physical effort with stretching.
3. Rapid weight gain.
4. Pregnancy.
5. Systemic and topical corticosteroid therapy.
6. Protease inhibitors.
7. Underlying endocrinopathies of the adrenal cortex (rare).

Self-Medication

Self-treatment with agents such as cocoa butter and vitamin E may occasionally trigger a contact allergy. In general, self-therapy is not a problem.

Supplemental Review From General History

When striae are wider and longer than usual, or are more extensively distributed, a general history, physical examination, and screening evaluation for an underlying endocrinopathy are indicated.

Dermatologic Physical Exam

Primary Lesions

Parallel linear patches of discolored or white depressed skin (*see* Photo 50).

Secondary Lesions

Yellow papules of herniated adipose tissue in the base of the stretch mark beneath the epidermis. Although usually primary lesions, here papules may occur as secondary lesions.

Distribution

Microdistribution: None.

Macrodistribution: Striae of puberty occur on the thighs and lumbosacral regions in boys. In girls, they occur on the thighs, buttocks, breasts, and upper posterior calves (*see* Figs. 9,10). Striae of pregnancy are distributed over the lateral abdomen, hips, thighs, and breasts (*see* Fig. 11). Striae secondary to prolonged lifting or stretching during exercise

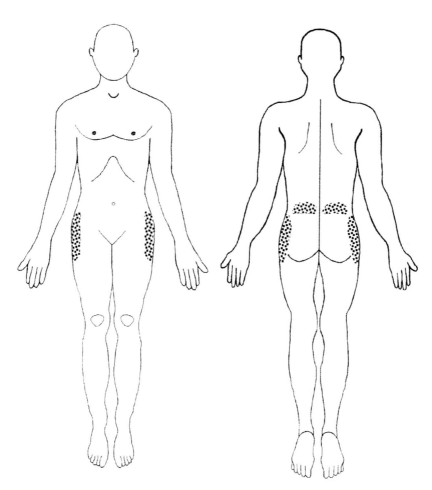

Figure 9: Macrodistribution of striae of puberty in boys.

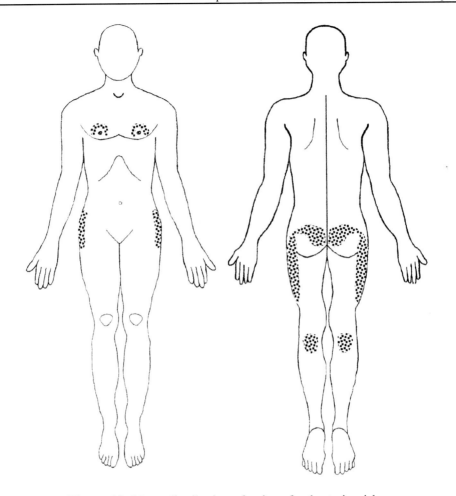

Figure 10: Macrodistribution of striae of puberty in girls.

are common over the lower back and are perpendicular to the gluteal cleft (*see* Fig. 12, Photo 50). Striae of endocrinopathy or from systemic corticoids involve similar areas but are usually individually longer, wider, and more extensive (*see* Photo 51). Striae induced by potent topical steroids or occlusive therapy are local at the site of application, and may be asymmetric (*see* Photo 52).

Configuration

Parallel linear lesions. Striae of endocrine origin may also have a fan-like configuration.

Indicated Supporting Diagnostic Data

When physical findings and history suggest a possible endocrinopathy, the patient should be appropriately tested. The most reliable screen is a dexamethasone suppression test. Alternative tests include 8 AM and 4 PM serum cortisol determinations, or a 24-hour urinary free cortisol.

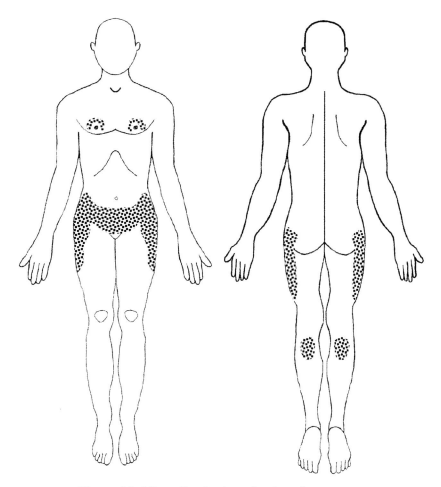

Figure 11: Macrodistribution of striae of pregnancy.

Therapy

Prevention

When possible, warn susceptible patients about, and advise how to eliminate, provoking causes. In adolescent patients, use systemic and topical corticosteroids with great caution. Avoid use of the more potent fluorinated topicals, and use them sparingly over skin regions that are prone to striae formation.

Topical Tretinoin

Uncontrolled reports of cosmetic benefit from applications of topical 0.1% tretinoin cream have been published. Results are encouraging following experience with only a few patients. Double-blind studies with photographic controls are needed. Early experience would suggest this is worth trying, as there is no other effective treatment. Tretinoin should not be used during pregnancy or breastfeeding.

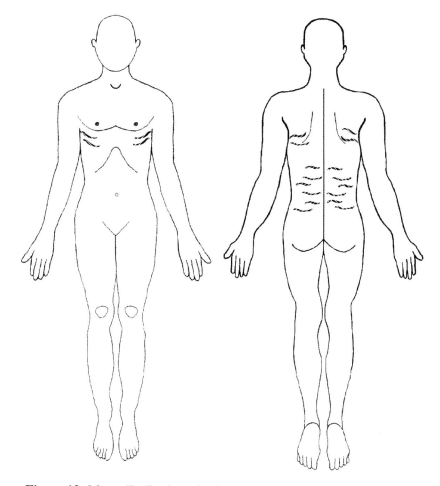

Figure 12: Macrodistribution of striae secondary to lifting or stretching.

Conditions That May Simulate Striae Distensae

None.

ANSWERS TO CLINICAL APPLICATION QUESTIONS

History Review

An obese, middle-aged, diabetic woman presents with a complaint of worsening stretch marks over the past year. She gives a history of marginal blood pressure readings in the past, but has never been on medication for hypertension. Exam reveals numerous wide purple-red stria beneath the breasts, in the folds of her panniculus, and on the proximal thighs just distal to the inguinal creases.

1. **What underlying causes should be of concern regarding her stria?**

Answer:
   a. Rapid weight gain.
   b. Pregnancy.
   c. Systemic or local corticosteroid therapy.
   d. Underlying endocrinopathy, e.g., Cushing's disease or syndrome.

2. **History reveals stable weight for 5 years, no recent pregnancy, no history of systemic steroid therapy, and normal wound healing. The patient was diagnosed with intertriginous monilia 12 months ago by another practitioner, and was given a refillable prescription for a potent antiyeast/steroid cream, which she has continued to use. What is the most likely cause of her stria?**

Answer: Iatrogenic stria from prolonged used of a potent topical corticosteroid.

3. **What laboratory data are indicated?**

Answer: There is enough reason in this patient to warrant screens for adrenal hypersecretion, despite the history of topical corticoid usage.

4. **What is the appropriate treatment?**

Answer: Stop the topical steroid and consider treatment with a topical retinoid.

5. **What should the patient be told regarding the appearance of her stria?**

Answer: The stria will fade, soften, and become less noticeable. They will never completely disappear.

REFERENCES for Part IV

1. Champion RH, Burton JL, Ebling FJG. Textbook of Dermatology. 5th ed. Oxford: Blackwell Scientific Publications, 1992 pp. 2164–2225, 675–676, 598–610, 1767–1769.
2. Braun-Falco O, Plewig G, Wolff HH, Winkelmann RK. Dermatology. Berlin-Heidelberg: Springer-Verlag, 1991 pp. 563–574, 348–357, 519, 546.
3. Braverman IM. Skin Signs of Systemic Disease. Philadelphia: W.B. Saunders Company, 1970 pp. 144–163.
4. Drug Facts and Comparisons. St. Louis: Wolters-Kluwer Co. 2003 ed.
5. Pavlidakey GP, et al. Chlorpromazine induced lupus-like disease. J Am Acad Dermatol 1985;13:109–115.
6. Provost TT, Reichlin M. Antinuclear antibody-negative lupus erythematosus. J Am Acad Dermatol 1981;4:84–89.
7. Trozak DJ. Topical Corticosteroid Therapy in Psoriasis. Cutis 1990;46:341–350.
8. Sontheimer RD, et al. Subacute Cutaneous Lupus Erythematosus. Arch Dermatol 1979;115:1409–1415.
9. Furner BB. Treatment of Subacute Cutaneous Lupus Erythematosus. Internat J Dermatol 1990;29:542–547.
10. Furner BB. Subacute Cutaneous Lupus Erythematosus Response to Isotretinoin. Internat J Dermatol 1990;29:587–590.
11. Callen JP, et al. Collagen-vascular disease: An update. J Am Acad Dermatol 1993;28:477–484.
12. Mitchell-Sams W, Huff JC. Practical Management of Cutaneous Lupus Erythematosus, Vasculitis, and Erythema Multiforme. Progress in Dermatology 1984;18:1–3.
13. Gilliam JN, Sontheimer MD. Distinctive cutaneous subsets in the spectrum of lupus erythematosus. J Am Acad Dermatol 1981;4:471–475.
14. Provost TT. Subsets in Systemic Lupus Erythematosus. J Invest Dermatol 1979;72:110–113.
15. Wechsler HL, Stavrides A. Systemic lupus erythematosus with anti-Ro antibodies: Clinical, Histologic, and immunologic findings. J Am Acad Dermatol 1982;6:73–83.
16. Provost TT, et al. The Relationship Between Anti-Ro (SS-A) Antibody-Positive Sjogren's Syndrome and Anti-Ro (SS-A) Antibody-Positive Lupus Erythematosus. Arch Dermatol 1988;124:63–71.
17. Estes D, Christian CL. The Natural History of Systemic Lupus by Prospective Analysis. Medicine 1971;50:85–95.
18. Callen JP. Serologic and clinical features of patient with discoid lupus erythematosus: Relationship of antibodies to single stranded deoxyribonucleic acid and of other antinuclear antibody subsets to clinical manifestations. J Amer Acad Dermatol 1985;13:748–755.
19. Provost TT. The relationship between discoid and systemic lupus erythematosus. Arch Dermatol 1994;130:1308–1310.
20. Ziering DO, et al. Antimalarials for children: Indications , toxicities and guidelines. J Amer Acad Dermatol 1993;28:764–770.
21. Potter B. Hydroxychloroquine. Cutis 1993;52:229–231.
22. Olansky AJ. Antimalarials and ophthalmologic safety. J Amer Acad Dermatol 1982;6:19–23.
23. Mitchell J, Rook A, Botanical Dermatology. Vancouver B.C.: Greengrass Ltd., 81–97.
24. Fisher AA. Contact Dermatitis. 2nd. ed. Philadelphia: Lea & Febiger, 1973 pp. 260–266.
25. Adams RM. Occupational Skin Disease. New York: Grune & Stratton Inc. 1983 pp. 331–337.
26. Goldstein N. The Ubiquitous Urushiols. Cutis 1968;4:679–685.
27. Guin JD, Gillis WT, Beaman JH. Recognizing the toxicodendrons (poison ivy, poison oak, and poison sumac). J Amer Acad Dermatol 1981;4:99–114.

From: *Current Clinical Practice: Dermatology Skills for Primary Care: An Illustrated Guide*
D.J. Trozak, D.J. Tennenhouse, and J.J. Russell © Humana Press, Totowa, NJ

28. Hanifin JM, Schneider LC, Leung DYM, et al. Recombinant interferon gamma therapy for atopic dermatitis. J Amer Acad Dermatol 1993;28:189–197.
29. Lobitz WC, Dobson RL. Physical and physiological clues for diagnosing eczema. JAMA 1956;161:1226–1229.
30. The guide to drug eruptions. 6th ed. Amsterdam: Free University Amsterdam; File of Medicines, 1995, p. 6.
31. Colon D. Stellate spontaneous pseudoscars: Senile and presenile forms, especially those caused by prolonged corticoid therapy. Arch Dermatol 1972;105:551–554.
32. Chernosky NE, Knox JM. Atrophic striae after occlusive corticosteroid therapy. Arch Dermatol 1964;90:15–19.
33. Macrae-Gibson NK. Red lineae distensae. Br J Dermatol 1952;64:315–323.
34. Elson ML. Treatment of striae distensae with topical tretinoin. J Dermatol Surg Oncol 1990;16:267–270.
35. Nesher G, Osborne TG, Moore TL. Parvovirus infection mimicking systemic lupus erythematosus. Semin Arthritis Rheum 1995;24:297.
36. Tan BB, Weald D, Strickland I, Friedmann PS. Double-blind controlled trial of effect of housedust mite allergen avoidance on atopic dermatitis. Lancet 1996;347:15–18.
37. Marks JG, Fowler Jr. JF, Sheretz EF, Rietschel. Prevention of poison ivy and poison oak allergic contact dermatitis by quaternium-18 bentonite. J Amer Acad Dermatol 1995;33:212–216.
38. Gravelink SA, Murrell DF, Olson, EA. Effectiveness of various barrier preparations in preventing and/or ameliorating experimentally produced Toxicodendron dermatitis. J Amer Acad Dermatol 1992;27:182–188.
39. Provost TT. The cutaneous spectrum of lupus erythematosus. Presentation Annual Meeting Sacramento Dermatologic Society, October 18, 2003, Napa California.
40. Mutasim DF, Adams BB. A practical guide for serologic evaluation of autoimmune connective tissue diseases. J Amer Acad Dermatol 42, #2, part 1: 159-170.
41. Srivastava M, Rencic A, Diglio G, et al. Drug induced, Ro/SSA-positive cutaneous lupus erythematosus. Arch Dermatol 2003;139:45-49.
42. Williams JV, Light J, Marks JG, et al. Individual variations in allergic contact dermatitis from urushiol. Arch Dermatol 1999;135:1002-1003.
43. Physicians Desk Reference. Thomson 57th. ed., 2003.
44. Wolverton SE. Comprehensive Dermatologic Therapy. W B Saunders Company, 2001.
45. Bornhovd E, Burgdorf WHC, Wollenberg A. Macrolactam immunomodulators for topical treatment of inflammatory skin disorders. J Amer Acad Dermatol 2001;45:736-743.
46. Topical pimecrolimus (Elidel) for treatment of atopic dermatitis. The Medical Letter 44, issue 1131, 48-50, 2002.
47. Darvay A, Acland K, Lynn W, et al. Stria formation in two HIV-positive persons receiving protease inhibitors. J Amer Acad Dermatol 1999;41:467-469.
48. Borkowski TA, Sampson HA. A combined dermatology and allergy approach to the management of suspected food allergy. Dermatological Therapy 1996;1:38-50.
49. La Grenade L, Manns A, Fletcher V, et al. Clinical, pathologic and immunologic features of human T-lymphotropic virus type 1-associated infective dermatitis in children. Arch Dermatol 1998;134:439-444.

Part V: Pigmented, Pre-Malignant, and Common Malignant Skin Lesions

IMPORTANT ABBREVIATIONS USED IN THIS PART:

AcpN	Acquired "congenital pattern" melanotic nevus/nevi
AK	Actinic keratosis
ALMM	Acral lentiginous mucosal melanoma
ANS	Atypical nevus syndrome
BCC	Basal cell carcinoma (epithelioma)
CMN	Congenital melanotic nevus/nevi
ELND	Elective lymph node dissection
KA	Keratoacanthoma
LCMN	Large congenital melanotic nevus/nevi
LM	Lentigo maligna
LMM	Lentigo maligna melanoma
LN2	Liquid nitrogen
MCMN	Medium congenital melanotic nevus/nevi
MM	Malignant melanoma
NM	Nodular melanoma
SCC	Squamous cell carcinoma
SCMN	Small congenital melanotic nevus/nevi
SK	Seborrheic keratosis
SLNB	Sentinel lymph node biopsy
SPF	Sun protection factor
SSMM	Superficial spreading malignant melanoma

25 Seborrheic Keratosis *(Old Age Spots, Liver Spots)*

CLINICAL APPLICATION QUESTIONS

A 70-year-old man is seen at your office for multiple raised pigmented lesions over his back and chest. These have developed gradually over several years. There are two lesions on the mid-lower back that intermittently itch intensely and are somewhat larger and much darker than the other lesions, which number 50 or more. Physical examination of the entire region reveals multiple seborrheic keratoses. Except for the two lesions in question there are no other suspect lesions. The patient is very worried about melanoma.

1. Should the two darker lesions be biopsied for melanoma?
2. If you determine that one or both of the darker lesions are seborrheic keratoses, what should you tell the patient about them?
3. What are the primary lesions that you would expect to find with seborrheic keratoses?
4. What are the secondary lesions that you would expect to find with seborrheic keratoses?
5. If you determine that one or both of the darker lesions are seborrheic keratoses, how should you treat them?

APPLICATION GUIDELINES

Specific History

Onset

These very common benign lesions normally begin insidiously during early or mid-middle age. This gradual onset is very typical. The sudden onset of multiple rapidly growing seborrheic keratuses (SKs) associated with pruritus is known as the sign of Leser-Trélat, and may indicate an underlying visceral malignancy, a leukemia, or lymphoma.

Evolution of Disease Process and Skin Lesions

Seborrheic keratoses are most often evident during the fifth decade, but may be present as early as the third decade. They begin as flat, tan, superficial 1- to 3-mm papules with a dull surface, and in their early stages may be very difficult to distinguish from flat warts. Over many years, certain lesions increase in size and thickness, then become increasingly keratotic, but retain their superficial character. SKs are described as appearing to have been "pasted" or "stuck on" normal-appearing skin (*see* Photo 1). Common coloration is gray-tan, yellow-tan, pink-tan, or medium brown. Color can vary from grey-white to black.

From: *Current Clinical Practice: Dermatology Skills for Primary Care: An Illustrated Guide*
D.J. Trozak, D.J. Tennenhouse, and J.J. Russell © Humana Press, Totowa, NJ

Crypts of keratotic debris sometimes cause the formation of comedones (plugs) over their surface. Developed lesions have an uneven surface and a soft, waxy character when palpated. Average size of developed lesions is 1 to 2 cm; however, some lesions may reach several centimeters, especially on the temple and scalp regions. Around the neck and on the eyelids they are often pedunculated (*see* Photo 10). While certain lesions grow and thicken, others may disappear after trauma or episodes of inflammation. The general trend is for the lesions to become larger, thicker, and more noticeable with advancing age. Rare reports in the dermatology literature document the combined presence of an SK with a common basal or squamous cell carcinoma. SKs are so common and these reports are so infrequent that it would seem best to consider these as the coincidental occurrence of two lesions at the same site. SKs are considered benign without significant risk of malignant degeneration.

Provoking Factors

SKs appear to be a dominantly inherited trait with marked variation in genetic penetrance. Occasionally, patients present with lesions strikingly limited to sun-exposed skin, raising the possibility of ultraviolet light being a provoking factor. Many patients, however, have lesions only on covered regions, and no proven provoking factors have been identified.

Self-Medication

Self-treatment is not a problem.

Supplemental Review From General History

Sudden development of large numbers of rapidly growing seborrheic keratoses, especially when associated with itching (Leser-Trélat sign), is an indication for an in-depth history and physical exam.

Dermatologic Physical Exam

Primary Lesions

1. Dull 1- to 3-mm papules (*see* Photo 1).
2. Keratotic "stuck on" plaques 0.5 to 2 cm (*see* Photo 2), occasionally larger (*see* Photo 3)

Secondary Lesions

Usually none.

Distribution

Microdistribution: None.

Macrodistribution: SKs are seen primarily on the face, upper back, and central chest. They can occur at almost any site. Only the palms, soles, and mucous membranes are spared (*see* Fig. 1).

Configuration

Occasionally SKs will follow lines of cleavage (*see* Photo 2). This may produce a "Christmas tree" pattern. Generally they are randomly distributed.

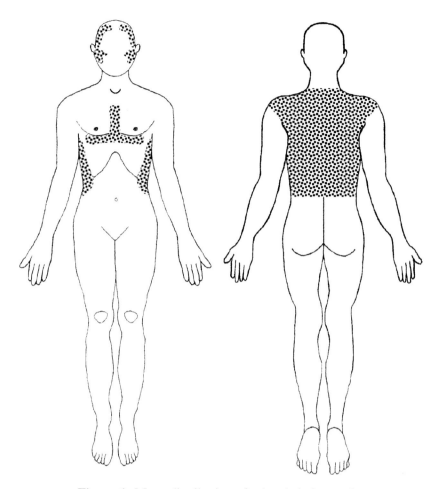

Figure 1: Macrodistribution of seborrheic keratosis.

Indicated Supporting Diagnostic Data

Biopsy

The vast majority of SKs can be diagnosed by physical inspection. Depending on their stage of evolution, there are times when SKs may be difficult to distinguish clinically from a pigmented basal cell carcinoma, lentigo maligna, or a malignant melanoma. In these rare instances the lesion should be referred to a dermatologist for evaluation and a decision regarding the appropriate type of biopsy if one is indicated.

Therapy

Seborrheic keratoses are benign lesions and treatment is elective. Exceptions include instances where they are symptomatic because of location, due to inflammation, or after trauma. These benign growths can be treated by nonscarring techniques. Except under very unusual circumstances, surgical excision of these lesions is inappropriate treatment. When the clinical diagnosis is uncertain, referral to a dermatologist is necessary and usually cost-effective.

Cryosurgery

Light applications of liquid nitrogen sufficient to produce a 0.5- to 1-mm rim of freeze at the perimeter of the base of the SK is usually sufficient for total removal. The advantage of this technique is the absence of scarring. Heavily pigmented persons must be warned about the possibility of posttreatment hyper- or hypopigmentation. This is especially important when working on the facial area. When patients express concern in this regard, we encourage treatment of one or two test lesions in an inconspicuous location before proceeding. During the sunny season, we strongly urge sun avoidance and the use of a sunscreen with makeup to prevent posttreatment darkening. Cryosurgery is the appropriate way to treat these lesions.

Shave Excision With Light Curettage and Electrodesiccation

On rare occasions one encounters an SK that simply will not respond to cryotherapy. When this occurs, the lesion must be biopsied to be certain it is not a more aggressive type of pigmented lesion. Once the lesion is found to be benign, therapy should consist of shave excision and gentle curettage followed by electrodesiccation at a very low setting. This procedure almost always leaves some superficial scarring and permanent pigment loss, and the patient should be forewarned.

Chemical Removal

Removal of SKs can also be accomplished with trichloroacetic acid or concentrated preparations of various α-hydroxy acids. Chemical removal usually also involves some use of curettage or combined use of liquid nitrogen, and should be performed only by a skilled operator.

Conditions That May Simulate Seborrheic Keratosis
Planar Warts

Early SKs on the dorsal forearms and hands can be virtually indistinguishable from planar warts except on biopsy. Generally, planar warts present in children or young adults, and tend to group asymmetrically in certain locations. SKs usually occur a decade or more later and are typically symmetrical.

Solar Lentigo

Differentiation between an early facial SK and a chronic solar lentigo can be difficult clinically. Usually with careful examination the raised edge of the SK is evident, whereas the lentigo is macular. Biopsy will distinguish them but is rarely relevant since both are benign lesions and both respond to liquid nitrogen (LN_2).

Actinic Keratosis and Squamous Cell Carcinoma

Usually SKs can be distinguished from premalignant sun-induced actinic keratoses (AKs) by their thicker "stuck-on" appearance and waxy surface feel. AKs may be brown in color, but there is usually a surface scale, a background of erythema, and the surface is rough and abrasive to the touch. Squamous cell carcinomas often have a keratotic surface, but unlike the SK they have an indurated base.

Malignant Melanoma and Pigmented Basal Cell Carcinoma

Usually the stuck-on appearance and waxy surface will serve to distinguish SKs. When there is doubt as to the diagnosis, referral to a dermatologist is indicated. This may avoid a needless scar, or prevent inappropriate handling of a potentially dangerous growth. If biopsy or excision is indicated, someone fully conversant with pigmented tumors should make that decision.

ANSWERS TO CLINICAL APPLICATION QUESTIONS

History Review

A 70-year-old man is seen at your office for multiple raised pigmented lesions over his back and chest. These have developed gradually over several years. There are two lesions on the mid-lower back that intermittently itch intensely and are somewhat larger and much darker than the other lesions, which number 50 or more. Physical examination of the entire region reveals multiple seborrheic keratoses. Except for the two lesions in question there are no other suspect lesions. The patient is very worried about melanoma.

1. Should the two darker lesions be biopsied for melanoma?

Answer: Despite its darker color, if the lesion has a waxy keratotic surface and a typical "stuck-on" appearance, it is clinically consistent with a benign SK. The lesion should not be biopsied at this time. If you strongly suspect the lesion is an SK but are uncertain that it has a superficial "stuck-on" character or that its surface is not waxy and keratotic, either obtain a dermatologic consultation or perform a punch biopsy for the purpose of identification.

2. If you determine that one or both of the darker lesions are seborrheic keratoses, what should you tell the patient about them?

Answer: Seborrheic keratoses are benign lesions. Treatment is optional. If specific lesions are sufficiently symptomatic that removal is desired, the appropriate approach is cryotherapy, which is almost always successful.

3. What are the primary lesions that you would expect to find with seborrheic keratoses?

Answer: Dull 1- to 3-mm papules, and waxy keratotic "stuck-on" appearing plaques that are 0.5 to 2 cm in size but occasionally larger. Color may vary from gray-white to black.

4. What are the secondary lesions that you would expect to find with seborrheic keratoses?

Answer: Usually none.

5. If you determine that one or both of the darker lesions are seborrheic keratoses, how should you treat them?

Answer: Cryotherapy is appropriate, with immediate follow-up if the lesions have not resolved in 30 days.

26 Ephelides *(Freckles)*

CLINICAL APPLICATION QUESTIONS

An attractive 20-year-old woman is seen at your office for multiple freckles over her face, shoulders, and dorsal surfaces of her upper extremities. They are limited to areas exposed to the sun. She desires their removal.

1. What are the primary lesions that you would expect to find in ephelides?
2. What should you tell the patient about removing ephelides?
3. What should you tell the patient about her prognosis?
4. Should this patient be warned about skin cancer?

APPLICATION GUIDELINES

Specific History

Onset

Ephelides are physiologic areas of increased pigment production that are first seen following solar exposure during the first decade of life. They are most common in people with reddish-blond hair and blue or green eye color.

Evolution of Disease Process and Skin Lesions

With increased outdoor activity freckling occurs and is limited to sun-exposed skin. The spots blossom in the spring and summer and tend to fade during the fall and winter. Usually the extent and density of ephelides reach a peak during adolescence. In middle life, they become less prominent, possibly merging with general background pigmentation.

Provoking Factors

Natural sunlight or ultraviolet light in the UVA and UVB spectrum.

Self-Medication

Self-treatment is not a problem.

Supplemental Review From General History

None indicated.

Dermatologic Physical Exam

Primary Lesions

One- to 3-mm reddish-tan macules of variable size and irregular shape (*see* Photo 4).

From: *Current Clinical Practice: Dermatology Skills for Primary Care: An Illustrated Guide*
D.J. Trozak, D.J. Tennenhouse, and J.J. Russell © Humana Press, Totowa, NJ

Secondary Lesions
     None.

Distribution
     Microdistribution: None.

     Macrodistribution: Symmetrically present on sun-exposed skin.

Configuration
     None.

Indicated Supporting Diagnostic Data
     None.

Therapy
     Ephelides are physiologic areas of enhanced melanin production and are a response to a natural stimulus. They are dominantly inherited and will recur with solar exposure. They can be lightened with various bleaching preparations, but this is usually successful only when combined with a monastic indoor existence. Provide these fair-skinned, skin cancer prone patients with support, a kindly explanation, and a discussion of proper sun avoidance and protection with a high SPF Parsol® containing sunscreen. Although there are methods for removing ephelides, the risks outweigh the potential benefits.

Conditions That May Simulate Ephelides
Lentigines
     Ephelides are usually tan or a light reddish-brown, color as opposed to the dark brown of a lentigo. They are found on sun-exposed regions, are tightly grouped, and are sometimes so dense they become confluent. Lentigines are sparse, scattered, and are not strictly found on sun-exposed skin. Lentigines may occur on mucous membranes. Unlike ephelides, lentigines do not regress in the absence of solar exposure.

ANSWERS TO CLINICAL APPLICATION QUESTIONS

History Review
     An attractive 20-year-old woman is seen at your office for multiple freckles over her face, shoulders, and dorsal surfaces of her upper extremities. They are limited to areas exposed to the sun. She desires their removal.

1. What are the primary lesions that you would expect to find in ephelides?

Answer: One- to 3-mm reddish-tan macules of variable size and irregular shape.

2. What should you tell the patient about removing ephelides?

Answer: Freckles can be lightened with certain skin-bleaching preparations. This effect is temporary and depends on almost total sun avoidance. Most patients cannot comply. It is more reasonable to emphasize that freckles are often considered an attractive feature.

3.   What should you tell the patient about her prognosis?

Answer: Freckles are a genetic trait. Sun avoidance is the only way to prevent additional freckling. Freckling often becomes less prominent with time.

4.   Should this patient be warned about skin cancer?

Answer: People who freckle are more prone to develop common skin cancers including malignant melanoma. This is an appropriate time to discuss sun avoidance, protective clothing, and use of sunscreen.

27 Lentigines

CLINICAL APPLICATION QUESTIONS

A 44-year-old man requests evaluation of an irritated brown lesion on his left shoulder. Evaluation reveals a typical 5-mm "stuck on" seborrheic keratosis. He also has multiple lentigines of various sizes in a solar distribution over his upper back, shoulders, and upper chest. An asymmetric multicolored 4 × 8 mm lesion is present on his left anterior shoulder. It has a notched margin and stands out from the other lesions.

1. Should the multicolored lesion be biopsied?
2. What are the primary lesions that you would expect to find in solar lentigines?
3. What are the secondary lesions that you would expect to find in solar lentigines?
4. What should you tell the patient about the solar lentigines?
5. Is there any relationship between lentigines and melanoma?
6. How are solar lentigines treated?

APPLICATION GUIDELINES

Specific History

Onset

A lentigo is a focal area of numerically increased, but benign, nonproliferating melanocytes at the dermoepidermal junction. There are two common types: small nonsolar lentigines and larger sun-induced lentigines. Most nonsolar lentigines arise during the first decade, but they may increase in number into adulthood or occasionally arise later in life. Solar lentigines begin in the second decade of life, except with intense solar exposure, when they may appear even earlier.

Evolution of Disease Process and Skin Lesions

Once present, nonsolar lentigines are quite stable. They do not change in color or number with solar exposure. Spontaneous disappearance has been recorded. This type of lentigo is usually dark brown and tends to be more discrete, symmetrical, and less densely grouped than ephelides. They show fewer tendencies toward confluence. Even confluent lentigines rarely exceed 0.5 cm in size.

A solar lentigo is microscopically identical to its nonsolar counterpart. This type is usually 0.5 to 1 cm or more in size and appears after acute or chronic sun exposure. The margins are irregular, but like nonsolar lentigines, the normal skin lines can be readily followed across the lesion's surface. Both are absolutely macular.

From: *Current Clinical Practice: Dermatology Skills for Primary Care: An Illustrated Guide*
D.J. Trozak, D.J. Tennenhouse, and J.J. Russell © Humana Press, Totowa, NJ

Provoking Factors

Nonsolar lentigines have no provoking factors. The stimulus for solar lentigines is intense ultraviolet light exposure.

Self-Medication

Self-treatment is not a problem.

Supplemental Review From General History

The presence of widespread small nonsolar lentigines may signal one of the rare multisystem syndromes, such as Leopard, Lamb, or Name syndromes. Periorificial and oral mucous membrane lesions may be a sign of Peutz-Jeghers syndrome. Appropriate historical review and exam are then indicated.

Dermatologic Physical Exam
Primary Lesions

Nonsolar lentigines: These are macules of medium to dark-brown pigmentation that retain normal skin markings over their surface. Even when confluent, their size rarely exceeds 5 mm. They may be clinically indistinguishable from a junctional nevus. They are generally darker, sharper, and more regular than ephelides (*see* Photo 5).

Solar lentigines: These are macules of light- to medium-brown pigmentation tht retain normal skin markings over their surface. Color is often uneven, and the margins are irregular and fuzzy. Size varies from 0.5 to 1 cm or more (*see* Photo 6).

Secondary Lesions

None with either type.

Distribution

Microdistribution: None with either type.

Macrodistribution: Nonsolar lentigines may be randomly present anywhere on the skin or mucous membranes. Solar lentigines may be seen in areas of intense sun exposure, especially in youths who sunburn easily. Face, upper back, and shoulders are common locations. These are also common in adults after chronic exposure, usually in their fifth decade or older. Facial eminences and dorsum of hands are the most common sites (*see* Fig. 2).

Configuration

None with either type.

Indicated Supporting Diagnostic Data

None, unless irregularity or size suggests another more aggressive type of pigmented lesion. In this case, dermatologic consultation or a diagnostic biopsy may be prudent.

Therapy

In general, no therapy other than an explanation and reassurance is indicated. On occasion, specific cosmetically bothersome lesions can be removed, but the practitioner

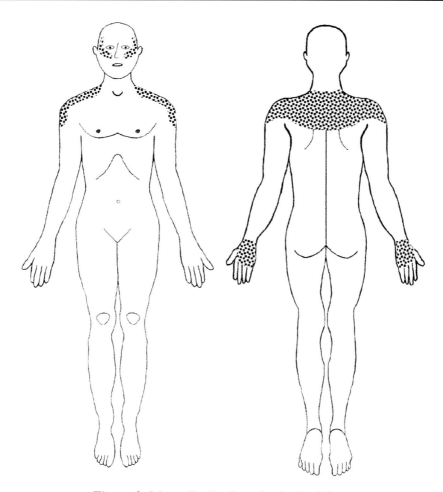

Figure 2: Macrodistribution of solar lentigines.

must carefully balance the benefits against any potential scarring. Cryotherapy with LN_2 is often successful with the solar type, but mild scarring and residual hypopigmentation can result. The patient must be forewarned. In some locations, such as the vermilion of the lip, punch excision gives an acceptable result. With invasive removal, site and skin type must be carefully assessed. A recent report cites solar lentigines as a significant independent risk factor for malignant melanoma. The risk factor is significant enough to warrant a total body pigmented-lesion check, instruction on monthly self-exam, and yearly follow-up.

Conditions That May Simulate Lentigines

Junctional Nevi (Moles)

A benign nonsolar lentigo may be absolutely indistinguishable on clinical exam from a benign junctional nevus. Unless either lesion is irregular or changing, the distinction is academic. Solar lentigines are larger and more irregular, and are not easily confused with nevi.

Ephelides

Benign nonsolar lentigines may be difficult to distinguish from ephelides. These lentigines tend to be more sparse and scattered than ephelides and are generally darker in color. In addition, they do not darken or multiply with sun exposure and show little tendency to become confluent. Solar lentigines are larger and are not easily confused with ephelides.

Seborrheic Keratosis

Solar lentigines and early SKs in older persons may be hard to distinguish. The SK will, on close inspection, show a subtle raised "stuck-on" appearance and a dull surface. The lentigo will retain the normal skin markings and light reflectance.

Actinic Keratosis

Solar lentigines and pigmented AKs are also hard to distinguish. The AK usually has a scale that is clinically evident or can be raised with light scraping. Like the SK, its surface is dull due to disordered surface formation.

Lentigo Maligna

Solar lentigines may enter into the differential diagnosis of this type of *in situ* malignant melanoma seen in older persons. Both lesions occur in similar solar-exposed areas and both are irregularly shaped areas of macular pigmentation. In general, lentigo maligna is a much larger and more irregular lesion, and shows irregular tan, brown, and dark-brown pigment within a given lesion. Most benign lentigines tend to be about 1 cm or less in size and show uneven tan pigment.

ANSWERS TO CLINICAL APPLICATION QUESTIONS

History Review

A 44-year-old man requests evaluation of an irritated brown lesion on his left shoulder. Evaluation reveals a typical 5 mm "stuck on" seborrheic keratosis. He also has multiple lentigines of various sizes in a solar distribution over his upper back, shoulders, and upper chest. An asymmetric multicolored lesion 4 × 8 mm is present on his left anterior shoulder. It has a notched margin and stands out from the other lesions.

1. Should the multicolored lesion be biopsied?

Answer: The multicolored lesion may be a melanoma, and conservative excisional biopsy is indicated.

2. What are the primary lesions that you would expect to find in solar lentigines?

Answer: Light to medium-brown macules that retain normal skin lines. Color is often uneven. Usually the lesions are 5 to 10 mm in size but occasionally may be slightly larger.

3. What are the secondary lesions that you would expect to find in solar lentigines?

Answer: Usually none.

4. What should you tell the patient about the solar lentigines?

Answer: Widespread solar lentigines are the result of chronic sun exposure, and generally are not treated. The patient should be warned about a small increased lifetime risk of melanoma, and should be counseled regarding sun avoidance, protective clothing, and use of sunscreen. Monthly self-examination based on the ABCD (**A**symmetry, irregular **B**orders, variegated **C**oloration, large **D**iameter) system should be advised along with yearly office follow-up and immediate follow-up for a changing lesion.

5. Is there any relationship between lentigines and melanoma?

Answer: Large numbers of solar lentigines have been reported as a significant independent risk factor for malignant melanoma. There is no established relationship between nonsolar lentigines and melanoma.

6. How are solar lentigines treated?

Answer: Generally solar lentigines are not treated.

28 Melanocytic Nevi

INTRODUCTION

The term *nevus*, used in its broadest sense, refers to any abnormality or irregularity attributed to heredity or embryonic development related to conception, gestation, or post-natal development. Within the discipline of dermatology, the term refers to a large number of congenital and acquired hamartomas of different tissue types, although it is used most often in the context of benign melanocytic neoplasms composed of pigment cells. Discussion will focus on the common mole or nevocellular nevus, and its most frequently encountered variants. This book will not attempt to cover all melanocytic nevi or even the entire spectrum of nevocellular nevi. The term *nevus* will be used interchangeably with the term *mole*.

CLINICAL APPLICATION QUESTIONS

A 34-year-old white roofer requests evaluation of a pigmented spot on his back, which he states is larger than his other moles. Although he currently practices reasonable sun avoidance and protection, in his youth he often worked without a shirt. Examination reveals a total of approximately 25 nevi scattered over his back, shoulders, and chest. These nevi show varying stages of maturation but nevi of similar stage resemble one another. The larger lesion is on his right scapular area. It is oval and measures 7 × 8 mm. The margin is sharp and even. The color is a uniform red-brown. The center is slightly raised on palpation but the skin lines are retained over the surface. There is no scale or other epidermal change.

1. What history questions should you ask this patient?
2. What should you ask this patient about the evolution of the larger lesion?
3. What are the primary lesions that you would expect to find in common benign nevi?
4. What are the secondary lesions that you would expect to find in common benign nevi?
5. Does this patient's physical exam suggest a form of atypical mole syndrome, and if so, why?
6. What should you tell the patient about the larger nevus?
7. Should the larger lesion be biopsied?

From: *Current Clinical Practice: Dermatology Skills for Primary Care: An Illustrated Guide*
D.J. Trozak, D.J. Tennenhouse, and J.J. Russell © Humana Press, Totowa, NJ

APPLICATION GUIDELINES: ACQUIRED MELANOCYTIC NEVI (MOLES)—COMMON BENIGN NEVI

Specific History

Onset

Common pigmented moles follow a defined evolution. At birth, only 1 to 2% of infants have an identifiable pigmented nevus. During the first decade of life, the number of moles increases rather slowly. At puberty and in the first half of the second decade, it is normal for this process to accelerate, and many new nevi appear. This proliferation often causes concern on the part of teenagers and their parents but is, in fact, a normal event provided the lesions themselves are clinically benign. New pigmented nevi also are common during pregnancy, and when combined with the physiologic darkening of preexisting moles during gestation, may cause patients to become unduly alarmed. All lesions of concern should be carefully evaluated and the patient advised and reassured.

Evolution of Disease Process and Skin Lesions

The common mole is composed of cells of neural crest origin, called nevus cells, which proliferate at the dermoepidermal junction, producing a benign neoplasm. Nevus cells have many of the properties of dendritic epidermal melanocytes but they also show distinctive morphological and functional differences. Like the dendritic melanocyte, they possess the organelles and enzyme systems to produce melanin pigment, which allows their presence to be distinguished from the adjacent epidermal surface. Unlike epidermal melanocytes, junctional nevus cells have an epithelioid-like appearance and lack dendrites.

The earliest stage in mole formation is a proliferation of nevus cells at the epidermal interface, which indents the epidermal base but does not raise, alter, or disturb its surface characteristics. The melanin produced defines the size and site of the lesion. Most acquired nevi in the first decade of life appear as small (5 mm or less) macular pigmented spots and are termed *junctional nevi.*

Some remain junctional for years, but in most instances the nevus cells continue to proliferate into the dermis and gradually push up on the overlying epidermis, effacing the skin lines or in some instances accentuating them. During this stage, the nevus will develop a raised component that may be visible and is definitely palpable. Nevus cells still form nests at the junction of dermis and epidermis, but with the added dermal component, this structure is now referred to as a *compound nevus.* This change, when it occurs in a gradual and orderly fashion, is reassuring and part of a benign evolutionary process. Compound nevi are typically dome-shaped with a smooth, shiny, or mammillated surface. As this maturation advances, the surface area of the nevus enlarges. In addition, the rate of pigment production in the dermal nevus cells may diminish; this combined effect often produces an overall lightening of the nevus. The effect is much like that seen when blowing up a red balloon. The balloon is still an even red, but the color has a lighter tint and appears more diluted due to the increased surface relative to the same amount of red pigment. The progression of moles from junctional to compound types may begin during the first decade of life and is usually firmly established by the middle of the second decade. This process continues well into middle life.

By the fourth and fifth decades, many nevi mature even further into dermal nevi. Within a dermal nevus, the cellular proliferation at the dermal–epidermal junction disappears and the nevus cells are predominantly, if not exclusively, intradermal. Dermal moles may be clinically indistinguishable from compound moles. With time, dermal nevi mature and often become flaccid, soft, and pedunculated. They may then resemble a common skin tag.

Nevi normally increase in number until the end of the fourth decade of life, when they reach a peak average of 43 per person in men and 27 per person in women of light skin type. There is considerable normal variation among individuals, and degrees of moliness are often consistent within family units. Heavily pigmented skin types have fewer moles per person. Except for the familial atypical mole syndromes (*see* section on atypical nevus syndromes, below), specific inheritance patterns and markers have not been determined. From the fourth decade of life on, nevi gradually undergo spontaneous resolution and mole counts of patients in their eighth decades of life and beyond are quite low. Most nevi resolve without a visible trace, while others fibrose into lesions clinically and microscopically indistinguishable from fibrous skin tags.

Provoking Factors

Puberty, pregnancy, and exogenous hormone administration have all been associated with rapid proliferation of nevocellular nevi. Mole-prone families usually exhibit greater numbers on sun-exposed skin with a relative paucity of nevi on covered and doubly covered regions. It is reported that heavy childhood sun exposure is a factor in the development of some moles.

Self-Medication

Self-treatment is seldom a problem in regard to pigmented nevi.

Supplemental Review From General History

Personal and family history relative to malignant melanoma should be obtained when evaluating pigmented nevi. History regarding pregnancy and recent hormonal therapy may also be relevant. When evaluating facial nevi in female subjects, history regarding hair growth and attempts at plucking or removing hair from the mole may be important. Traumatic epilation of hair can produce benign inflammatory changes that are more easily confused with malignancy.

Dermatologic Physical Exam

Primary Lesions

Junctional nevi: These are pigmented macules usually, 5 mm or less, which vary from tan to very dark brown. Skin surface lines are retained and the margins are even. Color is uniform and the shape is round to oval (*see* Photos 7,17).

Early compound nevi: These are dome-shaped papules that may retain skin lines or may have a smooth effaced surface. In early lesions, the macular junctional origin is evident at the margin of the central papular compound portion. Color in the raised region may be uniformly lighter because of relative dilution of pigment over the larger surface area (*see* Photo 8).

Developed compound nevi: These are minimally raised plaques, round to oval in shape. They are evenly colored tan to dark brown, and may have diminished, normal, or accentuated skin markings. Margins are usually smooth and distinct. Size is usually 6 mm or less (*see* Photo 7).

Mature compound and developed dermal nevi: Both types of moles may have a clinically identical appearance consisting of round or oval dome-shaped sharply demarcated papules with a smooth shiny surface and effaced skin lines. Color may vary from white to flesh-toned to medium brown. Shades of light tan are most common (*see* Photo 8).

Mature dermal nevi: These are pedunculated, soft papules with a wrinkled, flaccid appearance. Color may vary from flesh tones to medium tan, with light tan shades most common. Distinction from fleshy skin tags may not be possible on clinical grounds alone (*see* Photos 9,10).

Secondary Lesions

Papillomatosis: Some compound nevi have a pebbly or mammillated surface due to distortion of the epidermis by the dermal nevus cells. In its extreme form, this can cause clefting and give a cerebriform appearance. This surface change is especially common with compound nevi located on the scalp (*see* Photo 11).

Scale: A fine hyperkeratotic scale may be a normal finding in some compound moles (*see* Photo 12).

Hair growth: The presence of coarse, dark hairs longer than those in the adjacent skin is a normal finding and indicates a mature nevus (*see* Photo 13).

Comedo: Comedo formation in hair follicles may produce surface irregularity and speckling, but is a benign incidental change (*see* Photo 14).

Distribution

Microdistribution: None.

Macrodistribution: Moles may show some predilection for areas of heavy solar exposure in certain persons; however, usual distribution is generalized and random.

Configuration

None.

Indicated Supporting Diagnostic Data

Microscopic Examination

Whether a pigmented lesion is biopsied because of irregularity or removed for cosmetic purposes, the tissue should always be submitted for microscopic examination. Neglecting the microscopic examination is an open invitation to a future malpractice action simply because the practitioner is unable to prove what was removed. In addition, benign-appearing nevi may, on rare occasions, have clinically inapparent foci of malignant change; the microscopic examination then becomes a potentially lifesaving action. Be certain someone trained in cutaneous pathology examines the tissue. If a report is hedgy or uncertain, request a reading by several fully trained dermatopathologists. Most skin pathologists will automatically seek a consensus on pigmented lesions that are difficult to assess.

Therapy

Pigmented nevi are removed for basically three reasons: (1) elective cosmetic excision, (2) elective excision because of an inconvenient location or persistent but otherwise benign symptoms, or (3) nonelective removal for features suggesting possible malignant transformation. Techniques vary depending on the indication, location, type of lesion, and the patient's preference.

Elective Cosmetic Excision

This is accomplished by several techniques. Because of the elective nature of the procedure, the patient must be fully informed of the pros and cons of each method and the small risk that the result may be less satisfactory than the existing lesion.

Shave or tangential excision: This is rapid and produces minimal scarring when properly performed. This method is useful only on raised compound or dermal nevi, and is best reserved for fairly mature lesions to minimize the risk of clinical recurrence. The nevus is anesthetized with 1% lidocaine and is then carefully shaved off at the base with a no. 15 scalpel. With the hyfrecator at its lowest setting, the raw base is gently desiccated and then very gently contoured with a small sharp dermal or ear curette to match the adjacent epidermis. The resulting crust should be left to separate on its own, and in time most of these scars are barely visible. This technique is not recommended in preteen or midteen patients because their nevi are usually still actively growing and the recurrence rate is high. Shave removal is also not ideal in facial moles where the patient's desire is to remove the mole and the unsightly hairs. Often the follicle root extends lower than the base of the lesion and the hairs then promptly recur. Whenever a hair-bearing mole is superficially removed the patient should be warned about this possibility. Because shave excision is a partial removal, the patient must be carefully informed. If desire is total excision, then another technique should be used.

Punch excision and suturing: This is a second alternative, which offers the advantage of total removal and minimal scarring if the location is properly chosen. This method works best on areas of lax skin, and is especially useful in crease lines and in loose skin on the face. A circular biopsy punch is chosen that is 1 to 2 mm larger than the lesion. The lesion is then punched out in its entirety removing the full thickness of the dermis and 2 to 3 mm of the upper subcutaneous fat. The resultant circular defect is sutured into a straight line and, if the site is properly chosen, minimal puckering will result. With a small lesion in a lax area, a larger punch can be chosen, and by stretching the skin during the punch, an oval defect will result, which is even easier to close. The direction of the defect should be oriented to fit the surgical lines of election or the anatomy of the specific site. Best results are obtained with 3- to 6-mm punches. On occasion, in very lax regions, a reasonable closure can be obtained from an 8-mm punch. Beyond this size, elliptical excision is recommended. Properly performed, this method totally removes the nevus and any coarse hair follicles. Junctional or minimally raised compound nevi can also be removed by this procedure. The disadvantages are a somewhat more noticeable scar and a greater risk of thick scarring because of the degree of injury. On the chest, back, and abdomen, scars with this method have a tendency to spread.

Elliptical excision with a complex layered closure: When total removal is desired and the techniques described above are not applicable, elliptical excision with a complex layered closure to minimize scarring is indicated. With benign lesions, a 1- to 2-mm clinical margin is acceptable. Elective removal is also frequently performed when moles are inconveniently located or subject to repeated injury. Examples would be a raised nevus on the mid-nose interfering with conjugate vision, a lesion on the beard area subject to nicking while shaving, or a mole at the beltline that is raised and subject to chronic friction. There is no evidence to support claims in the older literature that repetitive trauma causes malignancy. The methods and precautions are essentially the same as for cosmetic removal.

Subneval folliculitis treatment: Subneval folliculitis is a frequently encountered and misunderstood change that occurs in raised, hair-bearing nevi. Follicular rupture, pimple formation, or ingrown hairs from plucking can cause rapid apparent growth in a nevus, which is usually accompanied by tenderness, erythema, and occasionally discharge of purulent matter and a small amount of blood. This change, although alarming, is perfectly benign and is rarely a reason for excision provided the mole returns to its original size and appearance within 3 to 4 weeks. If the patient has been plucking terminal hairs, an alternate method of removal, such as shaving or clipping, should be encouraged. If there is substantial acne present, it should be treated. In rare instances where there are frequent recurrent episodes, elective removal is justified for the patient's peace of mind. When subneval folliculitis is suspected but the mole fails to settle back to normal within a month, conservative excisional biopsy and microscopic examination are indicated.

Nonelective Excision

Nonelective removal of an atypical or suspicious pigmented lesion should always aim at total excision with a conservative clear margin. Specifics are discussed in the therapy section for primary melanoma. Exceptions to this rule are suspected lentigo maligna melanoma and acral lentiginous mucosal melanoma. Both will also be discussed later. Because melanoma prognosis correlates well with Breslow levels of microscopic invasion, subsequent surgical treatment recommendations are made from those readings. Microscopic assessment depends on examination of the entire lesion, and shave or punch biopsy specimens do not provide an optimal specimen. A shave biopsy of a suspect lesion can destroy the anatomic features needed for that evaluation. In the rare instance when a punch biopsy from a suspected melanoma may be indicated, a dermatologic consultant should make that decision. Despite warnings in the older literature, there is a body of evidence that punch biopsy or incision into a melanoma does not alter the patient's prognosis.

Conditions That May Simulate Common Nevi
Benign Nonsolar Lentigo

A benign nonsolar lentigo may be absolutely indistinguishable on clinical exam from a benign junctional nevus. Unless either lesion is irregular or changing, the distinction is academic. Solar lentigines are larger and more irregular, and are not easily confused.

Seborrheic Keratosis

SKs can almost always be distinguished from nevocellular moles on clinical exam. Their surface is dull and waxy or soft to the touch. They have a pasted or stuck-on appearance, and colors tend toward gray-tan or yellow-tan rather than the tan and true browns of the nevus. On rare occasions, the two cannot be separated except by biopsy.

Basal Cell Carcinoma

Small nodular basal cell carcinomas and small minimally pigmented dome-shaped compound or dermal nevi may be difficult to distinguish clinically. Helpful (but not absolute) signs are the translucency of the basal cell and the small dilated vessels that often course irregularly over its surface. A centrally located indentation or "dell" favors the basal cell carcinoma. In addition, there is an uncommon type of pigmented basal cell carcinoma that can sometimes simulate a pigmented nevus or melanoma. A dermatologic consultant can usually tell on clinical exam or advise as to the appropriate approach.

Dermatofibromas

These common fibrous growths occur at frequent sites of blunt trauma such as the shins, shoulders, and upper back. They are usually 6 mm or less in size, and often develop a smudgy tan pigmentation over their surface. They can be distinguished clinically from true moles by their firm feel, "like a button under the skin surface." Also they often show a positive "pucker" sign: with lateral compression between the examining fingers, the lesion puckers downward. A variant, the sclerosing hemangioma, has irregular blue-black pigmentation, and can be clinically confused with a nevus or melanoma.

APPLICATION GUIDELINES: ACQUIRED MELANOCYTIC NEVI (MOLES)—HALO NEVI (SUTTON'S NEVI)

Specific History

Onset

This variant of the common mole is striking in its appearance and evolution. Uncommon but not rare, they are seen most often in preteens and teenagers, and less frequently in young adults. Appearance of a halo nevus past age 30 is an indication for careful observation and excisional biopsy of the pigmented nevus portion if there is an irregularity of the nevus or the surrounding halo.

Evolution of Disease Process

A halo of pink or white depigmentation suddenly develops around one or occasionally several established nevocellular nevi. The area of pigment loss is absolute and usually surrounds the mole in a symmetric fashion. Edges of the halo are regular and smooth. It extends several millimeters from the edge of the nevus and stabilizes in size. Over the next few months the nevus will become fuzzy and indistinct and will gradually fade and disappear, often without a trace either clinically or microscopically. The halo may persist or gradually repigment, and there may ultimately be no trace of the event.

Evolution of Skin Lesions

See Evolution of Disease Process section.

Provoking Factors

None.

Self-Medication

Self-treatment is not a problem.

Supplemental Review From General History

A personal or family history of melanoma, atypical (dysplastic) nevi, or other nevi that are changing or symptomatic should spur careful observation.

Dermatologic Physical Exam

Primary Lesions

A common nevocellular, usually compound type (papule), surrounded by a symmetric halo (macule) of totally depigmented but otherwise normal skin that is white or pink, depending on the degree of inflammation (*see* Photo 15).

Secondary Lesions

Macular depigmentation (*see* Photo 16).

Distribution

Microdistribution: None.

Macrodistribution: May occur at any site of a pre-existing nevocellular nevus. This nevus is most common over the back and shoulders.

Configuration

Iris (e.g., concentric rings).

Indicated Supporting Diagnostic Data

None.

Therapy

Halo nevi are benign moles in the process of undergoing an immunologically induced regression. No therapy is indicated unless the nevus or halo shows distinct irregularities. There have been case reports of halo melanomas, but these are exceedingly rare. A personal or family history of melanoma or atypical (dysplastic) nevi should prompt careful observation to be certain the lesion follows the usual course. Similar precautions should be followed when a halo mole presents in a person over 30 years of age.

Conditions That May Simulate a Halo Nevus
Halo Melanoma

Halo nevi usually develop fuzzy edges and gradually fade from brown to tan to pink as they regress. Despite these changes, they remain round or oval in shape and the halo tends to mimic the shape of the evolving nevus. A halo around a melanoma tends to mimic the irregular shape of the tumor.

APPLICATION GUIDELINES: ACQUIRED MELANOCYTIC NEVI (MOLES)—ATYPICAL NEVI AND ATYPICAL NEVUS SYNDROMES

Introduction

Alternate terms for atypical nevus syndromes include B-K mole syndrome, familial atypical multiple mole melanoma syndrome, dysplastic nevus syndrome, and sporadic dysplastic nevus syndrome.

This concept was first introduced into the literature in 1978 with independent and simultaneous reports by two different investigators. The multiple designations are a result of a disease concept that is in evolution. A National Institutes of Health (NIH) conference has settled on the clinical term "atypical" rather than the histologic term "dysplastic," which was felt to be confusing and poorly defined. Whether these syndromes will eventually be defined as a group of distinct entities with the common feature of an atypical melanocytic nevus, or a continuum of disease with a variable risk for malignant melanoma, remains to be seen.

Specific History

Onset

During the second and third decades, patients with "classic" atypical mole syndrome (AMS) acquire large numbers of nevocellular nevi (100 or more). In addition to the conspicuous numbers, these moles are strikingly different from one another in their clinical appearance. These atypical nevi are variable because they exhibit many of the clinical warning signs of malignant melanoma, referred to as the "ABCD"s. They often:

A. Are **A**symmetric.
B. Have irregular **B**orders.
C. Display irregular variegated **C**oloration.
D. Are usually greater than 6 mm in **D**iameter, the size of a pencil eraser.

Their surfaces are mammillated and, unlike most mature common moles, they retain a macular component at the margins. Atypical nevi are also microscopically different and display a constellation of microscopic features and an absence of maturation, which distinguishes them from the common benign nevus. It should be noted that clinically atypical nevi are not always microscopically atypical, and vice versa. Any patient who, on physical exam, displays a striking mole pattern or has individual moles with these characteristics should be evaluated with this diagnosis in mind. The number of persons in the white population with these atypical nevi is estimated at 2 to 8%, and they may contribute disproportionately to the incidence of malignant melanoma.

Evolution of Disease Process

Unlike the person with an abundance of common moles, patients with "classic" atypical mole syndrome continue to develop new pigmented nevi past middle age. Most of their clinically atypical moles remain stable, while a small number gradually increase in size and show increased atypicality. Some lesions have been documented by serial photography to regress and disappear, and there have been a number of instances in which changing atypical nevi have been excised and confirmed to be malignant melanomas. Despite these reports, there has been ongoing debate as to the actual biologic potential of these atypical nevi. Whatever the true potential of the atypical mole as an actual precursor lesion, there is no question that they identify a significant population of persons with a substantially elevated risk of malignant melanoma.

As noted at the beginning of this section, this entity has been reported under a number of designations and there is a continuum of involvement with differing degrees of melanoma risk. At the low end of the spectrum are patients with a single or a few sporadic atypical moles but without an abnormal mole pattern, a personal or family history of melanoma, or relatives with an abnormal mole pattern. These individuals appear to have an increased risk of melanoma over the general population of approximately four- to sixfold.

At the high end are patients with "classic" changes with or without a personal history of melanoma, but with a family history of others with the nevus pattern and melanoma in two or more first- or second-degree relatives. Some investigators estimate their lifetime risk of melanoma as approaching 100%. "Classic" atypical mole syndrome is currently defined with the following criteria:

1. One hundred or more nevi.
2. One or more nevi 8 mm or larger.
3. One or more atypical nevi showing the clinical features mentioned above.

These patients appear to have approximately a 100- to 200-fold risk of melanoma compared to similar populations without atypical moles. Patients with "classic" features but without a family history are felt to be at a lower but still very significant risk. Patients with smaller numbers of moles, smaller diameter moles, or moles that exhibit lesser degrees of clinical atypicality are probably at intermediate risk. It will be several years before the risk factors and categories are definitively worked out. It is important to note also that persons with melanoma in this setting are at substantial risk of developing additional primaries.

Evolution of Skin Lesions

See Evolution of Disease Process section.

Provoking Factors

In some patients, AMS is unquestionably a hereditary trait. Solar exposure might be a factor in stimulating increased numbers of atypical moles or subsequent malignant change.

Self-Medication

Self-treatment is not a problem in AMS.

Supplemental Review From General History

Personal and family history for atypical (dysplastic) moles and melanomas should be recorded. Family history of other malignancies should also be recorded, although at present this is not clearly established as an added risk factor. Other features that should be recorded are tendency to sunburn, lifetime tendencies for solar exposure, and use of sunscreens and solar protection.

Dermatologic Physical Exam
Primary Lesions

The primary lesions of atypical mole syndrome consist of irregular pigmented macules, macules with a papular component, or plaques with a macular periphery. The nevi are strikingly dissimilar in shape and size and have variegated colors of reds, tans, blacks, and browns. Many are larger than the usual 6 mm, often 1.5 cm or larger. The raised component is minimal compared to the diameter, and the irregular macular margin blurs with the adjacent skin. One, several, or a hundred or more nevi may be present. The surface is typically rough or mammillated (*see* Photos 17,18).

Secondary Lesions

Secondary changes of scaling, crusting, erosion, ulceration, or scarring would suggest malignant change in an atypical nevus.

Distribution

Microdistribution: None.

Macrodistribution: Atypical moles may be widely distributed, but show a predilection for the upper and mid-truncal regions (*see* Photos 19,20).

Configuration

In some patients with large numbers of moles, there is suggestion of a dermatome pattern.

Indicated Supporting Diagnostic Data
Biopsy

It has been recommended that the diagnosis of AMS be confirmed by the microscopic examination of two of the clinically atypical nevi. In clinically typical cases, especially those with a strong family history, this seems excessive. Recent papers have argued that in many patients the diagnosis can be reliably made on the basis of clinical features alone. When there is doubt, biopsy of the most atypical lesions should be performed. This should be a conservative but complete excisional biopsy. The lateral margins usually contain the most characteristic histology. Whenever changes occur that suggest possible evolution to melanoma, a similar complete excisional biopsy is indicated.

Therapy
Education

Patient education is the most important tool in the prevention of melanoma deaths with this syndrome. Despite intensive physician follow-up, informed patients performing regular self-examinations have a much better chance of identifying a developing melanoma simply because of their proximity to the problem.

Atypical mole patients should be carefully instructed in methods of monthly self-examination of all pigmented lesions. Prompt action and the reasons for it must be made very clear. To aid in this education process, there are color brochures available from the American Academy of Dermatology with life-size photos of melanomas, a review of the ABCDs, and self-examination directions. During follow-up physician exams, hidden moles or those in locations likely to be overlooked should be pointed out to the patient so that they will be evaluated during self-examination.

Proper sun avoidance and physical protection with a hat and clothing should be discussed and emphasized, and the patient should be given a sample of an effective sunscreen. A product that contains the UVA blocking agent Parsol® and an SPF number of at least 30 is recommended. Since the vast majority of these patients survive their melanomas, it is critical to approach this situation in a positive fashion and enlist their help rather than discourage or frighten them.

Where history suggests a familial link, first- and second-degree relatives should be advised to have an examination and should forewarn the examiner of the reason. Children from these families should be taught how to minimize sun exposure and use a sunscreen regularly. In their early teen years they should be assessed, and if the syndrome is present, they should also be placed on regular follow-up.

Early manifestation of the syndrome may be marked by an increased number of banal-appearing nevi toward the end of the first decade. During the second decade of life, nevi in patients with atypical mole syndrome will acquire their striking characteristics. Even in the absence of signs, persons from these families should practice careful sun avoidance and protection, and promptly seek advice for any changing pigmented lesions.

Follow-Up

Atypical nevus patients are worrisome and inherently difficult to follow. Unless a practitioner has special expertise in this area, follow-up is best deferred to a dermatologic consultant. High-risk patients should receive a head-to-toe total mole examination on a 3- to 4-month basis. Intermediate-risk patients should be similarly examined every 6 months, whereas low-risk patients should be seen every 12 months. Irrespective of grouping, all atypical mole patients are instructed to come in immediately with any rapidly changing mole. There are reports in the literature of an increased risk of ocular and mucosal melanomas in these patients. Exams should include an external eye exam and examination of easily accessible mucous membranes. Patients should be advised to alert their ophthamologist and obtain periodic funduscopic exams. Female patients should be offered the option of a speculum exam or alert their gynecologist to watch for changing pigmented lesions of the vaginal mucosa.

Excision

Any pigmented lesions that show rapid growth or decisive changes that suggest malignancy should be excised with a clear clinical margin in all directions. It is very important to include the peripheral macular portion, which may be fairly indistinct. This margin can often be defined by a Wood's lamp exam in a darkened room. Although some physicians will remove these nevi by deep shave excision, we discourage this procedure for any suspect pigmented lesion. Elliptical excision with margins up to, but not through, the superficial fascia is the recommended technique. It is too easy to miss a deep margin with shave excision, and, in the event that a melanoma is removed, the deep component is needed for the Breslow measurement, which determines prognosis. Failure to perform an adequate biopsy may needlessly commit the patient to a more mutilating reexcision. Wholesale excision of large numbers of atypical but otherwise stable nevi is not recommended for the following reasons:

1. There is no way at present to tell which lesions will progress to melanoma.
2. In patients with large numbers of lesions, the process of excision would be mutilating and extremely expensive.
3. At present, it is uncertain what proportion of melanomas arise from the atypical moles versus those that form *de novo*.
4. Because these patients develop new nevi throughout their lives, wholesale excision will not resolve the problem.
5. The statistical risk of an individual atypical mole turning into melanoma is estimated at 1 in 10,000.

Conditions That May Simulate Atypical Nevi

Solar Lentigines/Common Nevi

Persons with large numbers of solar lentigines or an abundance of common nevi over their upper torso may, on initial inspection, appear to have this syndrome. Solar lentigines are monotonous and show similar size and coloration. In addition, color tends to be constant throughout each individual lesion. Common nevi also tend to resemble one another in a given individual. They do not show the variable warning signs (ABCDs) of melanoma. Common nevi generally are 6 mm or less in size.

Although the risk is not as high as in atypical nevus syndrome, there is evidence that the presence of large numbers of uniform, small, darkly pigmented nevi, the "cheetah phenotype," is also a marker for increased melanoma risk.These moles individually resemble nonsolar lentigines, but the profusion of lesions is very striking.

APPLICATION GUIDELINES: CONGENITAL MELANOCYTIC NEVI AND ACQUIRED "CONGENITAL PATTERN" MELANOCYTIC NEVI

Introduction

During the past two decades there has been a great deal of discussion and investigative effort expended regarding the definition and role of congenital moles as precursor lesions for malignant melanoma in children. Contrary to reports in the older literature, 0.3 to 0.5% of all melanomas occur in children under age 13 years. Although childhood melanoma is rare, there is no absolute safe age range. About two-thirds of childhood melanomas arise *de novo* and these tumors have a biological course and potential similar to adult melanomas of similar thickness, level and staging. Approximately 3% of childhood melanomas arise in a large congenital melanocytic nevus (also called "giant nevus," "garment nevus," and "bathing trunk nevus"), and half of these occur by age 3 years. Because the malignancies often arise deep in the nevus, clinical signs are often absent until after spread has occurred, and the overall 5-year survival figures are abysmal. The focus on these large precursor lesions has spawned a raging debate over the lifetime malignant potential of more commonly occurring small and medium-sized congenital melanotic moles that are clinically and histologically similar to the larger ones. Subsequent studies have identified an even more common acquired childhood nevus that shares clinical and microscopic features with those that are present at birth. These acquired "congenital pattern" moles may, because of their frequency, be more important as an overall lifetime melanoma precursor. This is a complicated issue, which must be handled in an open yet sensitive fashion. At this time the potential of the large congenital nevi is fairly well established. Statistics regarding the true malignant threat from small and medium congenital nevi and the acquired lesions are still speculative. Therefore, there are no hard and fast answers in regard to treatment. Because these are often striking lesions, the question regarding their proper treatment will arise with some frequency in any practice that sees a significant pediatric population.

Specific History

Onset

Congenital nevi are by definition present at birth; multiple studies confirm the presence of a pigmented mole in 1% of the newborn population. The vast majority of congenital nevi are the small type. In clinical practice, isolated medium-sized lesions are rarely encountered. Large congenital moles are very rare, and are estimated to occur in 1 of every 20,000 live births. Current nomenclature is based on their size during infancy.

- Large congenital melanotic nevus (LCMN): >20 cm diameter
- Medium congenital melanotic nevus (MCMN): 1.5 to 20 cm diameter
- Small congenital melanotic nevus (SCMN): <1.5 cm diameter

As moles are basically benign hamartomas composed predominantly of nevus cells, it is not surprising that congenital nevi have an acquired counterpart. Some of the other benign hamartomas of skin first appear after birth. In a population of newborns who were examined and found to be free of pigmented nevi at birth, a reevaluation at 2 to 3 years revealed moles in 25%, and half of these "acquired" lesions showed a "congenital pattern" on microscopy. These acquired congenital-pattern melonotic nevi (AcpN) were also clinically different from common acquired moles, tending to be larger in size and with speckles and variegated color. This report has established AcpN as a distinct entity. At the present time their true incidence is unknown because it is uncertain how late in life they may continue to appear. Other benign hamartomas, such as Becker's nevus, for example, may not become clinically apparent until well into early adulthood.

Evolution of Disease Process

LCMN are striking lesions, which often cover major anatomic areas. This explains the many descriptive eponyms listed above. These nevi usually change during infancy and childhood. After birth, the lesions may extend, but for the most part their growth is concordant with that of the child. It is common for them to become thickened and rugose; these features are especially common when they occur over the scalp. Several small or medium-sized satellite CMN are common in the same infant, and these may be spread over wide anatomic areas. As the child matures, the color of the LCMN often lightens;

however, at puberty the hairs on their surface become coarser, darker, and more noticeable. About 20% of patients experience varying degrees of chronic pruritus. Nodular and lobular areas may develop due to growth of the nevus or the occurrence of other hamartomas within the mole. In a small percentage of cases, total regression has been reported; one of the authors has personally seen two cases of regressed MCMN and is following a patient with a LCMN where several medium-sized satellites have regressed along with substantial regression of the main lesion.

LCMN are without question potential precursor lesions for malignant melanoma. The incidence of malignant change is quoted from 5 to 20% over a lifetime. At present the true incidence appears to be 5 to 15%. Half of these melanomas occur before age 3 years. Malignancies often arise deep in the mole, masking the early clinical signs for melanoma. The benign evolutionary changes described, and the presence of other benign tumors arising inside the nevus, make these lesions extremely difficult to follow.

Small and medium-sized CMN generally grow concordantly with the individual. These are often striking lesions and the majority of teen-aged and adult victims consider them "ugly" or embarrassing. Like the large version, they tend to become hairier, coarser, and more noticeable with age. These nevi may lighten in color, but also may become more raised and mammillated. Confirmed reports of melanoma arising in these smaller CMN are published, and although the lifetime risk appears to be much smaller than with the large type, the risk is not nonexistent. One study calculated a 21-fold lifetime risk based on historical information regarding a preexisting birth lesion. The same report calculates a 3- to 10-fold increased lifetime risk based on histologic findings. All previous attempts at quantifying the incidence fail to take into account the more common AcpN. Some investigators suggest that malignant change in a SCMN is very rare in the first two decades of life. Again, however, reports of such change exist and it should be recalled that it was only a few decades ago that the common wisdom considered all childhood melanoma to be nonexistent.

Evolution of Skin Lesions

See Evolution of Disease Process section above.

Provoking Factors

None.

Self-Medication

Self-treatment is not a problem.

Supplemental Review From General History

None indicated.

Dermatologic Physical Exam

Primary Lesions

Plaques of pigmented skin lesions are generally palpably raised above the adjacent normal skin. Color may vary from light brown to brown-black. Dark brown is usual. The surface may be smooth, mammillated, lobulated, or thrown into deep folds (rugose). Areas of speckling are common, especially with small CMN, medium CMN, and the acquired type. Margins are usually distinct. Sizes of CMN were discussed earlier. AcpN tend to be between 0.4 and 1.2 cm in size (*see* Photos 21–24).

Secondary Lesions

Hypertrichosis in the form of longer more terminal type hair growth is usually noted even in the early course of CMN. This hair growth tends to become coarser, darker, and more prominent with age (*see* Photo 21). Hairiness is not always present (*see* Photo 22). Hairiness is not mentioned as a clinical feature of AcpN (*see* Photo 24).

Diffuse erythema that is most evident at the nevus margin occurs with active regression (*see* Photo 25).

Diffuse induration throughout the nevus may occur during periods of active regression (*see* Photo 25).

Erosions may occur from excoriation due to pruritus from regression or may signal malignant changes.

Secondary nodules, tumors, or ulcerations may signal the presence of melanoma or other benign or malignant hamartomas within the nevus. Hamartomas of nonnevus cell derivation are reported with the LCMN.

Distribution

Microdistribution: None.

Macrodistribution: SCMN, MCMN, and AcpN are randomly distributed on the skin surface and may occur at any site. LCMN are often distributed over a large region, such as on the scalp, upper neck, and shoulders, or on the lower back, buttocks, genitalia, and proximal thighs. They may also cover a major anatomic structure such as a limb. This is the source of eponyms such as "shawl nevi," "bathing trunk nevi," and "garment nevi" (*see* Photo 25).

Configuration

None.

Indicated Supporting Diagnostic Data

Biopsy

LCMN are clinically self-evident; tissue examination is done only at the time of definitive excision or when changes within them suggest the possibility of malignancy. In addition to malignant melanoma, benign and malignant hamartomas and active nevus regression can produce symptomatic change in these lesions. A well-placed punch or small wedge biopsy may be indicated before a major procedure is undertaken.

SCMN, MCMN, and AcpN can occasionally be confused with other benign pigmented lesions. In most instances a dermatologic consultant can tell the difference on physical examination. If this is not possible on physical examination alone, a punch biopsy and tissue exam are indicated provided the differential is between benign lesions.

MRI Scans

LCMN located over the scalp, upper back, or spinal column may involve portions of the spinal cord and central nervous system (CNS). Proliferation of nevus cells can, in rare instances, cause hydrocephalus and seizures. In addition, melanoma can arise in the CNS portions of the mole. Magnetic resonance imaging (MRI) can delineate this involvement and explain these neurologic findings. Furthermore, when making a decision regarding removal of one of these lesions, the presence of CNS involvement may, for the family, be an important part of the decision process.

Therapy

Removal of LCMN

The only definitive treatment for any pigmented nevus is complete surgical excision. Since LCMN are clearly significant precursor lesions, there is currently general, but not universal, agreement that these lesions should, if possible, be totally excised at the earliest feasible time. New tissue expansion techniques now allow coverage and closures that were not possible a few years ago. Some authorities have proposed dermabrasion or shave removal of the upper parts of the mole as a means of reducing the tumor load and the risk of melanoma. They also report substantial cosmetic improvement in the appearance of the lesions. Since many of the melanomas arise deep in the nevus, this type of procedure should be reserved for technically nonresectable lesions, or, if used for partial removal, parents should be carefully and fully informed.

The decision to remove an extensive CMN is a difficult one, and is a substantial monetary and emotional burden on the family. It is important to first relieve the parents of any personal guilt feelings and to make it clear to them that there is no "ideal" solution. Because melanoma often occurs deep in these lesions, the most meticulous clinical follow-up may not detect change soon enough. Parents must be informed regarding the risks of surgical complications versus malignant change, and they must be advised there is no absolute "safe" waiting period. It is important to identify any CNS involvement, as its presence may affect the overall decision. Emotional aspects of extensive surgery on an infant must be balanced against the long-term emotional burden of the appearance of the nevus and the lifelong threat of malignant change. If a family decides against removal, they should be given strong support for having made a wrenching and courageous decision.

When a decision is made to defer or avoid removal, regular follow-up exams should be established. These may be frequent at first while the parents are being educated in regard to changes, and may be spread out to yearly exams when the mole is stable and the parents are informed and more comfortable with it. Any sudden change or symptom should be reported, and the mole examined as soon as possible.

Removal of SCMN, MCMN, and AcpN

Removal of SCMN, MCMN, and AcpN is at the present time a very controversial issue. Although the contribution of these nevi to the sum total of all melanomas may be far greater than that of LCMN, the risk of an individual lesion changing appears to be much lower. One school argues that this is an emotional issue and that the same parameters are not applied to other potential precursor lesions. Another school argues that the lifetime follow-up of these lesions exceeds the cost of excision, and if one adds the morbidity and cost of even a few melanomas, the difference is even greater. At the present time there are no definitive statistics on which to base the decision.

Try to inform parents regarding the controversy and the issues involved. They need to know that the overall risk is low but continues as long as the mole is present. It is essential that they understand the gravity and urgency of a malignant change and the reasons why clinical follow-up could fail. Accurately document this discussion. Although melanoma seems to occur later in these smaller nevi, there is no safe waiting period. It is also important to discuss with the parents the cosmetic issues, which can be a significant deciding factor. Adequate discussion will allow the parents to make an intelligent and informed decision. In the future there will be better definition, clearer statistics, or other markers available to predict malignant potential. This will allow us to be more selective in this process. Do not criticize parents who wish to defer active intervention. Follow-up should then be similar to that with a LCMN, and should consist of a combination of practitioner observation and parental education.

Conditions That May Simulate CMN/AcpN

LCMN are clinically diagnostic. The following differential applies mainly to SCMN, MCMN, and AcpN.

Common Benign Nevi (Moles)

Common moles are usually smaller than congenital-type nevi and generally have lighter shades of tan or brown color. They rarely exceed 5 mm in size during childhood and are symmetric and sharply demarcated. Visible hair growth is absent until adulthood, and even then consists of a few terminal hairs. The distinction is mainly between SCMN and AcpN. The histology pattern is different.

Café-au-Lait and Coast of Maine Spots

Both of these pigmented spots are light tan, macular, and evenly pigmented. The café-au-lait spots are usually multiple but when single could be confused with a lightly colored SCMN or an AcpN. They are usually oval with smooth sharp borders. Coast of Maine spots are larger and could be confused with a MCMN. These lesions are irregular in shape and typically have irregular or serrated borders. Neither lesion shows nevus cells on biopsy.

Mongolian Spot, Nevus of Ota, and Nevus of Ito

The distribution of these three melanocytic birthmarks is similar to that of a LCMN. All three of these lesions share common histology consisting of dendritic melanocytes in the mid-dermis. Nevus cells are not present. Borders are irregular and indistinct and the color is blue-gray to blue-black. Mongolian spots occur on the low back and presacral region. Nevus of Ota involves skin in the distribution of the first and second branches of the trigeminal nerve, and the ocular conjunctiva and iris. Nevus of Ito is found in the skin over the shoulder and upper chest.

Epithelial Nevi

Hamartomas of epidermal elements also can produce tan or brown raised surface lesions that could resemble the congenital-type nevi. These lesions are usually linear and follow the lines of Blaschko. The borders are distinct and the surface is raised and rough. Biopsy shows a proliferation of epithelial elements. Nevus cells are absent.

ANSWERS TO CLINICAL APPLICATION QUESTIONS

History Review

A 34-year-old white roofer requests evaluation of a pigmented spot on his back which he states is larger than his other moles. Although he currently practices reasonable sun avoidance and protection, in his youth he often worked without a shirt. Examination reveals a total of approximately 25 nevi scattered over his back, shoulders, and chest. These nevi show varying stages of maturation but nevi of similar stage resemble one another. The larger lesion is on his right scapular area. It is oval and measures 7 × 8 mm. The margin is sharp and even. The color is a uniform red-brown. The center is slightly raised on palpation but the skin lines are retained over the surface. There is no scale or other epidermal change.

1. What history questions should you ask this patient?

Answer: The patient should be asked if there is any personal or family history of malignant melanoma.

2. What should you ask this patient about the evolution of the larger lesion?

Answer: The patient should be asked if there was any recent or sudden change in appearance of the lesion (size, shape, border, or color) or symptoms (bleeding, crusting, etc.).

3. What are the primary lesions that you would expect to find in common benign nevi?

Answer: Uniformly colored macules, dome-shaped papules that are smooth and have retained skin lines, uniformly colored plaques, and pedunculated soft papules may all be found in common benign nevi.

4. What are the secondary lesions that you would expect to find in common benign nevi?

Answer: Papillomatosis, fine hyperkeratotic scale, hypertrichosis, and comedones may all be found in common benign nevi.

5. Does this patient's physical exam suggest a form of atypical mole syndrome, and if so, why?

Answer: No. Family and personal history for melanoma is negative. The number of nevi on the patient's torso falls within expected parameters for common benign nevi. Furthermore, his nevi are similar to one another and do not exhibit the variability of atypical nevi.

6. What should you tell the patient about the larger nevus?

Answer: Despite its larger size, at the present time this mole shows no other irregularity in regard to either history or physical evaluation. There is no medical indication at this time for intervention. If the mole changes, the patient should return immediately for reevaluation.

7. Should the larger lesion be biopsied?

Answer: Although the lesion in question exceeds 6 mm in size, it otherwise shows normal clinical parameters for a common benign nevus. Furthermore, it resembles other benign nevi of similar maturity on this patient. Unless it has recently undergone a specific change (size, shape, border, or color) or symptom (bleeding, crusting, etc.), biopsy is not indicated.

29 Malignant Melanoma

INTRODUCTION

Malignant melanomas are derived from cells of melanocytic origin. The question of dual origin from both epidermal melanocytes and nevus cells versus origin from epidermal melanocytes alone, remains an area of active controversy. This section will be limited to discussion of the major clinical forms of cutaneous melanoma, including superficial spreading malignant melanoma (SSMM), nodular melanoma (NM), acral lentiginous mucosal melanoma (ALMM), and lentigo maligna melanoma (LMM). Uncommon variants will not be covered.

Despite dramatically improved 5-year survival statistics, deaths from this tumor continue to rise because of an even greater increase in incidence. This increased incidence amounts to 4 to 6% per year in the United States alone. The rise is faster than that of any other human malignancy.

CLINICAL APPLICATION QUESTIONS

A 35-year-old woman is seen at your office for a rapidly changing pigmented lesion on her right upper hip. Although she tans easily, she has had extensive sun exposure surfing and lounging on the beach. The lesion is located in an area that is usually sun-protected, below her bathing suit line. The patient is very worried about melanoma.

1. What additional history should you elicit from this patient?
2. What characteristics of the lesion found on physical examination would suggest malignant melanoma?
3. What are the primary lesions that you might find in malignant melanoma?
4. What are the secondary lesions that you might find in malignant melanoma?
5. Should the lesion be biopsied for melanoma, and if so, what type of biopsy should be done?
6. If you determine that biopsy is not mandatory at this time, what should you tell the patient?

APPLICATION GUIDELINES

Specific History

Onset

Melanoma is an uncommon tumor during the first two decades of life. It is important to stress, however, that childhood melanoma can and does occur. Depending on the series of cases under consideration, about 10 to 40% of childhood melanomas arise in a congenital melanotic nevus (CMN) or acquired congenital-pattern melanotic nevus (AcpN).

From: *Current Clinical Practice: Dermatology Skills for Primary Care: An Illustrated Guide*
D.J. Trozak, D.J. Tennenhouse, and J.J. Russell © Humana Press, Totowa, NJ

The remainder arise either from acquired common nevi or *de novo* (on the skin without a preexisting pigmented lesion). It is generally agreed that with equivalent depths of invasion, childhood melanomas behave biologically like adult lesions. A 1995 retrospective report of melanomas in children under age 16 suggests a more favorable prognosis. This, however, needs further investigation.

From the third decade of life onward, the incidence of MM steadily, increases with a median age at diagnosis of 53 years. In certain parts of Europe, there is a 2:1 gender preponderance of females to males. This ratio becomes equal in regions of high incidence and is thought to be due to an overriding effect of ultraviolet light exposure. Melanoma is one of the most common malignancies of light-skinned young adults. There were an estimated 88,000 cases of melanoma in the United States alone in 2002, 92,000 cases in 2003, and a projected 96,000 cases in 2004. Almost 8000 deaths occur yearly. The projected lifetime risk of this tumor rose from 1 in 1500 in 1935 to 1 in 123 by 1987. In 2002, lifetime risk was estimated at 1 in 41.

1. Superficial spreading malignant melanoma (SSMM) is the most common type, comprising 70% of all melanomas. In male victims the trunk is the most frequent site, while in women the legs predominate. These lesions may develop *de novo* as an area of irregular pigmentation or in conjunction with a preexisting pigmented nevus, or an atypical nevus at which time the precursor lesion shows growth and irregularity. A clinical characteristic of SSMM is a significant radial (horizontal) growth phase prior to vertical invasion. This phase may last several months or a few years. The radial component presents as a centrifugally spreading macular or minimally raised stain, while the vertical component usually presents as a papule, a nodule, or an area of distinctly darker color (*see* Fig. 3).

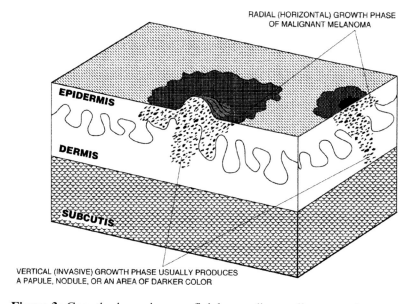

Figure 3: Growth phases in superficial spreading malignant melanoma.

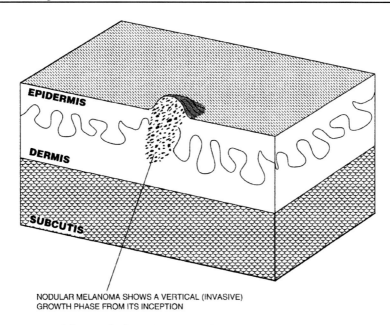

NODULAR MELANOMA SHOWS A VERTICAL (INVASIVE)
GROWTH PHASE FROM ITS INCEPTION

Figure 4: Growth phase of a nodular melanoma.

2. Nodular melanoma (NM) is more common in men and occurs frequently on the head, neck, and trunk. A 1995 series in the British literature reported a striking preponderance of nodular melanomas in children (70%). Comprising about 15% of all melanomas, NM may occur within a preexisting lesion or may arise *de novo* as a rapidly growing and often symmetrical dome-shaped nodule. The radial growth phase is absent; these lesions are invasive from their inception. The growth rate is usually striking and occurs over a period of weeks or months (*see* Fig. 4). This is of particular concern in pediatric cases where other, more common, rapidly growing benign lesions such as acquired common nevi, Spitz nevi, or pyogenic granulomas may mimic NM. Although the incidence of melanoma in children is very low, a rapidly growing papule or nodule should be conservatively removed and examined microscopically without delay. This becomes even more pressing if there is a history of bleeding without significant trauma.

3. Lentigo maligna melanoma (LMM) typically begins a full decade or more later than the other common forms of melanoma. This type makes up 4 to 10% of all melanomas and is usually preceded by a lesion with a radial growth phase that can last for years before vertical invasion begins. Typically located on heavily sun-exposed areas of the face and limbs, the precursor lesion consists of a gradually enlarging area of macular brown-black pigmentation, which may reach several centimeters in size and becomes increasingly irregular in shape and color. LMM is located most often on the face, followed by the sun-exposed areas of the arms and legs. The precursor lesion, known as a lentigo maligna or melanotic freckle of Hutchinson, is now generally considered an *in situ* melanoma. Because of the

prolonged radial growth phase, this type of melanoma was once considered biologically less aggressive than the other forms. Once invasion occurs, however, the
prognosis for a given level of vertical invasion appears to be the same as in the
other types.

4. Acral lentiginous mucosal melanoma (ALMM) affects the palms, soles, nail beds,
    and mucous membranes. It is the most common form of melanoma in African-
    Americans, Asians, and persons with heavily pigmented skin. This variant has a
    significant radial growth phase and usually begins as a macular discoloration of
    irregular shape and shading. Skip areas are common, and the location of ALMM
    in hidden anatomic sites, plus the occasional occurrence of minimal histologic
    findings, can delay the diagnosis until the tumor is advanced. These features
    account for the overall poor prognosis. Anorectal and vulvar locations have a par-
    ticularly low 5-year survival rate. ALMM comprises an estimated 2 to 8% of
    melanomas in white persons.

Evolution of Disease Process

The single most important concept in regard to the prognosis and treatment of cutaneous melanoma is recognition of the radial (horizontal) versus vertical growth phases.
With the separation of melanomas into the four major clinicohistologic subtypes discussed
above, it became apparent that SSMM and LMM had a much better overall prognosis. The
next critical advance was the concept of levels of dermal invasion by Clark and cowork-
ers (Table 1).

When the different subtypes were compared on the basis of Clark's levels, it became
apparent that SSMM and LMM melanomas, which have a prolonged radial growth phase
(Clark's level I), showed significantly less dermal invasion at the time of excision than
tumors of the NM subtype. This finding suggested that the depth of dermal invasion and
proximity of the tumor to the larger dermal blood vessels and lymphatics was a critical
factor.

This work was further refined by the introduction of the Breslow measurement of
tumor thickness, which is now a standard when reading a melanoma. Depth of invasion
into the dermis is measured from the base of the granular cell layer using an ocular
micrometer. The Breslow measurement provides numerical breakpoints that define sur-
vivor subgroups, and is an invaluable aid in management and determining prognosis
(Table 2).

Table 1
Clark's Levels

Clark's Level	Lesion Characteristics	Possible Metastasis
I	*In situ,* above epidermal basement membrane	No
II	Invasion to papillary dermis only	Yes
III	Invasion to interface of papillary and reticular dermis	Yes
IV	Distinct invasion of reticular dermis	Yes
V	Invasion into subcutaneous tissue	Yes

Table 2
Breslow Breakpoints

Tumor Thickness	Risk	5-Year Survival Rate
<0.75 mm	Minimum	96% (95–99%)
0.76–1.49 mm	Low	87% (80 to 95%)
1.50–2.49 mm	Intermediate	75% (60–75%)
2.50–3.99 mm	Intermediate	66% (60–75%)
>4.00 mm	High	47% (<50%)

Table 3
Traditional Three-Stage Melanoma Staging System

Stage	Lesion Characteristics	5-Year Survival
I	Skin only	79%
II	Nodal metastasis	36%
III	Distant metastasis	5%

Breslow levels correlate with, and have for the most part, supplanted the use of Clark's levels. In areas of very thin dermis (eyelids, ears) or with ulcerated tumors, however, the Clark's levels are still useful. Over the years, it has become evident that the depth of invasion is the dominant factor in predicting risk of metastatic disease. When the clinical variants of melanoma are compared on the basis of equivalent depth of dermal invasion, the apparent prognostic differences between melanoma subtypes disappear. This would also explain the poor outlook for melanomas arising in a CMN, where the malignancy can arise in the depth of the nevus in immediate proximity to larger vessels and lymphatics.

The crucial factors in any melanoma are therefore the transition from the nonmetastasizing radial growth phase to the vertical growth phase, where the incidence of metastasis correlates as a linear function with depth of invasion. Early treatment should be aimed at removal during the *in situ* phase when possible (SSMM, LMM, ALMM); or with the least level of dermal invasion (all forms). Once melanoma has spread beyond the primary site, to lymphatics or other organs, the survival rates drop precipitously (Table 3).

Since the mid-1980s, staging of malignant melanoma has undergone several revisions. The most current system (American Joint Committee on Cancer [AJCC] 2002 Revised Melanoma Staging, Table 4) has four major stages and multiple substages. This more complicated system takes into account Breslow measurements, Clark's levels, ulceration, sentinel-node biopsy results, number of positive nodes, and metastases (both local and distant). Vascular invasion is likely to be added soon. This system is primarily of value to tertiary melanoma clinics dealing with more advanced disease, to oncologists making decisions regarding adjunctive treatment, and for research, but only the first stages are useful to clinicians dealing with primary lesions.

With the introduction of sentinel-node biopsy for melanoma, lesions staged IB or greater should be referred to an established tertiary melanoma clinic for consideration regarding sentinel-node biopsy and evaluation for additional and adjunctive treatment. Since this complicated new staging system is not otherwise relevant to this book, the other

Table 4
AJCC 2002 Revised Melanoma Staging System (Partial)

Stage	Characteristics
0	Intraepithelial/*in situ* melanoma (TisN0M0)
IA	<1 mm invasion without ulceration and Clark level II/III (T1aN0M0)[a]
IB	<1 mm invasion with ulceration or Clark level IV/V (T1bN0M0) or 1.01–2 mm invasion without ulceration (T2aN0M0)
IIA	1.01–2.0 mm invasion with ulceration (T2bN0M0) or 2.0–4.0 mm without ulceratin (T3aN0M0)

T = tumor thickness; N = lymph node status; M = metastasis
[a] Breslow break points were revised to whole numbers in this system. Up to 6% of patients with primary tumors 0.76–0.99 mm may harbor metastatic disease on sentinel-node evaluation. Inquire as to which break-point your referral clinic is using to determine candidacy for sentinel-node exam.

stages are not listed here. The survival figures make it clear that prompt recognition on physical exam and early removal prior to spread beyond the primary tumor are of paramount importance.

Evolution of Skin Lesions

See Evolution of Disease Process section, above.

Provoking Factors

Ultraviolet radiation appears to be the most important provoking factor for some, but not all, melanomas. The high incidence of this cancer among Caucasian populations living in regions of intense solar exposure, and an increasing incidence per population in latitudes near the equator, are cited as proof. The relationship of melanoma to solar radiation is more complex than that of the more common basal and squamous cell skin cancers. With melanoma, short periods of intense exposure rather than chronic cumulative exposure appears to be the trigger. Melanoma is not increased in persons with outdoor occupations but is more often seen in those with indoor occupations who get intermittent weekend or vacation exposure. Repeated severe sunburns during childhood and adolescence are also felt to predispose to melanoma. Early evidence suggests that tanning-parlor UVA exposure may also contribute. An exception is LMM, where patients are typically a decade or more older and typically have had intense long-term solar exposure.

Self-Medication

Self-treatment is not a problem.

Supplemental Review From General History

Additional risk factors include:

1. Fair complexion with a tendency to sunburn easily.
2. Presence of atypical moles with or without a family history of melanoma.
3. Higher than average number of pigmented nevi.

4. History of melanoma in a first-degree relative.
5. Prior personal history of melanoma.
6. Immunologic suppression for any reason.

Therefore a careful personal history regarding solar exposure, tanning-bed usage, and prior pigmented lesions is important. Family history should include any history of relatives with unusual moles or mole patterns.

Dermatologic Physical Exam

ABCD Technique

Physical examination of pigmented lesions is a difficult task and is best approached by using the ABCD technique mentioned earlier in the chapter on atypical nevi (*see* Chapter 28). If a lesion is abnormal by these criteria, and especially if there is also a history of distinct change or evolution over the prior 6 to 12 months, there is a high probability of melanoma. Many benign moles will have one of these changes. A melanoma usually shows several or all.

Asymmetry: In Chapter 28, benign nevi are described as usually round or oval in shape. The disordered growth of melanoma cells tends to produce distinct variations in the symmetry of the lesion. This is particularly true with SSMM, LMM, and ALMM (*see* Photos 26–30,32).

Border: Benign moles usually have distinct, smooth, regular borders, which are easily marked. Melanoma margins are irregular, pseudopod-like, or grossly notched. This is typical of SSMM (*see* Photos 26,29,30,32,33). Indistinct margins that fade into the adjacent skin may be seen with all types, but are especially common with LMM and ALMM (*see* Photos 27,28).

Color: Benign nevi are generally flesh, tan, or brown shades, and are usually evenly pigmented. Some variants of a benign mole, such as the Spitz nevus and blue nevi, are blue-black or black because the melanin is deep in the dermis. Therefore blue-black or black color does not necessarily equate with malignancy. The color of MM can vary from white to red to shades of gray, blue, brown, blue-black, and pitch black. In general, the intense darker colors are seen more often in malignant tumors. NM tends to exhibit even coloration that varies from flesh-colored to red to dark browns or black. The other three major types (SSMM, LMM, and ALMM) tend to show variegated colors within the individual lesion, and this, along with speckling of pigment, is an important diagnostic sign. If an otherwise benign-appearing pigmented lesion shows irregular color, the examiner should look for an explanation such as terminal hairs or surface comedones, which can cause such a change (*see* Photos 26,27,31–33).

Diameter: Benign nevi are usually 6 mm or less in diameter; however, many perfectly normal moles exceed this size. If the lesion is stable in size by history and does not offer other signs or symptoms of malignancy, the odds are very strong that it is benign. MM is usually larger than 6 mm, which is roughly the size of a pencil eraser. Change in diameter is also important. Most melanomas will have visibly increased in size in the previous 6 to 12 months (*see* Fig. 5).

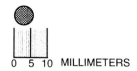

0   5   10   MILLIMETERS

Figure 5: Melanoma size. A 6 mm circle, roughly the diameter of a lead pencil eraser. Most benign nevi are this size or smaller. Most malignant melanomas exceed this size.

Other Signs

Other important signs of MM include secondary surface changes (listed in the Secondary Lesions section). Rapid elevation of a previously flat lesion, sudden pigment loss, or inflammation at the base of the lesion all are cause for concern.

Unfortunately, NM does not fit well into the ABCD approach. This type of melanoma usually presents as a rapidly growing symmetrical papule or nodule with even color. The lesions are often exophytic and the margins may not be visibly notched or may simply not be visible. NM can have significant depth of dermal invasion before exceeding 6 mm in diameter. Therefore any rapidly growing pigmented lesion that has arisen *de novo* and cannot otherwise be identified, should be biopsied (*see* Photos 34,35). A recent paper on the early diagnosis of melanoma presents evidence supporting the addition of a fifth criterion to the diagnosis of melanoma. The authors propose expanding to an ABCDE approach, where the E represents "evolving" change in a pigmented lesion.

Primary Lesions

1. Irregularly shaped and irregularly pigmented macules or patches (*see* Photos 27,28,33). SSMM: 0.5 to 3 cm. LMM and ALMM: 1 to several cm.
2. Irregularly shaped and irregularly pigmented plaques (*see* Photos 26,29–32). SSMM: 0.5 to 3 cm. LMM and ALMM: 1 to several cm.
3. Papules (*see* Photo 34). NM: only a few millimeters in size.
4. Nodules. NM: 1 to several cm.
5. Exophytic or pedunculated nodules (*see* Photo 35). NM: 1 to several cm.

Secondary Lesions

1. Secondary papules or nodules within a macular or plaque lesion indicate an area of vertical growth (*see* Photos 26,30,32).
2. Areas of pigment loss may indicate areas of regression or an area that is amelanotic (*see* Photo 32).
3. Scale develops as the epidermis is invaded (*see* Photo 26).
4. Erythema at the pigmented border.
5. Very late secondary signs: erosions, crusting, ulceration, or bleeding.

Distribution

Microdistribution: None.

Macrodistribution: Melanoma can occur at any site on the skin or mucous membranes. In men they are more common on the back, neck, and scalp (*see* Fig. 6). In women they are more common on the legs (*see* Fig. 7).

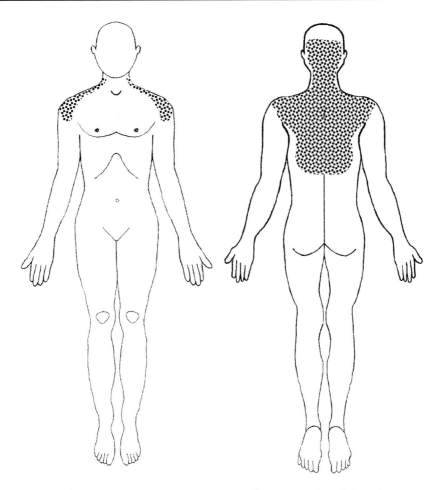

Figure 6: Favored sites for malignant melanoma in adult males.

Configuration

Melanoma has no special configuration.

Indicated Supporting Diagnostic Data

Biopsy

Microscopic examination is the only definitive laboratory study that will diagnose MM. Small suspect lesions should be completely but conservatively removed so that the whole lesion can be evaluated. Some authors suggest either elliptical excision or saucerization to the level of the subcutaneous tissue.

We recommend complete conservative total excision with 1- to 2-mm lateral margins extending to the superficial fascia drainage (*see* discussion of sentinel node biopsy, below). Whenever possible, the excision should be oriented parallel to the anticipated lymphatic.

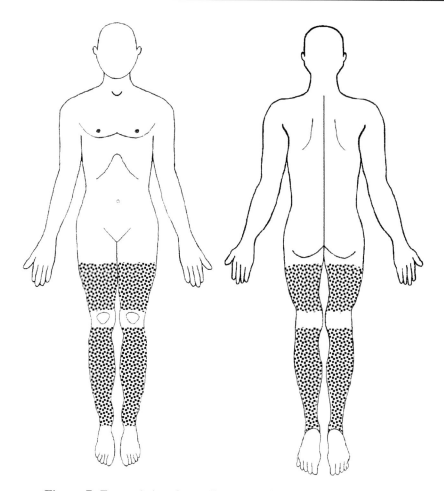

Figure 7: Favored sites for malignant melanoma in adult females.

Saucerization usually leaves a wide, unattractive scar. Also, it is very easy to fail to go deep enough in the dermis and thereby destroy the areas needed for the Breslow measurement. This procedure may save time for the practitioner, but we do not recommend it for a suspect melanoma.

Lesions that are too large for simple excisional biopsy or are located in an anatomic site where the biopsy would be needlessly deforming can be sampled by an incisional biopsy. Despite cautions raised in the older literature, incisional biopsy does not worsen the prognosis of melanoma. Incisional biopsy can be done by punch or elliptical incision. In the authors' opinion, an elliptical specimen 2 to 3 mm wide from one interface of the lesion to the other and extending into the subcutis is preferred. Punch incision can also be employed, but this technique may be misleading if a skip area or an area of minimal irregularity is biopsied. This limited specimen gives less reliable information on which to base definitive excision margins.

The following features should be carefully documented before biopsy is carried out of any suspect melanoma:

1. Anatomic location, preferably accompanied by a drawn map.
2. Color(s), and presence of variegation or speckling.
3. Size, measuring the two greatest dimensions at right angles.
4. Surface character, including scale, pebbling, papules, nodules, and especially erosions or ulceration.
5. Character of the border.
6. Presence or absence of satellite lesions.
7. Status of regional lymph nodes.

Pathology Report

The pathology report of a melanoma should include the following essentials: diagnosis, melanoma subtype (SSMM, LMM, etc.), tumor thickness in millimeters (Breslow measurement), and a statement regarding margins. Ideally it should also include the anatomic site, Clark's level (with ulcerated lesions or lesions where the dermis is thin, such as the eyelids), mitotic rate, growth phase (radial/vertical), and the presence or absence of ulceration, microscopic regression, inflammatory response, angiolymphatic spread, neurotropism, microsatellites, and any precursor lesion.

Table 5
Current Recommended Margins Based on AJCC Staging and Breslow Thickness in Millimeters

Stage	Tumor Thickness	Margin
0	*in situ* (no invasion)	0.5 cm
IA(T1a)	<1.0 mm (low risk)	1.0 cm
IB(T1b)	<1.0 mm (ulcerated or Clark's IV,V)	1–2 cm
IB(T2a)	1.01–2.0 mm (no ulceration)	1–2 cm
IIA(T2b)	1.01–2.0 mm (ulcerated)	1–2 cm
IIA(T3a) and above	over 2.1 mm	2.0 cm

Therapy

Discussion of treatment will be limited to stages 0 and IA primary melanoma. With the advent of sentinel node examination, primary lesions graded IB or greater should be referred to a tertiary multidisciplinary melanoma clinic for review and recommendations.

Surgery

Complete excision with adequate margins remains the only definitive treatment of cutaneous melanoma limited to the skin. Over the past three decades, the margins recommended for excising these tumors have been refined based on the work of many investigators using the principles put forth by Clark and Breslow (Table 5). Today margins are determined by a number of factors, but are determined primarily by the depth of invasion into the dermis. These margins should be obtained in every direction from the lateral margin of the melanoma. Excision should be carried to, but not through, the muscular fascia. Reexcision of the primary site should be undertaken only after the biopsy tissue has been examined and it has been determined that the lesion falls into a Stage 0 or IA category and does not require melanoma clinic referral.

The presence of vital anatomic structures or unusual risks may supersede the recommended margins, and somewhat narrower margins may be acceptable. Conversely, in the presence of ulceration, microsatellites, microscopic neurotropism, microscopic vessel invasion, high mitotic index, or significant microscopic regression, consider using wider margins than those listed above. With intermediate-thickness lesions showing 1 to 2 mm depth of invasion, obtain the widest margin from 1 to 2 cm that will allow a primary or nondeforming closure.

Additional Therapy for MM Limited to Skin

Sentinel lymph node biopsy (SLNB) is a mapping technique that employs the use of vital dyes and radioisotopes to define the sentinel lymph node or direct lymph node chain draining the site of a primary melanoma. The procedure requires the interaction of a highly trained team of surgeons, dermatopathologists, and nuclear medicine specialists. Techniques are employed, especially in the pathology evaluation, that are not commonly available to the regular medical community. At present, this procedure should be performed only at tertiary care centers where it can be done accurately. Consideration for SLNB is given to patients with primary melanomas Stage IB or greater using a Breslow breakpoint of 0.76 or 1.0 mm of dermal invasion, depending on the criteria of the tertiary clinic (*see* Table 4). SLNB has now been adopted as a standard; hence the current specific recommendations regarding biopsy technique. This also means that currently all primary lesions graded IB or greater should be sent forward for evaluation before any additional therapy is rendered. Performed properly, SLNB can identify the lymph drainage and status of the nodes with a high degree of accuracy. If the lymph nodes examined are negative, it has a high degree of prognostic value. Compared to elective lymph node dissection, it is a minimally invasive operation with low morbidity. To date, SLNB has not been shown to have any therapeutic value, and it remains a staging and investigative tool that should be reserved for use at centers with ongoing investigative studies.

Elective lymph node dissection (ELND) involves removal of clinically negative lymph node basins, and is a procedure that has generated heated controversy for several decades. Critics point to the significant morbidity (40%) and the fact that 80% of patients subjected to ELND were found to be metastasis-negative. Another criticism is the unpredictable lymph drainage on sites such as the trunk, leading to invasion of the wrong node chain. The strongest evidence against ELND are numerous studies that have failed to show any clear benefit. SLNB has now essentially eliminated the 80% of cases that would have been ELND-negative. Although some recent studies suggest that ELND may benefit a small number of selected patients, the value of this surgery remains unproven. Taking into account the proven tendency of melanoma to spread hematogenously, and the lack of evidence that ELND or other adjunctive therapies alter the course of metastatic melanoma, a noted authority has given cogent reasons for abandoning both SLNB and ELND. For now, however, SLNB remains a standard procedure.

Adjunctive therapies consisting of vaccines and various chemotherapy regimens have come and gone. At present, the only approved adjunctive treatment for advanced melanoma is a prolonged course of high-dose interferon-α2b. The beneficial effects have been

Table 6
Follow-Up

Stage	Initial Work-up	Follow-Up
0	No routine	S & N exam every 3 mo; TE/6 mo × 1 yr, then TE yearly thereafter
IA	No routine	S & N exam every 3 mo; TE/6 mo × 3 yr, then TE yearly thereafter
IB and above	B-Cxr, LFT[a], addl. imaging as indicated	S & N exam every 3 mo; TE/6 mo × 3 yr, then TE every 6 mo × 2 yr then yearly thereafter. Other lab and imaging studies as indicated

[a] Optional

B-Cxr, baseline chest X-ray; LFTs, liver function tests; S & N, site and node exam; TE, total pigmented lesion exam.

modest, and many patients cannot tolerate the side effects for the entire recommended course. Decisions in this regard are made at the tertiary clinic and are usually carried out by a community oncologist.

Follow-Up

Once a diagnosis of MM has been made, every patient should have a head-to-toe examination of skin and mucous membranes, palpation of regional and all other node chains, and an abdominal exam looking for organomegaly or masses. Regular follow-up is recommended as shown in Table 6. Patients with atypical mole syndrome require more rigid follow-up that must be maintained on a lifelong basis.

Education

Melanoma patients, even those without atypical mole syndrome, are at increased risk of developing a second primary melanoma. Patient education is their best and first line of protection. Like atypical mole patients, melanoma patients should be carefully instructed in methods of monthly self-examination of all pigmented lesions. Prompt action and the reasons for it must be made very clear. Document this instruction. To aid in the education process, there are color brochures available from the American Academy of Dermatology with life-size photos of melanomas, a review of the ABCDs, and self-exam directions.

During follow-up physician exams, hidden moles or those in locations likely to be overlooked should be pointed out so that they can be evaluated during self-examination. Proper sun avoidance and physical protection with a hat and clothing should be discussed and emphasized, and the patient should be given samples of an effective sunscreen with a minimal SPF value of 30 and a UVA-blocking ingredient such as Parsol®. As the vast majority of patients survive their melanomas, it is essential to approach them in a positive fashion and enlist their help, rather than discourage or frighten them.

Routine imaging studies and lab tests are not required for the staging of patients with primary cutaneous melanoma with less than 4 mm invasion. Imaging studies and lab tests should be ordered based on symptoms or follow-up findings. Special studies such as positron emission tomography for high-risk situations are best recommended by the tertiary melanoma clinic.

Conditions That May Simulate Malignant Melanoma
Pseudomelanoma

Partially excised melanocytic nevi can produce a disturbing clinical and histologic picture when partial regrowth occurs. It is essential that the examining pathologist be aware of the prior procedure so that the original tissue sections can be obtained and a frightening error avoided.

Spitz's Nevus

The Spitz or epithelioid nevus is a benign mole that occurs predominantly in children and has clinical and microscopic features that mimic MM. It is essential that a fully trained dermatopathologist examine worrisome pigmented lesions in children.

Pigmented Basal Cell Carcinoma

MM and nodular pigmented basal cell carcinoma may look quite similar. When there is a question, a dermatologist can often distinguish the two on physical exam. Biopsy will clearly separate the two.

Pyogenic Granuloma

These are rapidly growing lesions that often occur after a history of discrete trauma. They are usually cherry-red, friable, and show a constricted or pedunculated base. Sometimes when the surface layer is thick they have a blue-gray color. Unfortunately, amelanotic nodular MM can have an identical appearance. Excision and microscopic exam will distinguish them.

Dermatofibromas

These reactive fibrous growths are found on the distal limbs and upper back, which are sites of blunt skin trauma. The dermatofibroma often shows irregular tan pigmentation and a fuzzy border. Palpation will reveal a firm button-like tumor in the dermis and, with lateral compression, the lesion will depress downward (a positive "pucker" sign). A variant of dermatofibroma known as a "sclerosing hemangioma" typically shows irregular blue-black color changes and may be very difficult to distinguish clinically from a melanoma.

Thrombosed Capillary Aneurysm

These lesions appear rapidly, have a purple-black color, and may simulate early NM. Because of the thrombosis, they will not blanch with pressure. These lesions are small and can usually be punch-excised with margins for microscopic examination.

Nail Bed Hemorrhage

This benign condition occurs after trauma and may simulate ALMM of the nail unit. When there is a history of trauma, or this benign condition appears likely, a short period of observation is indicated. The hemorrhage should move distally as the nail grows while the color clears at the base. If clearing does not begin in 6 weeks, a biopsy is needed. If pigment extends from the nail unit into the adjacent skin (Hutchinson's sign; *see* Photo 28), melanoma is almost certainly present.

ANSWERS TO CLINICAL APPLICATION QUESTIONS

History Review

A 35-year-old woman is seen at your office for a rapidly changing pigmented lesion on her right upper hip. Although she tans easily, she has had extensive sun exposure surfing and lounging on the beach. The lesion is located in an area that is usually sun-protected, but is below her bathing suit line. The patient is very worried about melanoma.

1. What additional history should you elicit from this patient?

Answer: Was there a stable preexisting pigmented lesion at the site? If so, how has its shape, color, size, and border changed, and over what time period? If there was no preexisting lesion, how long has the patient been aware of the lesion in question, and what changes were seen during that time period? Has there been any open sore or bleeding consistent with an ulceration? Is there any personal or family history of malignant melanoma?

2. What characteristics of the lesion found on physical examination would suggest malignant melanoma?

Answer: ABCD—**A**symmetry, **B**order irregularity, **C**olor variation, **D**iameter exceeding 6 mm. Also look for secondary papules or nodules, focal areas of hypopigmentation, scale, border erythema, erosions, crusting, ulceration, and/or bleeding.

3. What are the primary lesions that you might find in malignant melanoma?

Answer:
   a. An irregularly shaped and/or irregularly pigmented macule, patch, or plaque (SSMM, LMM, and ALMM).
   b. A rapidly growing papule or nodule (NM).
   c. An exophytic or pedunculated nodule (NM).

4. What are the secondary lesions that you might find in malignant melanoma?

Answer: Secondary papules or nodules within a macule or plaque, pigment loss, scale, and border erythema. Late secondary changes can include erosions, crusting, ulceration, and/or bleeding.

5. Should the lesion be biopsied for melanoma, and if so, what type of biopsy should be done?

Answer: If the lesion shows two or more of the ABCD parameters for malignant melanoma described in the answer to question 2, combined with the history of rapid change, this is an indication for diagnostic biopsy. If the lesion shows only one of the ABCD parameters, all facets of the history and physical findings should be considered when making a decision whether or not to biopsy the lesion. The appropriate type of biopsy is an elliptical excisional biopsy that removes the entire lesion with a conservative margin.

6. If you determine that biopsy is not mandatory at this time, what should you tell the patient?

Answer: The patient should be warned about the vagaries and potential of malignant melanoma. The patient should be offered the option of dermatologic consultation, biopsy, or monthly reassessment of the lesion.

30 Actinic Keratosis *(Solar Keratosis)*

CLINICAL APPLICATION QUESTIONS

A 65-year-old white man is seen at your office for multiple scaling lesions over his face, ears, neck, and the V of the chest. These have developed gradually over several years. He is an outdoor sportsman. He is concerned about the character and potential of these lesions, and would like to have them removed because they are itchy and irritable. Physical examination of the involved regions reveals multiple actinic keratoses (AKs). Careful examination reveals no lesions that appear overtly malignant.

1. What are the primary lesions that you would expect to find in actinic keratoses?
2. What are the secondary lesions that you would expect to find in actinic keratoses?
3. What should you tell the patient about actinic keratoses?
4. How should you treat actinic keratoses in this patient?

APPLICATION GUIDELINES

Specific History

Onset

This type of keratosis is seen with increased incidence in patients from the fifth decade of life onward. The individual lesions begin insidiously as erythematous patches of vasodilation that are often more apparent after solar exposure. Early lesions are usually otherwise asymptomatic.

Evolution of Disease Process

AKs develop after a long latency period (one to two decades), and are caused primarily by solar radiation in the UVB or sunburn range from 2900 to 3200 Å. They occur in groupings and are limited to sun-exposed skin. The early erythematous lesions can progress to forms that (1) scale (keratotic type), (2) thicken dramatically (cutaneous horn type), (3) develop a brown branny scale (pigmented type), or (4) become violaceous, slightly indurated, and inflamed to resemble papules of lichen planus (lichenoid type). The last type is uncommon and probably represents an AK with an immune response aimed at rejection. These more developed forms are often mildly symptomatic and patients will complain of intermittent itching and prickling, especially after solar exposure. Following a lengthy latent period some AKs evolve into squamous cell carcinomas, usually of low metastatic potential. Patients will occasionally report spontaneous clearing of specific lesions, possibly a consequence of the histologic changes seen in the lichenoid type.

From: *Current Clinical Practice: Dermatology Skills for Primary Care: An Illustrated Guide*
D.J. Trozak, D.J. Tennenhouse, and J.J. Russell © Humana Press, Totowa, NJ

Thickening at the base of an AK, the presence of a cutaneous horn, or failure to respond promptly to proper cryotherapy should suggest the possibility of malignancy.

Evolution of Skin Lesions

See Evolution of Disease Process section, above.

Provoking Factors

Extensive sun exposure obtained during recreation or in outdoor occupations is the major cause. Climates with predominantly warm sunny days, increased proximity to the equator, and exposure at higher altitudes all increase the injury, which is of a cumulative nature. These lesions occur primarily in persons of Celtic heritage with types I and II complexions, who sunburn easily.

Self-Medication

Inappropriate self-treatment with topical 5-fluorouracil (5-Fu) obtained from relatives or prescribed by misguided practitioners can alter lesions or hide established malignancies without effectively removing them. Patients will also attempt to treat themselves with various cosmetics and patent medications, but soon discover that this is fruitless.

Supplemental Review From General History

A history of lifetime sun exposure, ease of burning, and regular use of sunscreens and protective clothing should be reviewed.

Dermatologic Physical Exam

Primary Lesions

1. Erythematous macules and patches 0.5 to 1 cm across (*see* Photo 36).
2. Thin plaques 0.5 to 1 cm across with secondary changes (*see* Photo 37).

Secondary Lesions

1. Adherent white, yellow, or brown scale that is removed with difficulty, and upon removal may leave a depressed bleeding base (*see* Photos 36–39).
2. A cutaneous horn that is firmly attached and may extend a centimeter or more above the normal skin surface (*see* Photo 38).
3. Erosions (*see* Photo 39).
4. Ulcerations (*see* Photo 39).

An indurated base, cutaneous horn, or the presence of erosions or ulceration should raise the possibility of malignant transformation within an AK. If a lesion of this type is treated without biopsy, it should be followed up within 4 to 6 weeks to be certain there has been a complete response.

Distribution

Microdistribution: Follicular: AKs will occasionally occur at the ostium of a hair follicle. Follicular AKs are most often seen on the upper facial area and nose. Because the cellular changes extend down the follicular infundibulum, they usually recur after cryotherapy.

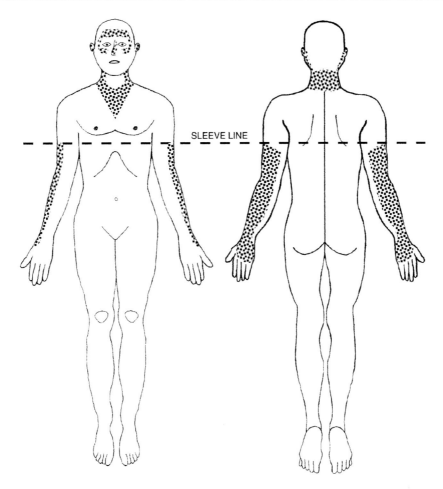

SLEEVE LINE

Figure 8: Macrodistribution of actinic keratosis.

Macrodistribution: AKs are distributed on sun-exposed skin such as the upper face, malar and zygomatic eminences, ears, dorsal forearms, and the V area of the upper chest (*see* Fig. 8).

Configuration

Configuration is grouped.

Indicated Supporting Diagnostic Data

Biopsy

The vast majority of AKs can be diagnosed and treated based on clinical examination. When there is a question about intervening malignancy, a punch biopsy should distinguish them.

Therapy

Cryosurgery

Light applications of liquid nitrogen (LN$_2$) sufficient to produce a 0.5- to 1-mm rim of freeze at the perimeter of the base of the AK are usually satisfactory for total removal. The advantage of this technique is the absence of scarring. Persons with olive complexions must be warned about the possibility of posttreatment hyper- or hypopigmentation. During the sunny season, warn patients about sun exposure and the use of a sunscreen with makeup to prevent posttreatment darkening, and for future prevention. Cryosurgery is the technique of choice in patients with a small number of lesions or in patients who cannot comply with, or who refuse, topical therapy. Patients should be warned to return if any lesion fails to resolve within 4 to 6 weeks.

Topical Chemotherapy

The advantage of topical chemotherapy is the ability to destroy actinic damage that is otherwise invisible and would be missed with cryotherapy. Patients with large numbers of keratoses or a great deal of latent injury, who are reliable and will follow through, are ideal candidates. Topical chemotherapy should be started only after the intended treatment sites have been examined for overtly malignant lesions. This therapy can remove the surface signs of an established cancer while it continues to spread beneath the epidermal surface.

5-fluorouracil: 5-FU selectively seeks out and destroys AKs with little or no effect on the adjacent normal skin. This medication is available as a 0.5% cream with time-releasing microsponges incorporated into the vehicle. It is also marketed as a 1% water-washable cream and as 2% and 5% solutions in propylene glycol. All of the products work in a similar fashion and have excellent efficacy. The 0.5% cream has the advantage of a single daily application, which improves patient compliance. Patients are instructed to apply the agent to the affected area in a thin layer morning and evening or once daily, depending on the preparation chosen. Careful instructions are needed or the reaction may be very disconcerting to the patient. Within 5 to 6 days, selected areas of damage and visible keratoses will become red, itchy, angry, and irritable. Different patients show different tolerance, and fair-skinned persons seem more reactive. Lesions should be treated until they are inflamed and some of the thinner lesions are coming off. Some lesions may erode and bleed, and patients will need reassurance that this is not a complication. After this point is reached, the treatment is stopped and patients are switched to a low-potency steroid preparation such as topical 0.05% desonide in a soothing lubricating cream base. This product should be used morning and evening until the redness and irritation has resolved; then it should be discontinued. Follow patients up 6 weeks from the time the 5-FU is stopped. At that time, there are usually scattered thick lesions that have not responded, and these are removed with LN$_2$. During 5-FU treatment, patients should be warned to minimize solar exposure. Significant sun can rapidly accelerate the reaction, and although no permanent injury will result, the effect is frightening and uncomfortable.

A second method of using 5-FU is the "treat through" technique. The drug is continued until the reaction ceases as the AKs are eliminated. Few patients will put up with this duration of irritation, and occasional patients who show nonspecific irritation to 5-FU would not fare well with this technique.

A third method is to use 5-FU and a topical steroid together over a longer period of time. The intent is to reduce irritation and increase compliance. Although reported effective, there is no substantial body of evidence to show that this method has equivalent efficacy.

Diclofenac sodium: This medication is prepared as a 3% gel and is applied twice daily to the affected sun-damaged areas morning and evening. Treatment is recommended for 60 to 90 days, and patients should then have a follow up visit at 6 weeks to freeze any lesions that have not responded. During therapy patients should be warned to minimize sun exposure. This medication is a safe alternative for patients allergic to 5-FU. Head-to-head comparisons with long-term follow-up between the two agents has not been reported. The prolonged treatment course raises questions regarding patient compliance. Despite claims to the contrary, patients do experience erythema and irritation with diclofenac sodium similar to that seen with 5-FU.

Imiquimod: Imiquimod cream 5%, an immune modulator that has been available for several years for treatment of genital and perianal warts, is also approved for the treatment of actinic keratosis. Like topical 5-FU, it selectivley destroys malignant keratinocytes but leaves normal ones alone. It is applied twice weekly for a period of 16 weeks. Applications are done at bedtime and left on for 8 hours. Efficacy appears excellent, with 75% or greater reduction of lesions. Drawbacks to this treatment are the prolonged treatment time, which would diminish compliance, and the current cost, which is five or six times the cost of other products.

Curettage and Electrodesiccation

Removal by this technique should be undertaken only with the rare lesions that fail to respond to topical or cryotherapy. Although effective, this method of destruction leaves superficial scarring, which is seldom justified. The patient should be forewarned.

Prevention

Solar avoidance and covering up with adequate clothing prevents these premalignant lesions. In female patients, the daily use of makeup that contains or is used over a sunscreen provides substantial protection from keratosis and from the chronic aging effects of the sun. High SPF sunscreen (30 or greater), (preferably containing Parsol), used on a daily basis has been shown to substantially reduce their occurrence.

Conditions That May Simulate Actinic Keratosis

Seborrheic Keratosis (SKs)

Pigmented AKs can appear quite similar to early SKs. Actinic lesions are thin and do not show a defined edge or the "stuck-on" appearance of the seborrheic type. In addition, AKs show telangectasia and an adherent scale that often leaves bleeding points when removed.

Solar Lentigo

Pigmented AKs can also be confused with solar lentigines. The latter lesion is usually macular with normal skin markings, whereas the actinic lesion has a scale, and the surface markings are lost.

Discoid Lupus Erythematosus (DLE)

Large AKs can be confused with plaques of DLE because of the telangectasia, adherent white scale, and solar distribution. AKs have a more adherent scale, are usually grouped, and do not show the scarring seen with DLE. The scale of DLE, when removed, shows "carpet-tacking" (*see* Chapter 19).

Squamous Cell Carcinoma

Differentiation from this malignant tumor is discussed in the chapter on squamous cell carcinoma.

ANSWERS TO CLINICAL APPLICATION QUESTIONS

History Review

A 65-year-old white man is seen at your office for multiple scaling lesions over his face, ears, neck, and the V of the chest. These have developed gradually over several years. He is an outdoor sportsman. He is concerned about the character and potential of these lesions, and would like to have them removed because they are itchy and irritable. Physical examination of the involved regions reveals multiple actinic keratoses. Careful examination reveals no lesions that appear overtly malignant.

1. What are the primary lesions that you would expect to find in actinic keratoses?

Answer: Erythematous macules, patches, and thin plaques 5 to 10 mm in size.

2. What are the secondary lesions that you would expect to find in actinic keratoses?

Answer:
   a. Adherent white, yellow, or brown scale.
   b. Erosions.
   c. Ulcerations.

3. What should you tell the patient about actinic keratoses?

Answer: Actinic keratoses are the result of chronic sun exposure and are precancerous lesions. Over a period of time, some of them may change into skin cancers. Removal is recommended because of their malignant potential.

4. How should you treat actinic keratoses in this patient?

Answer: This patient may be treated with topical chemotherapy. Because he has large numbers of lesions, this approach is cost-effective. Cryosurgery is appropriate for patients with a small number of actinic keratoses, for patients who cannot comply with a topical chemotherapy regimen, or for patients who simply refuse topical chemotherapy. Cryosurgery is also indicated for the removal of any lesions that do not respond to topical chemotherapy. Topical agents are of marginal value for thick actinic keratoses on the dorsum of the hands and forearms. Cryotherapy is more cost-effective in these locations.

31 Keratoacanthoma *(Molluscum Sebaceum)*

CLINICAL APPLICATION QUESTIONS

A 35-year-old farmer is seen at your office for a rapidly growing nodule on his right upper lip near the vermilion margin. This was first noticed 4 weeks ago. He is concerned about the character and potential of this lesion. Physical examination of the involved region reveals a lesion suggesting a keratoacanthoma (KA).

1. What are the primary lesions that you would expect to find in keratoacanthoma?
2. What are the secondary lesions that you would expect to find in keratoacanthoma?
3. Keratoacanthoma is most commonly mistaken for what other condition?
4. What should you tell the patient about keratoacanthoma?
5. Should you treat keratoacanthoma in this patient, and if so, how?

APPLICATION GUIDELINES

Specific History

Onset

KAs are common tumors that are first encountered in middle-aged patients and are frequently seen from age 60 onward. Onset is usually sudden, with rapid growth, and most patients give definite timing regarding the onset and progression.

Evolution of Disease Process

A typical KA begins as a solitary firm papule on sun-damaged but otherwise normal skin. Early lesions may resemble a molluscum wart or a verrucous wart; however, rapid growth and large size usually offer a clue as to the true nature of the tumor. A typical KA measures 1 to 2 cm across at the base, and is elevated 0.5 to 1.0 cm above the adjacent skin surface.

The initial *rapid growth phase* lasts 1 to 2 months, and the lesions then typically become stable in size. This *stationary phase* may last from a few to several months, and is the stage during which patients most often present for evaluation. After a period of stability, and frequently after biopsy, some KAs will enter a *regressive phase,* which may last for 6 months. Following spontaneous regression, there is almost always some residual scarring at the site, which consists of a depression with papules and elevated tags at the margin. Recurrence after spontaneous resolution has been reported.

Special forms of keratoacanthoma include (1) a generalized eruptive type, (2) a multiple type (following cutaneous carcinogen exposure), (3) a giant type (up to 15 cm in

From: *Current Clinical Practice: Dermatology Skills for Primary Care: An Illustrated Guide*
D.J. Trozak, D.J. Tennenhouse, and J.J. Russell © Humana Press, Totowa, NJ

diameter), and (4) a dominantly inherited self-healing variant. There is disagreement over the precise classification of this variant.

Evolution of Skin Lesions

See Evolution of Disease Process section, above.

Provoking Factors

Because of the preference of keratoacanthoma for sun-exposed skin, and because KAs are seen most often in persons with severe solar damage, there is no question that UV radiation is a major factor in their etiology. As a corollary, fair-skinned Caucasians who sunburn readily and are subject to solar injury are the persons who present with these tumors most frequently.

Occurrence of a KA shortly after penetrating, but minor, physical trauma to the site is common. Other provoking factors include topical carcinogens (such as tar compounds) and natural or iatrogenic states of immunologic suppression.

Self-Medication

Self-treatment is not a problem.

Supplemental Review From General History

The occurrence of giant, atypical, or multiple KAs is an indication for review of family history, possible chemical carcinogen exposure, and any factors or concomitant conditions that might cause general immune suppression.

Dermatologic Physical Exam

Primary Lesions

1. A rapidly growing dome-shaped papule with a central dull pebbly core (*see* Photo 40).
2. A rapidly growing dome-shaped nodule with a central dull pebbly core (*see* Photos 41,42).

The initial lesion is a papule with a central depression or dell. The peripheral epithelial lip can vary from flesh-colored to pink or orange-red depending on the degree of inflammatory reaction and the number of dilated (telangiectatic) vessels. There is no infiltration of the skin peripheral to the margins of the lesion. The central cavity develops as the KA matures, and becomes increasingly larger as the epithelial rim thins. The central keratotic material has a gray-yellow color. In the early papule/nodule stage with the dell there can be considerable resemblance to a basal cell carcinoma. Small lesions with an early keratotic core can simulate a large molluscum wart.

Secondary Lesions

1. Giant lesions form a rough, pebbly central vegetation. The epithelial margin may become quite diminutive and difficult to recognize.
2. Scarring with a depression and peripheral epidermal tags are usually left after spontaneous regression (*see* Photo 43).

Distribution

Microdistribution: Some keratoacanthomas develop from the upper epithelium of the hair follicle; however, this distribution is not clinically evident.

Macrodistribution: 90% of KAs occur on the sun-exposed skin of the face, hands, and forearms. They can also occur on covered sites and have been reported on the vermilion margin of the lip, the buccal mucosa, in the anogenital regions, and beneath nails (*see* Fig. 9).

Configuration

Grouped in the case of multiple KAs.

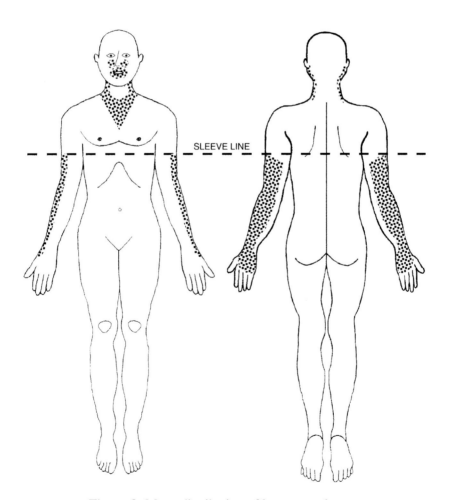

Figure 9: Macrodistribution of keratoacanthomas.

Indicated Supporting Diagnostic Data

Biopsy

The histology of a keratoacanthoma is very similar to that of a well-differentiated squamous cell carcinoma of the skin. KAs commonly contain squamous cells with atypical mitosis, individual cell keratinization, and other histologic signs of malignancy. The microscopic differentiation is dependent on both the cellular detail and the low-power configuration of the lesion. At each margin, a narrow spur of dermal connective tissue separates the normal epidermis from the lesion at the transitional junction between the normal and proliferating cells. For this reason, marginal punch biopsy is not adequate to distinguish between the two. Excisional biopsy or an incisional biopsy that contains a cross-section of the lesion into the adjacent normal skin is needed.

Therapy

Surgery

Because keratoacanthomas are difficult to separate clinically and microscopically from squamous cell carcinoma, and since substantial scarring occurs after spontaneous involution, small- to moderate-sized lesions are usually removed by excisional surgery. Giant lesions, or those in locations where removal would be mutilating or require extensive reconstruction, should be referred to a dermatologic consultant for consideration of alternative treatment. Recurrences of keratoacanthoma can occur after any type of therapy, and after apparent spontaneous involution.

Alternative Therapy

Other modalities used in the destruction of KAs include curettage and electrodesiccation, cryosurgery, intralesional injections of triamcinolone or 5-FU, highly fractionated soft X-irradiation, and the use of oral retinoids for multiple lesions.

Conditions That May Simulate Keratoacanthomas

Molluscum Contagiosum

An early KA lesion with a keratotic core may resemble a giant molluscum wart. The solitary lesion, rapid growth, and ultimate size will usually serve to distinguish the two.

Basal Cell Carcinoma

Early KA lesions with a central dell, a flesh-colored margin, and prominent vessels can be confused with a BCC. Basal cells are slow-growing, however, and are distinguishable as the central keratin core of the KA develops.

Squamous Cell Carcinoma

Both tumors can develop rapidly and show great clinical and microscopic similarities. They must be distinguished microscopically; however, this is not always possible.

Other Vegetating Lesions

Some deep fungal diseases produce vegetating lesions that could be confused with a giant highly keratotic KA. A punch biopsy with appropriate special stains should distinguish the two.

ANSWERS TO CLINICAL APPLICATION QUESTIONS

History Review

A 35-year-old farmer is seen at your office for a rapidly growing nodule on his right upper lip near the vermilion margin. This was first noticed 4 weeks ago. He is concerned about the character and potential of this lesion. Physical examination of the involved region reveals a lesion suggesting a keratoacanthoma.

1. What are the primary lesions that you would expect to find in keratoacanthoma?

Answer: A rapidly growing dome-shaped papule or nodule with a central dull pebbly core.

2. What are the secondary lesions that you would expect to find in keratoacanthoma?

Answer: Central vegetation and/or scarring.

3. Keratoacanthoma is most commonly mistaken for what other condition?

Answer: Squamous cell carcinoma resembles keratoacanthoma both on physical examination and microscopic evaluation. Distinguishing the two is not always possible.

4. What should you tell the patient about keratoacanthoma?

Answer: Keratoacanthoma is classified as a benign lesion but shows many signs and microscopic features of malignancy. Although true keratoacanthomas do not metastasize, they can cause significant scarring and alteration when they occur on a cosmetically sensitive site. Treatment is recommended to minimize scarring and to distinguish keratoacanthoma from squamous cell carcinoma.

5. Should you treat keratoacanthoma in this patient, and if so, how?

Answer: When a keratoacanthoma is small or occurs in an area that is not cosmetically sensitive, conservative elliptical excision or saucerization followed by curettage and desiccation is acceptable treatment. Giant keratoacanthomas or lesions on cosmetically sensitive areas such as the face should be referred to a dermatologic consultant for consideration of alternative treatments.

32 Common Skin Cancers

CLINICAL APPLICATION QUESTIONS

A 54-year-old tennis enthusiast is seen at your office for a lesion on the left side of her chin. The lesion has been present for 2 years and has increased in size about 50%. Two weeks ago, minor trauma caused bleeding and ulceration, which brought the lesion to her attention. Physical examination of the lesion reveals findings suggesting ulcerating basal cell carcinoma.

1. List the different types of basal cell carcinoma, and briefly describe the appearance of each.
2. What should you tell this patient about basal cell carcinoma?
3. Should you biopsy this lesion, and if so, how?
4. How should you treat this patient's basal cell carcinoma?

APPLICATION GUIDELINES: BASAL CELL CARCINOMA (BASAL CELL EPITHELIOMA)

Specific History

Onset

Basal cell carcinomas (BCCs) are the most common type of skin cancer and arise from pluripotential cells similar to those that make up the basal cell layer of the skin and appendages. BCCs occur most often in Caucasians aged 50 to 80 years with type I and II skin (Table 7). In localities with intense sun that are populated by large numbers of fair-skinned people, these tumors may be encountered in adolescents and younger adults. They begin with a focal lesion that may be a distinct papule, a nondescript relatively flat plaque, or in some cases a depressed discoloration.

Table 7
Skin Phototypes

Type	Skin Color	Response to Sun Exposure
I	Pale white	Do not tan; burn easily
II	White	Tan with difficulty; burn easily
III	White	Tan after initial sunburn
IV	Light bown	Tan easily
V	Brown	Tan easily
VI	Black	Become darker

From: *Current Clinical Practice: Dermatology Skills for Primary Care: An Illustrated Guide*
D.J. Trozak, D.J. Tennenhouse, and J.J. Russell © Humana Press, Totowa, NJ

Evolution of Disease Process

BCC is a tumor that is threatening because of its capacity to invade and destroy adjacent tissues. Metastasis is a rare event: only about 200 metastatic lesions have been recorded since the turn of the last century. Once spread occurs, the prognosis is grave. The main problem with BCC is the progressive invasion of adjacent tissues, causing destruction of vital anatomic structures and requiring extensive reconstruction. With invasion into areas such as the brain, death can occur from direct tumor extension. There are several clinical types of basal cell cancers, and the clinical types show some correlation with the tumor's aggressiveness.

Solid or **nodular type BCCs** present as translucent, smooth, gray to pink-gray papules or nodules that enlarge slowly over months to years. Prominent dilated (telangiectatic) blood vessels course over the surface of the lesion. With time, the lesion may ulcerate and deep local invasion may occur while peripheral extension continues. This form is common wherever BCC is found.

Ulcerating or **rodent ulcer type BCCs** form a central ulcer while the raised pearly border continues to extend peripherally. This type is common on the face and scalp, and local destruction of landmarks and vital structures such as the eyelids and canthal structures is the greatest problem.

Pigmented BCCs contain variable amounts of melanin, which is usually unevenly distributed. This variant may occur wherever BCC is found and may be confused with other benign and malignant pigmented growths. If BCC is suspected, a punch biopsy will readily distinguish it and does not worsen the prognosis should the lesion prove to be of melanocytic origin.

Morpheiform BCCs tend to occur over the central and upper face; they are difficult to diagnose because they are subtle lesions with few symptoms and they do not fit the usual clinical appearance of basal cell cancer. This type of basal cell lesion is flat to slightly raised, yellow or porcelain-white, and the surface shows discrete telangectasia. The margins are indistinct and they simulate a plaque of localized morphea. Ulceration and symptoms are rare, and these lesions can spread widely and deeply before detection. This is a more aggressive type of BCC and is more prone to recurrence.

Superficial BCCs occur frequently in areas with minimal light exposure, especially the trunk and lower extremities. Islands of basal cell lesions arise superficially in a multifocal fashion from the base of the epidermis. They are often multiple and are sometimes encountered in fair-skinned persons with minimal evidence of lifetime sun exposure. In some instances, there is a prior history of arsenic exposure. These tumors are usually relatively flat red or red-brown plaques that enlarge peripherally and may reach a diameter of several centimeters. They may easily be mistaken for plaques of psoriasis, nummular eczema, or a Bowen's epithelioma. Careful examination with a hand lens will usually reveal a thready or discontinuous pearly border that suggests the correct diagnosis. Although exophytic tumors and deep extension can occur within these lesions, both are uncommon even with longstanding growths. Large exophytic areas often have little or minimal deep invasion.

Giant or **mutilating BCCs** fortunately are uncommon. These are aggressive tumors which ulcerate and invade deeply, tend to recur, and are responsible for many of the metastatic and fatal cases. These lesions tend to occur on the central face and scalp.

Evolution of Skin Lesions

See Evolution of Disease Process section, above.

Provoking Factors

Chronic solar damage, X-ray and other forms of therapeutic radiation, trivalent inorganic arsenic exposure, burn scars, and vaccination scars have all been implicated as provoking factors for basal cell carcinoma. A dominantly inherited multisystem syndrome known as the "basal cell nevus syndrome" is responsible for a small number of cases.

Self-Medication

Self-treatment is occasionally a problem in patients who are self-medicating AKs from a home supply of 5-fluorouracil. Treatment of all but the most superficial of BCCs with this drug will remove the surface of the tumor while it continues to spread undetected in the dermis. Recurrence will give rise to a much more significant problem in regard to removal and repair. Patients should be carefully evaluated for malignant lesions before treating AKs with topical chemotherapy.

Supplemental Review From General History

In the case of multiple tumors, family history and history for possible arsenic exposure should be investigated.

Dermatologic Physical Exam

Primary Lesions

1. A dome-shaped translucent papule, flesh to pink-gray in color with dilated vessels over its surface. A central dell is common (*see* Photos 44,45).
2. A dome-shaped translucent nodule, flesh to pink-gray in color with dilated vessels over its surface (*see* Photos 46,47).
3. A yellow or porcelain-white plaque with dilated surface vessels, showing minimal elevation and having a shiny surface due to loss of skin lines (*see* Photos 48–50).
4. A red to red-brown plaque that is sharply demarcated, has a dull surface, exhibits a loss of skin lines, and usually shows a thready pearly margin (*see* Photos 51,52).
5. Pigmented variants may contain irregular flecks of melanin or may be so heavily pigmented that the lesion is predominantly gray-brown or brown (*see* Photos 53,54).

Secondary Lesions

1. Surface erosions are common (*see* Photos 51,52).
2. Central ulceration with peripheral spread is typical (*see* Photos 55–57).
3. Surface crusting (*see* Photos 52,57).
4. Eschar formation in late lesions (*see* Photo 57).
5. Scarring in areas of tumor regression (*see* Photos 53,57).
6. Sclerosis with the morpheiform type.

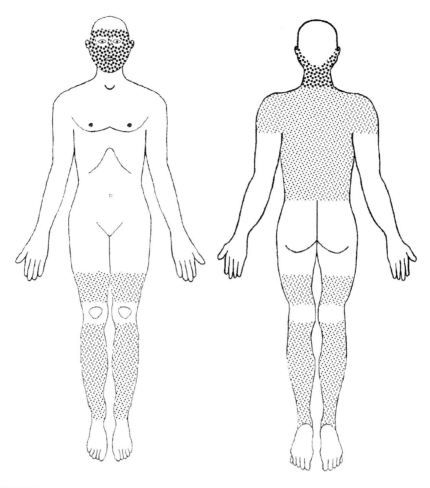

SOLID, ULCERATING, MORPHEIFORM, AND GIANT BASAL CELL CARCINOMAS MOST COMMON

SUPERFICIAL TYPE BASAL CELL CARCINOMAS MOST COMMON

Figure 10: Macrodistribution of basal cell carcinomas.

Distribution

Microdistribution: None.

Macrodistribution: Solid, ulcerating, morpheiform, and giant BCCs are more common over the sun-exposed skin of the central face and neck (*see* Fig. 10). Superficial BCCs are more common on the trunk and on the lower extremities (*see* Fig. 10).

Configuration

None.

Indicated Supporting Diagnostic Data

Biopsy

Punch biopsy of a suspect BCC is undertaken for purposes of diagnosis and also to look at the microscopic pattern of the tumor. Basal cell tumors have several histologic patterns. This pattern should be reported by the dermatopathologist because, along with the anatomic site, size, and patient's age, it will be a major factor in planning treatment.

Undifferentiated, adenoid, and superficial BCC histologic patterns tend to be very responsive to treatment and are less likely to recur. Micronodular, spiky, and metatypical (basosquamous) patterns are more likely to recur and should be treated more aggressively. Morpheiform or sclerosing patterns, tumors that are recurrent after initial therapy, tumors arising in old scar tissue, or tumors that show neural invasion should all be treated aggressively.

Therapy

Surgical Excision

Treatment of small, primary, uncomplicated basal cell carcinomas can be accomplished by excision. If the tumor has distinct margins and does not show any of the clinical or microscopic features associated with increased aggressiveness, a 3- to 5-mm margin of normal tissue should suffice. The specimen should be submitted for step sections to confirm complete surgical margins. After removal by any means, it is standard to follow the site every 3 months for the first year, and then on a yearly basis for the next 5 years.

When tissue exam shows an inadequate margin, then either reexcision of the site with repeat tissue examination should be done or the case should be referred to a dermatologic consultant. Because BCCs are stromal dependent growths, the recurrence rate is low even if a margin is clipped (about 30%). Depending on the site, histologic type of BCC, and the depth and the apparent amount of tumor based on evaluation of the tissue sections, dermatologists will inform the patient of the inadequate margin, explain the odds of recurrence, and offer a reexcision. If the patient declines, intensive follow-up is necessary. This is not a decision that should be undertaken by a primary care practitioner. Clinicians often underestimate the long-term potential of basal cell carcinoma. Remember, your best chance of eradicating these tumors is the first time around. Although most BCCs are indolent in their primary state, dealing with a recurrent or neglected lesion is an entirely different matter and may require substantial expense or disfiguring surgery. When complicated situations arise, dermatologists are the only physicians familiar with the entire biologic potential of these lesions and are the only ones familiar with all the techniques used to treat them.

Other Treatments

1. Excision with complicated flap and graft closures.
2. Curettage and electrodesiccation.
3. Cryosurgery.
4. Radiation.
5. Excision under frozen control, employed for complicated closures and lesions with indistinct margins.
6. Moh's fresh tissue microscopic excision, which is employed for problem tumors or where preservation of maximal amounts of uninvolved adjacent tissue is essential.

The decision as to which treatment method is best requires considering the lesion's size, site, and histologic pattern along with the patient's age, general health, and expectations in regard to the final cosmetic result.

Conditions That May Simulate Basal Cell Carcinoma

Molluscum Contagiosum

An early nodular BCC with a central dell could be confused with a large molluscum wart. The core of the wart is usually keratotic, and if expressed out and smeared, will show diagnostic molluscum bodies. In addition, molluscum lesions are usually multiple, while BCC is solitary. If the diagnosis cannot be determined on clinical exam, a biopsy will distinguish one from the other.

Common Compound Nevi

An early smooth-surfaced BCC can be very difficult to distinguish from a flesh-colored or lightly pigmented compound mole. Pigmented BCCs can also resemble small normally pigmented nevi. BCCs tend to be translucent, while nevi are opaque. Nevi often contain terminal hairs. The melanin in a pigmented BCC is often present in small, irregular, unevenly distributed clumps. Biopsy may be required to distinguish the two.

Sebaceous Hyperplasia

This is a common benign change that occurs in persons with coarse, oily, seborrheic complexions. The age of onset coincides with that of BCC. The clinical lesions consist of raised papules with a central dell 3 to 7 mm in size. The resemblance to BCC is striking. Sebaceous hyperplasia usually has an intense white or yellow color, which is helpful. In addition, close inspection will usually reveal several other similar lesions, and will sometimes show sebaceous debris at the central pore.

Nummular Eczema/Psoriasis

Superficial BCC can be difficult to distinguish from these inflammatory skin disorders and tends to occur in the same distribution. The latter usually show multiple lesions, and tend to move from one site to another. Nummular eczema is pruritic. There is almost always a thready pearly border at the expanding rim of the basal cell. Biopsy is best obtained from the rim, as superficial BCCs may have skip areas.

Bowen's Epithelioma

This is an *in situ* squamous cell cancer that is clinically distinguishable from superficial BCC only by the thready pearly border. Biopsy is often needed to separate the two.

Nodular Melanoma

Pigmented BCC can imitate NM. The BCC usually shows translucency and a pearly margin. When NM is seriously being considered, a dermatologic consultation is indicated.

Morphea

Morpheiform BCC is strikingly similar to scar tissue and to localized scleroderma. Careful inspection will often reveal a rolled translucent border. Biopsy will distinguish them.

APPLICATION GUIDELINES: SQUAMOUS CELL CARCINOMA OF SKIN

Specific History

Onset

Squamous cell carcinomas (SCCs) of skin are the second most common type of skin cancer and are about one-tenth as common as basal cell cancers. They are composed of malignant keratinocytes, which breach the normal barrier at the epidermal basement membrane and invade the underlying dermis. SCC, like BCC, is common in fair-skinned Caucasians with types I and II skin. Peak age of onset is about a decade later than that for BCC (age 60 to 80 years). Isolated lesions may be seen in much younger persons when specific provoking factors are present. Onset is earlier in fair-skinned populations living in subtropical climates. Incidence increases by a factor of five times in sunny versus temperate regions.

Persons of Asian descent and persons with very heavily pigmented skin have a low incidence of SCC on sun-exposed sites; studies, however, indicate that even persons with type III complexions who seldom burn are susceptible to these tumors once a certain cumulative threshold of solar damage is reached. All skin types are susceptible to SCC induced by chronic injury or irritation.

Evolution of Disease Process

Like basal cell carcinoma, SCC has the capacity to cause significant destruction of adjacent tissue. Unlike BCC, it can metastasize to other sites via the lymphatics. Squamous cell tumors arising on areas of chronic solar damage are usually well differentiated and have a low incidence of spread. Exceptions to this are the vermilion margin of the lip, external genitalia, and the skin of the external ear. Regional node spread from these three sites is fairly common. Tumors arising in chronic scar or at sites of injury other than chronic sun damage also seem to have a greater capacity for distant spread. The tendency to metastasize is also inversely related to the degree of cellular differentiation.

SCC begins as an area of thickening (induration), and may present as a papule, nodule, or plaque with a scaling, verrucous, keratotic, eroded, or ulcerated surface. They usually become quite exophytic, and commonly bleed when the adherent scale is removed or they are otherwise manipulated. These lesions fissure and split easily with any handling. Growth rate is variable and lesions may be indolent with slow growth over several months or quite rapid. Rare lesions can double in size in a month or less. These high-grade lesions can also metastasize within a few months of onset.

Evolution of Skin Lesions

See Evolution of Disease Process section, above.

Provoking Factors

Any site of chronic cicatricial scar formation or chronic irritation may be predisposed to SCC. The following provoking factors have been recorded:

1. Ultraviolet radiation.
2. Photochemotherapy with 8-methoxypsoralen followed by UVA radiation (PUVA) therapy for psoriasis.

3. X-irradiation.
4. Inorganic trivalent arsenicals.
5. Coal tar, tar derivatives, and other hydrocarbons.
6. Burn scars.
7. Vaccination scars.
8. Tight or cicatricial scars.
9. Certain strains of human papillomavirus.
10. Scarring from cutaneous tuberculosis and lupus erythematosus.
11. Immunosuppression, either natural or iatrogenic (SCCs are very common in transplant patients on chronic immune suppression).
12. Smoking and use of smokeless tobacco are common factors in men with lesions of the lips and oral cavity.
13. Heavy alcohol intake may combine with tobacco as a cofactor.

Self-Medication

Self-treatment is occasionally a problem in patients who are self-medicating actinic keratosis from a home supply of 5-fluorouracil. Treatment of SCCs with this drug will remove the tumor surface while it continues to spread undetected. Recurrence may give rise to a much more significant problem in regard to removal and repair.

Supplemental Review From General History

When lesions occur on the lips, a careful history for tobacco and ethanol intake is essential, along with a careful exam of the entire oral cavity and the regional nodes. When SCC arises in the absence of chronic sun damage, history should be reviewed for antecedent conditions, injuries, and old scars.

Dermatologic Physical Exam

Primary Lesions

1. Indurated papule (*see* Photo 58).
2. Indurated nodule (*see* Photo 59).
3. Indurated plaque.

The induration around papules and nodules is at the base. Surface character may be variable (*see* Secondary Lesions section). Color varies from gray to yellow-white to red. The surface is friable, and bleeds or splits easily with trauma. Lesions tend to be raised or exophytic.

Secondary Lesions

1. Hyperkeratotic adherent scale (*see* Photo 59).
2. Papillomatosis.
3. Cutaneous horn formation (*see* Photo 38).
4. Surface erosions.
5. Fissures.
6. Ulceration (*see* Photo 59).

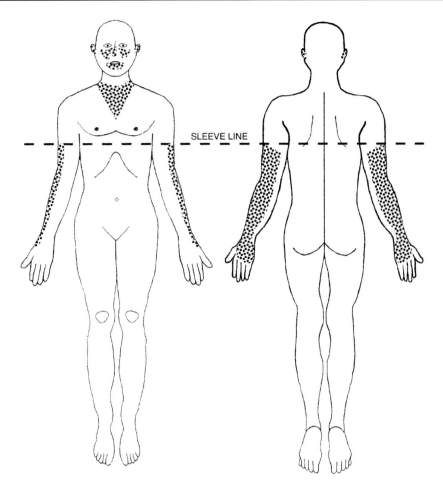

Figure 11: Macrodistribution of squamous cell carcinoma.

Distribution
   Microdistribution: None.

   Macrodistribution: Squamous cell carcinoma of skin almost always arises on previously damaged skin, and is most common on the central face, pinna, dorsal forearms, and the top of the hands (*see* Fig. 11). In these locations, chronic solar injury is the most common cause. Dark-skinned people are more prone to develop SCC at sites of chronic injury on the lower extremities. The vermilion margin of the lip, penis, and vulva are also common sites. A special site that is often overlooked is the nail bed. Chronic X-ray exposure in medical personnel was once a provoking factor in this location.

Configuration
   None.

Indicated Supporting Diagnostic Data
Biopsy

A punch, incisional, or excisional biopsy is the definitive laboratory study. The pathology report should specify whether the tumor is well, moderately, or poorly differentiated. This is determined by the number of atypical mitosis, degree of tumor cell adhesiveness, proportion of differentiated cells, and the tumor's overall general architecture. The older Broder's classification is seldom used today. Poorly differentiated tumors should be treated more aggressively because of a greater tendency to metastasize.

Therapy
Surgical Excision

Treatment of small primary uncomplicated squamous cell skin cancers can be best accomplished by surgical excision. Well-differentiated lesions in areas of chronic solar injury can be resected with a clear clinical margin of 5 mm, and should be submitted for step sections to confirm clear microscopic margins. Larger tumors or those exhibiting rapid growth or lesser degrees of differentiation should be removed more aggressively.

When tissue exam shows an inadequate margin, reexcision of the site should be undertaken promptly because of the greater tendency for SCC to spread into the lymphatics or to distant sites.

Follow-up, similar to that with BCC, should be every 3 months for the first year, then yearly for the next 5 years. Regional lymph nodes should be examined along with the primary excision site on each visit.

Other Treatments

Other treatment modalities employed are similar to those used for BCC. These include:
1. Excision with complicated flap and graft closures.
2. Curettage and electrodesiccation.
3. Cryosurgery.
4. Radiation.
5. Excision under frozen control, employed for complicated closures and lesions with indistinct margins.
6. Moh's fresh tissue microscopic excision, which is employed for problem tumors or where preservation of maximal amounts of uninvolved adjacent tissue is essential.

Here also, the decision as to which method is optimal involves consideration of the lesion's size, site, and histologic pattern along with the patient's age, general health, and expectations in regard to the final cosmetic result. When the tumor is large, poorly differentiated, or penetrates deeply into the dermis, consideration should be given to adjunctive postoperative radiation once complete excision has been achieved.

Conditions That May Simulate Squamous Cell Carcinoma
Molluscum Contagiosum

A giant, rapidly growing molluscum lesion as might occur in a person with immune suppression could be confused with SCC. The squamous cell lesion should have an indurated base. A molluscum smear or biopsy will distinguish the two.

Verruca Vulgaris

VV with rapid growth and formation of a cutaneous horn may mimic SCC. Again, the latter has a more indurated base. Biopsy may be needed to distinguish the lesions, especially those involving the nail bed. Any refractory lesion in this location should be promptly referred, especially when there is a history of radiation exposure.

Actinic Keratosis

Hypertrophic AKs or those with a prominent cutaneous horn may be confused with SCC. The diagnosis is more likely to be SCC if there is induration at the base. A biopsy is usually needed to distinguish them.

Seborrheic Keratosis

SKs can usually be distinguished clinically by their "stuck-on" appearance and waxy surface feel. SKs also do not have the indurated base seen with SCC.

Keratoacanthoma

Both tumors evolve rapidly and show similar clinical and microscopic features. Differentiation must made microscopically; however, this is not always possible.

Bowen's Epithelioma/Superficial Spreading BCC

Early invasive SCC developing in a Bowen's lesion may not show enough clinical induration to distinguish it from a preinvasive Bowen's or superficial spreading BCC except by biopsy.

Nodular Melanoma

Amelanotic NM and an exophytic SCC that has lost its keratotic surface may be very similar in appearance. Location on chronically sun-damaged skin favors the latter; however, this can be confirmed only by biopsy with microscopic examination.

ANSWERS TO CLINICAL APPLICATION QUESTIONS

History Review

A 54-year-old tennis enthusiast is seen at your office for a lesion on the left side of her chin. The lesion has been present for 2 years and has increased in size about 50%. Two weeks ago, minor trauma caused bleeding and ulceration, which brought the lesion to her attention. Physical examination of the lesion reveals findings suggesting ulcerating basal cell carcinoma.

1. List the different types of basal cell carcinoma, and briefly describe the appearance of each.

Answer:
   a. Solid or nodular basal cell carcinoma—smooth, translucent gray to gray-pink papules or nodules.
   b. Ulcerating basal cell carcinoma—nodules with a central punched-out ulcer and a raised translucent border.

   c. Pigmented basal cell carcinoma—papules, nodules, or plaques with flecks of brown pigmentation interspersed with gray translucent areas.
   d. Morpheiform basal cell carcinoma—patches or plaques that are yellow or porcelain white in color with dilated surface vessels.
   e. Superficial basal cell carcinoma—shallow plaques that are red-brown with a dull or scaling surface and a thready pearly border.

2. What should you tell this patient about basal cell carcinoma?

Answer: Basal cell carcinoma is the most common form of skin cancer. Metastasis is rare and usually associated only with tumors that have been neglected. Treatment is needed to prevent local destruction of normal tissue.

3. Should you biopsy this lesion, and if so, how?

Answer: A suspected basal cell carcinoma should be biopsied both to establish the diagnosis and to determine the microscopic pattern that can affect choice of treatment. Punch biopsy should be obtained from the translucent margin.

4. How should you treat this patient's basal cell carcinoma?

Answer: Excision followed by microscopic confirmation of clear margins is the treatment of choice. The type and complexity of the excision and repair are determined by the microscopic pattern of the basal cell carcinoma, the defect required to obtain clear margins, and the patient's desires regarding cosmetic results. Certain superficial basal cell carcinomas on the trunk and extremities are better treated by curettage and electrodesiccation. Following treatment, reevaluation of the surgical site every 3 months for the first year, then yearly for the next 5 years, is appropriate.

REFERENCES for Part V

1. Champion RH, Burton JL, Ebling FJG. Textbook of Dermatology. 5th. Ed. Oxford: Blackwell Scientific Publications, 1992, pp. 1465–1467, 1526–1527, 1527–1528, 2535, 1529–1533, 1535–36, 1543–1545, 1556–1557, 1545–1560, 1478–1479, 1470–1473, 1481–1483, 1488–1502.
2. Braun-Falco O, Plewig G, Wolff HH, Winkelmann RK. Dermatology. Berlin-Heidelberg: Springer-Verlag, 1991, pp. 987–989, 689, 692–694, 956–962, 705, 1036–1045, 999–1001, 1014–1015, 1018–1035.
3. Leider M, Rosenblum M. A Dictionary of Dermatological Words, Terms and Phrases. New York-Toronto-London-Sydney: Mc Graw-Hill, 1968, pp. 297.
4. Karvonen S, Vaajalahti P, Marenk M, et al. Birthmarks in 4,346 Finnish Newborns. Acta Derm Venereol 1992;72:55–57.
5. Alper JC, Holmes LB. The Incidence and Significance of Birthmarks in a Cohort of 4,641 Newborns. Ped Dermatol 1983;1:58–68.
6. Rhodes AR. Pigmented Birthmarks and Precursor Melanocytic Lesions of Cutaneous Melanoma Identifiable in Childhood. Ped Clin N Amer 30, 1883;#3:435–463.
7. Clark Jr. WH, Reimer RR, Greene M, et al. Origin of Familial Malignant Melanomas from Hereditable Melanocytic Lesions. Arch Dermatol 1978;114:732–738.
8. Lynch HT, Frichot RM, Lunch JF. Familial Atypical Multiple Mole Melanoma Syndrome. J Med Genet 1978;15:352–360.
9. Elder DE, Goldman LI, Goldman SC, et al. Dysplastic Nevus Syndrome: A Phenotypic Association of Sporadic Cutaneous Melanoma. Cancer 1980;46:1787–1794.
10. NIH Consensus Development Panel on Early Melanoma, Diagnosis and Treatment of Early Melanoma. JAMA 1992;268:1314–1319.
11. NIH Consensus Development Panel, Precursors to Malignant Melanoma. JAMA 1984;251:1864–1866.
12. Schneider JS, Moore DH, Sagebiel RW. Risk Factors for Melanoma Incidence in Prospective Follow Up, The Importance of Atypical (Dysplastic) Nevi. Arch Dermatol 1994;130:1002–1007.
13. Holly EA, Kelly JW, Shpall SN, et al. Number of Melanocytic Nevi as a Major Risk Factor for Malignant Melanoma. J Amer Acad Dermatol 1987;17:459–467.
14. Tiersten AD, Grin CM, Kopf AW, et al. Prospective Follow Up for Malignant Melanoma in Patients with Atypical-Mole (Dysplastic-Nevus) Syndrome. J Dermatol Surg Oncol 1991;17:44–48.
15. Marghoob AA, Kopf AW, Rigel DS, et al. Risk of Cutaneous Malignant Melanoma in Patients with "Classic" Atypical-Mole Syndrome. Arch Dermatol 1994;130:993–998.
16. Diagnosis and Treatment of Early Melanoma: report on the NIH consensus development conference January 27-29, 1992. The Melanoma Letter 10, #1: 1–4, 1992.
17. Kelly JW, Crutcher WA, Sagebiel RW. Clinical Diagnosis of Dysplastic Nevi, A Clinicopathologic Correlation. J Am Acad Dermatol 1986;14:1044–1052.
18. Special Symposia, The Management of Congenital Nevocytic Nevi. Ped Dermatol 1984; 2:143–156.
19. Roth ME, Grant-Kels JM, Kuhn MK, et al. Melanoma in Children. J Amer Acad Dermatol 1990;22:265–274.
20. Ceballos PI, Ruiz-Maldonado R, Mihm MC. Melanoma in Children. NEJM 1995;332: 656–662.

From: *Current Clinical Practice: Dermatology Skills for Primary Care: An Illustrated Guide*
D.J. Trozak, D.J. Tennenhouse, and J.J. Russell © Humana Press, Totowa, NJ

21. Rhodes AR. Pigmented Birthmarks and Precursor Melanocytic Lesions of Cutaneous Melanoma Identifiable in Childhood. Ped Clin N Amer 1983;30:435–463.
22. Trozak DJ, Rowland WD, Hu F. Metastatic Malignant Melanoma in Prepubertal Children. Pediatrics 1975;55:191–204.
23. Quaba AA, Wallace AF. The Incidence of Malignant Melanoma (0 to 15 Years of Age) Arising in "Large Congenital Nevocellular Nevi". Plast Reconstr Surg 1986;78:174–182.
24. Clemmenson OJ, Kroon S. The Histology of "Congenital Features" in Early Acquired Melanocytic Nevi. J Amer Acad Dermatol 1988;19:742–746.
25. Williams ML. Early-Onset Nevi. (Correspondence) Ped Dermatol 1993;10:198–199.
26. Walton RG, Jacobs AH, Cox AJ. Pigmented Lesions in Newborn Infants. Br J Dermatol 1976;95:389–396.
27. Alper JC, Holmes LB. The Incidence and Significance of Birthmarks in a Cohort of 4,641 Newborns. Ped Dermatol 1983;1:58–68.
28. Gari LM, Rivers JK, Kopf AW. Melanomas Arising in Large Congenital Nevocytic Nevi: A Prospective Study. Ped Dermatol 1988;5:151–158.
29. Rhodes AR, Wood WC, Sober AJ, et al. Nonepidermal Origin of Malignant Melanoma Associated with a Giant Congenital Nevocellular Nevus. Plast Reconstr Surg 1981;67:782–790.
30. From L. Congenital Nevi-Let's Be Practical. Ped Dermatol 1992;9:345–346.
31. Rhodes AR, Melski JW. Small Congenital Nevocellular Nevi and the Risk of Cutaneous Melanoma. J Pediatr 1982;100:219–224.
32. Elder DE. The blind men and the elephant: Different Views of Small Congenital Nevi. Arch Dermatol 1985;121:1263–1265.
33. Johnson TM, Smith JW, Nelson BR, Chang A. Current Therapy for Cutaneous Melanoma. J Amer Acad Dermatol 1995;32:689–707.
34. Koh HK. Cutaneous Melanoma. NEJM 325: 171–182, 1991.
35. Kopf AW, Bart RS, Rodriguez-Sains RS, Ackerman AB. Malignant Melanoma. New York: Masson Publishing USA, Inc, 1979. pp. 7–15.
36. Clark WH, From L, Bernadino EA, Mihm MC. The Histogenesis and Biologic Behavior of Primary Human Malignant Melanomas of Skin. Cancer Res 1969;29:705–727.
37. Breslow A. Thickness, Cross-Sectional Areas and Depth of Invasion in the Prognosis of Cutaneous Melanoma. Ann Surg 1970;172:902–908.
38. Ho VC, Sober AJ. Therapy for Cutaneous Melanoma: An Update. J Amer Acad Dermatol 1990;22:159–176.
39. Epstein E, Bragg K, Linden G. Biopsy and Prognosis of Malignant Melanoma. JAMA 1969;208:1369–1371.
40. Lederman JS, Sober AJ. Does Biopsy Influence Survival in Clinical Stage I Cutaneous Melanoma? J Amer Acad Dermatol 1985;13:983–987.
41. Naylor MF, Boyd A, Smith DW, et al. High Sun Protection Factor Sunscreens in the Suppression of Actinic Neoplasia. Arch Dermatol 1995;131:170–175.
42. Williams ML, Pennella R. Melanoma, Melanocytic Nevi and Other Risk Factors in Children. J Pediatr 1994;124:833–845.
43. Handfield-Jones SE, Smith NP. Malignant Melanoma in Childhood. Br J Dermatol 1995;134: 607–616.
44. Garbe C, Buttner P, Weiss J, et al. Risk Factors for Developing Cutaneous Melanoma and Criteria for Identifying Persons at 1994;Risk:Multi-Center Case Control Study of the Central Malignant Melanoma Registry of the German Dermatological Society. J Invest Dermatol 102; 695–699.
45. Berwick M. Reduction of Melanoma Mortality through Skin Self-Examination. The Melanoma Letter 14 1996;#2:1–4.
46. Tucker MA, Halpern A, Holley EA. et al. Clinically Recognized Dysplastic Nevi: A Central Risk Factor For Cutaneous Melanoma. JAMA 1997;277:1439-1444.

47. Snels DG, Hille ET, Gruis NA et al. Risk of Cutaneous Malignant Melanoma in Patients with Nonfamilial Atypical Nevi from a Pigmented Lesions Clinic. J Amer Acad Dermatol 1999; 40:686-693.

49. Naeyaert JM, Brochez L. Dysplastic Nevi. NEJM 2003;349:2233-2240.

50. Tremblay JF, O'Brian, Chauvin PJ. Melanoma in situ of the Oral Mucosa in an Adolescent with Dysplastic Nevus Syndrome. J Amer Acad Dermatol 2000;42:844-846.

51. Huynh PM, Glusac EJ, Alvarez-Franco M et al. Numerous, Small, Darkly Pigmented Melanocytic Nevi: The Cheetah Phenotype. J Amer Acad Dermatol 2003;48:707-713.

52. Sahin S, Levin L, Kopf A et al. Risk of Melanoma in Medium-sized Congenital melanocytic nevi: A Follow-up study. J Amer Acad Dermatol 1998;39:428-433.

53. Williams M. Melanoma, Melanocytic Nevi, and Other Melanoma Risk Factors in Children. J Pediatr 1994;124:833-845.

54. Ruiz Maldonado R, Orozoco-Covarrubias M. Malignant Melanoma in Children. Arch Dermatol 1997;133:363-371.

55. Richardson SK, Tannous ZS, Mihm Jr. MC. Congenital and Infantile Melanoma: Review of the Literature and Report of an Uncommon Variant, Pigment-synthesizing Melanoma. J Amer Acad Dermatol 2002;47:77-90.

56. Chen YJ, Wu CW, Chen JT et al. Clinicopathologic analysis of Malignant Melanoma in Taiwan. J Amer Acad Dermatol 1999;41:(45-949.

57. The Rationale Behind the 2002 AJCC Melanoma Staging Committee Recommendations. The Melanoma Letter 19 2001;#4:1-4.

58. Kashani-Sabet M, Sagibiel RW, Ferriera CMM et al. Vascular Involvement in the Prognosis of Primary Cutaneous Melanoma. Arch Dermatol 2001;137:1169-1173.

59. Perrott RE, Glass LF, Reintgen DS et al. Reassessing the Role of Lymphatic Mapping and Sentinel Lymphadenectomy in the Management of Cutaneous Malignant Melanoma. J Amer Acad Dermatol 2003;49:567-588.

60. Guidelines /Outcomes Committee AAD. Guidelines of Care for Primary Cutaneous Melanoma. J Amer Acad Dermatol 2001;45:579-586.

61. Guidelines /Outcomes Committee AAD. Draft Guidelines of Care for AAD Member Comment. Dermatology World: 1-24, Suppl. May, 2000.

62. Sentinel Node Biopsy: The Evolving Standard of Care for Melanoma Patients. The Melanoma Letter 21 2003;#1:1-2.

63. Johnson TM, Bradford CR, Gruber SB et al. Staging Workup, Sentinel Node Biopsy, and Follow-up tests for Melanoma. Arch Dermatol 2004;140:107-113.

64. Medalie N, AckermanAB. Sentinel Node Biopsy Has No Benefit for Patients with Primary Cutaneous Melanoma: An Assertion Based on Comprehensive, Critical Analysis. Dermatology 2002;101:1-50.

65. Physicians Desk Reference. Thomson 58th. Ed., 2004.

66. Wolverton SE. Comprehensive Dermatologic Drug Therapy. W.B. Saunders Company, 2001.

67. Rigel DS. The Effect of Sunscreen Use on Melanoma Risk. Derm Clin V20: #4, W.B Saunders Company, October 2002.

68. Imiquimod (Aldara) for Actinic Keratosis. The Medical Letter 2004;46:42-44.

69. Abbasi NR, Shaw HM, Rigel DS et al. Early Diagnosis of Cutaneous Melanoma: Revisiting the ABCD criteria. JAMA 2004;292:2771–2776.

70. The New NCCN Guidelines for Management of Melanoma. The Melanoma Letter. 2004; 1:1–4.

71. Fitzpatrick TB, Johnso RA, Wolff K. Color Atlas and Synopsis of Clinical Dermatology. 4th Ed. McGraw-Hill Medical Publishing Division, 2001, p. 212.

Part VI: Vesiculo-Bullous and Papulo-Pustular Disorders

IMPORTANT ABBREVIATIONS USED IN THIS PART:

HIV	Human immunodeficiency virus
HSV	Herpes simplex virus
HSV-1	Herpes simplex virus, type 1
HSV-2	Herpes simplex virus, type 2
HZV	Herpes zoster virus
LE	Lupus erythematosis
PCR	Polymerase chain reaction
PHN	Postherpetic neuralgia
RIF	Rapid immunofluorescence test
SPF	Sun protection factor

33 Impetigo *(Impetigo Contagiosa)*

INTRODUCTION

The following three clinical variants of impetigo are discussed in this chapter:

1. Nonbullous impetigo.
2. Bullous impetigo.
3. Secondary impetiginization superimposed on another primary dermatitis.

CLINICAL APPLICATION QUESTIONS

A 14-year-old girl presents at your afternoon clinic accompanied by her mother for evaluation of oozing blisters on the left upper thigh starting at the level of the gluteal crease. Onset was sudden with rapid progression over 3 days, and the lesions are both tender and pruritic. The mother is concerned about some sort of insect-bite reaction and about the rapid progression of the lesions. You suspect impetigo.

1. With what primary form of impetigo is this clinical course most consistent?
2. What provoking factors might account for this somewhat unusual anatomic location?
3. What are the primary lesions of bullous impetigo?
4. What are the secondary lesions of bullous impetigo?
5. What treatment should you start?

APPLICATION GUIDELINES

Specific History

Onset

Onset of impetigo on otherwise normal skin is abrupt. When impetigo occurs as a secondary complication of another skin disorder, the onset can be insidious and it can be difficult to recognize. Impetigo may affect any age group, but is most commonly encountered in preschool and school-aged children.

Evolution of Disease Process

There are two primary forms of impetigo: bullous and nonbullous. Both primary forms begin as localized disease and usually extend peripherally onto the adjacent skin. Localization to one or two sites is most common. Extensive disease may occur if early symptoms are neglected, or if there is an underlying pruritic skin disorder such as atopic

From: *Current Clinical Practice: Dermatology Skills for Primary Care: An Illustrated Guide*
D.J. Trozak, D.J. Tennenhouse, and J.J. Russell © Humana Press, Totowa, NJ

dermatitis or scabies. Cellulitis, osteomyelitis, septic arthritis, pneumonia, and septicemia may complicate either of the primary clinical forms of impetigo.

Nonbullous impetigo tends to be somewhat indolent with gradual extension, and may spontaneously resolve over a few weeks or may chronically extend for long periods. Since the early 1980s, the organisms most frequently cultured are phage group II, *Staphylococcus aureus*. The predominant organisms during the late 1960s and 1970s were Lancefield Group A, β-hemolytic streptococci. These organisms, and occasionally other Lancefield groups, are now encountered primarily in children ages 3 to 7 years. When nephritogenic strains of streptococci are involved, there is a significant incidence of post-streptococcal acute glomerulonephritis. Scarlet fever, but not rheumatic fever, has also been reported as a postimpetigo event. Lymphangitis, suppurative lymphadenitis, and onset of psoriasis vulgaris may follow a streptococcal impetigo.

The striking appearance and more rapid extension of the bullous-type impetigo usually compels victims or their parents to seek help promptly. Bullous impetigo can also spontaneously resolve. Typically, it spreads to adjacent skin and may jump to new sites while the original sites clear. The cause of this variant is a strain of staphylococcus, usually one of several group II phage types. These bacteria secrete epidermolytic toxins that bind to and split the epidermis just below the granular cell layer. Unrecognized or untreated in neonates, this form of impetigo can generalize resulting in pemphigus neonatorum, which carries a high mortality.

Secondary impetiginization is usually a chronic low-grade infection of a primary skin disease with an organism of low pathogenicity. Failure to recognize and treat this complication can materially interfere with the management of the primary dermatitis. The organisms involved are usually strains of *Staphylococcus aureus*.

Evolution of Skin Lesions

The nonbullous type begins with thin-walled vesicles that are transient and are seldom seen. The presenting clinical lesions are crusted, burnished, red macules. Lesions are grouped, and often coalesce while they extend in an irregular fashion. As they heal, the erythema fades, and the crusts and scales separate leaving transient hyper- or hypopigmentation. Normally there is no scarring with any type of impetigo.

Bullous impetigo begins with clear, fluid-filled bullae 1 to 2 cm in size, which may persist for some time prior to rupture. When the blisters are old the fluid may become turbid and occasionally gravity will localize the turbidity to the lower half of the bulla. As the blisters rupture, a moist central surface is uncovered. The blister roof at the point of attachment is retained, causing a peripheral scale with its free edge turned in toward the center. Lesions tend to heal centrally. This feature, combined with a tendency to coalesce, can produce striking patterns. Secondary impetiginization presents as serous exudative change and honey-colored crusting superimposed upon the primary skin condition.

Provoking Factors

Crowding, poor hygiene, intimate contact, and fomites predispose to epidemics of this disease. Subtropical humid climates favor the nonbullous variety, and both primary types are more common during the warm summer months. Abrasions, insect bites, or chafing from tight wet bathing suits can provide a portal of entry. In some third-world countries, insects are a significant vector. An underlying pruritic skin problem predisposes to secondary impetiginization and also widespread primary impetigo when more aggressive organisms are involved.

Self-Medication

Self-treatment with topical steroids can spread the disease. Self-treatment with topical antimicrobials such as neomycin or bacitracin is sometimes effective in localized nonbullous disease.

Supplemental Review From General History

Inquire regarding playmates, siblings, or preschool contacts that may have been the original source of the infection and could act as a source of reinfection.

Dermatologic Physical Exam

Primary Lesions

1. Nonbullous impetigo: Thin-walled, small, transient vesicles that rupture easily (*see* Photo 1); burnished, moist, deep-red macules 0.5 to 1.0 cm that may enlarge as they coalesce (*see* Photo 2).
2. Bullous impetigo: Bullae 1 to 2 cm in size that are clear at first and later become cloudy (*see* Photos 3,4); scaling and red plaques 1 to 2 cm or more in size that show central resolution (*see* Photo 5).

Secondary Lesions

1. Crusting, typically honey-colored, that may also be brown or hemorrhagic (*see* Photos 4–6).
2. Loose white scale that occurs in both types at the attachment point of the degenerated blister roof (*see* Photos 5,6).
3. Postinflammatory hyperpigmentation.
4. Postinflammatory hypopigmentation.

Distribution

Microdistribution: None.

Macrodistribution: Nonbullous impetigo favors the perinasal and perioral areas of the face (*see* Fig. 1), while the bullous type is more common in intertriginous regions (*see* Fig. 2). Impetigo may occur almost anywhere on the skin surface.

Configuration

1. Grouped lesions (both primary types) (*see* Photos 1,5).
2. Annular (bullous type) (*see* Photos 3,6).
3. Polycyclic (bullous type) (*see* Photo 1).

Indicated Supporting Diagnostic Data

Gram Stain of Blister Fluid

This simple test is positive in staphylococcal bullous impetigo, and shows clumps of Gram-positive cocci. In nonbullous impetigo, smears can be of value if early vesicles are still present. Chains of Gram-positive cocci may be seen.

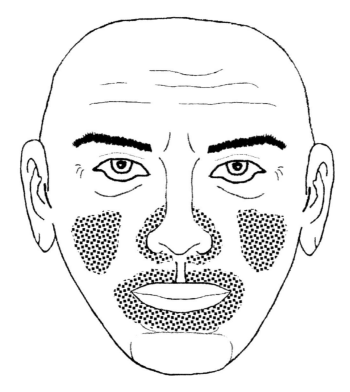

Figure 1: Macrodistribution of nonbullous impetigo.

Culture and Sensitivity

These studies are needed when the clinical circumstances suggest:

1. Another noninfectious blistering disorder.
2. The impetigo does not respond to antimicrobial treatment, suggesting a resistant organism.
3. Cases of bullous impetigo where therapy will be initiated with erythromycin because of penicillin allergy. If the organism recovered is erythromycin-resistant, then treatment can be promptly corrected.

Serology

ASO titers are weakly positive in streptococcal pyoderma and are of little value. Anti-DNAase B and hyaluronidase titers rise briskly and are of greater value in the serodiagnosis. In most instances, these are of only academic interest.

Microscopic Urinalysis

This cost-effective test should be done when streptococcal-type impetigo is diagnosed, and then repeated 2 to 3 weeks post-therapy to screen for any sign of acute glomerulonephritis. This is especially pertinent during epidemics.

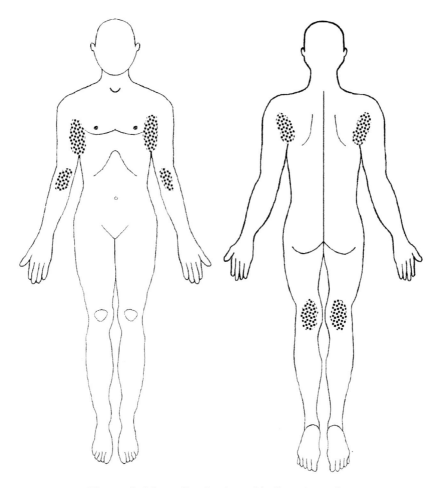

Figure 2: Macrodistribution of bullous impetigo.

Therapy

Hygiene

Minimal direct physical contact with the victim and avoidance of fomites will limit spread within family and school units. Separate hand towels and bath linens should be encouraged and disinfection of communal basins and tubs should be recommended. Preschool and school-aged children are best quarantined for a few days until treatment has rendered them noncontagious. If they remain in school, all contact activities or sports that involve common equipment that could serve as fomites should be suspended.

Topical Therapy

Topical 2% mupirocin ointment applied in a thin layer TID is effective in eradicating mild nonbullous impetigo and is active against streptococci and most of the staphylococcus organisms encountered. Mupirocin or bacitracin ointments can also be used to reduce communicability during the early stages of systemic treatment. This will add to the immediate cost, but may be cost-effective if other cases within a family or social unit are prevented. Because of the thickness and persistence of the blister roof, topical treatment of bullous impetigo is not recommended. Some mupirocin-resistant staphylococcus organisms have already been reported.

Recurrent impetigo may indicate chronic *S. aureus* colonization of the nasal vestibule, perineum, or axillae. Cultures are indicated. Topical mupirocin applied to the colonized carrier site QID for 5 to 7 days will be effective in most cases.

Systemic Therapy

Stains of *S. aureus* isolated from both clinical forms of impetigo have shown increasing resistance to penicillin and erythromycin. As a result, cephalexin, dicloxacillin, and amoxicillin/clavulanic acid are now the initial systemic agents of choice and should be administered in weight-adjusted doses. In both primary forms of impetigo, therapy should be continued for 7 to 10 days.

Secondary impetiginization of a primary skin disorder usually involves an antibiotic-sensitive Staphylococcus organism of low pathogenicity. Here, low-dose oral erythromycin for short periods over 7 to 14 days is often effective. If signs of superficial impetiginization persist, a culture and sensitivity study is warranted.

Conditions That May Simulate Impetigo

Herpes Labialis

Both diseases are common in the central facial region, and both begin with clear small vesicles on an inflammatory base. Herpetic lesions tend to remain fixed and singular, but may evolve secondarily into a bacterial impetigo. A smear with a Gram stain will often show bacteria with cases of impetigo. A Tzanck smear of a blister base will show herpes-virus cytopathic effect with herpes labialis. A rapid immunofluorescence (RIF) test is also positive in herpes (*see* Chapter 34). Bacterial and viral cultures are expensive and are seldom justified.

Varicella

The small vesicles of the initial stage of nonbullous impetigo could be confused with early varicella. The lack of constitutional and upper respiratory symptoms with impetigo, and the clustering of lesions, rapid rupture and ensuing crusting should differentiate them. A Tzanck smear of a blister base and a Gram stain of the fluid can distinguish impetigo from varicella. A RIF test is also positive in varicella (*see* Chapter 34).

Tinea Circinata

Annular tinea corporis can simulate the later phase of bullous impetigo when only the clearing blister base and marginal scale remain. In tinea of this type, blisters and bullae do not occur and a KOH prep should be definitive.

Bullous Pemphigoid

Localized or early bullous pemphigoid produces bullae on a noninflammatory base similar to early bullous impetigo. Gram stain or culture of blister fluid should be positive in impetigo and negative in bullous pemphigoid. Biopsy shows a distinctly different level of cleavage in each disease, and impetigo responds promptly to appropriate antibiotic therapy.

ANSWERS TO CLINICAL APPLICATION QUESTIONS

History Review

A 14-year-old girl presents at your afternoon clinic accompanied by her mother for evaluation of oozing blisters on the left upper thigh starting at the level of the gluteal crease. Onset was sudden with rapid progression over 3 days, and the lesions are both tender and pruritic. The mother is concerned about some sort of insect-bite reaction and about the rapid progression of the lesions. You suspect impetigo.

1. With what primary form of impetigo is this clinical course most consistent?

Answer: Bullous impetigo typically has an abrupt onset and a tendency toward rapid extension.

2. What provoking factors might account for this somewhat unusual anatomic location?

Answer: A pool scrape or other minor abrasion, an insect bite, or as occurred in this case, the lesions began as a chafe site from wearing a wet bathing suit after swimming.

3. What are the primary lesions of bullous impetigo?

Answer: Bullae 1 to 2 cm in size with clear or turbid contents. Ruptured bullae will appear as 1- to 2-cm red plaques with a peripheral scale and central resolution.

4. What are the secondary lesions of bullous impetigo?

Answer:
   a. Crusts, typically honey-colored, but sometimes brown or hemorrhagic.
   b. Loose white peripheral scale.
   c. Hyperpigmentation.
   d. Hypopigmentation.

5. What treatment should you start?

Answer:
   a. Discuss hygiene at home and school. Among other things, communal swimming should be restricted until treatment has taken effect.
   b. A topical antibiotic, either mupirocin or polysporin ointment BID, will prevent spread to others and gives some symptomatic relief from the itching.
   c. A 7- to 10-day course of systemic antibiotics is indicated. Cephalexin, diloxacillin, or amoxicillin/clavulanic acid are now considered first choice.

34 Herpes Simplex Recidivans *(Herpes Labialis, Cold Sores, Fever Blisters, Herpes Genitalis)*

INTRODUCTION

The most common clinical presentation of herpes simplex viruses (HSVs) are the recurring skin lesions of the facial and genital skin that follow a primary infection. Certain individuals have regular recurrences, while others who are infected never have overt clinical lesions. These secondary lesions occur because the herpesviruses have the ability to establish latent infection in sensory nerve ganglia despite measurable host immune response. Various triggers reactivate the latent virus, which then replicates and travels to the skin via the sensory nerve. The factors that determine individual susceptibility to recurrent herpetic lesions are, at this time, unknown. This chapter will focus on recognizable recidivans lesions; however, comments about the primary phase and asymptomatic shedding in the absence of overt lesions will be included.

CLINICAL APPLICATION QUESTIONS

A 45-year-old man seeks your advice regarding lesions on the penile shaft that have recurred four times over the preceding 6 months. He is recently divorced and has participated in unprotected sexual activity with two partners. He is concerned about possible genital herpes. Exam reveals a single lesion on the left mid-penile shaft with what appear to be dry crusted vesicles on an erythematous base. Regional lymph nodes are normal.

1. How is history helpful in the diagnosis?
2. You advise the patient that although the lesion present is in a late phase and is not diagnostic, the overall picture is consistent with genital herpes. He desires a definitive diagnosis if possible. What lab tests are indicated?
3. The rapid immunofluorescence (RIF) test for herpes is positive and confirms the presence of HSV-2, but a serologic test for syphilis is negative, as are the HIV titers. What counseling will you give the patient regarding future sexual activity?
4. What treatment is indicated for this patient?
5. If the clinical findings included one or more small painful ulcers and regional adenopathy, what would be the most likely diagnosis?

APPLICATION GUIDELINES

Specific History

Onset

Recurrent herpes labialis is seen with increased frequency starting in the mid-teen years, and peaks in the third and fourth decades. Sporadic recurrences are seen following

From: *Current Clinical Practice: Dermatology Skills for Primary Care: An Illustrated Guide*
D.J. Trozak, D.J. Tennenhouse, and J.J. Russell © Humana Press, Totowa, NJ

surgical procedures on the lips in older adults, but spontaneous cyclical attacks are uncommon. Recurrent herpes genitalis is associated with sexual activity, and is encountered mainly in young and middle-aged adults. Occasional cases are encountered in sexually active persons in the sixth and seventh decades.

Evolution of Disease Process

Most cases of labial and facial herpes are caused by HSV-1 and are acquired during childhood before the age of 4 years. The initial infection may be from droplet contact and takes the form of a viral gingivostomatitis. Diffuse inflammation is present along with numerous aphthous type ulcers in the anterior oral cavity. Primary inoculation from someone with an active shedding lesion is a second potential route of infection, and the skin lesions are similar to those seen with recurrent disease, but are more extensive and usually multiple. Regional adenopathy is common with primary infection, but is uncommon with the recurrent lesions. Primary infection may also be occult and asymptomatic. The incidence of asymptomatic shedding in oral HSV-1 infections is not well documented.

Herpes genitalis is generally caused by HSV-2, and is usually acquired during sexual activity. Primary infection may take the form of a severe vulvovaginitis in female patients. Infrequently male patients may develop a diffuse balanitis. Infection may occur as a primary inoculation lesion in either sex. Men have a lower incidence of symptomatic primary infection and recurrent lesions than women. Genital pain, papules, pustules, crusts, ulcers, or fissures with regional adenopathy may be signs of a primary episode. In male patients, bacteriologically negative cases of "nonspecific urethritis" have cultured both types of HSV. Other uncommon signs of a primary episode include dysuria, symptoms of cystitis, lumbosacral radicular pain, and aseptic meningitis. It is now established that a significant proportion of genital herpes infections are acquired from a partner without visible clinical lesions. Transmission among serologically discordant couples occurs 70% of the time during periods of asymptomatic viral shedding. Asymptomatic shedding is most frequent in the first year following primary infection, in the immediate prodrome period before a recurrent lesion, and in the week following a recurrence. Despite these statistics, transmission of HSV is much more efficient from an open lesion and there is evidence that concomitant transmission of other sexually transmitted disease (syphilis, HIV, etc.) is also increased. Recognition of these recurrent lesions is important in reducing the spread of herpes genitalis. Many asymptomatic carriers who are educated about herpes discover they are having active lesions.

Whether labial or genital, asymptomatic primary infection is common, and the first sign of infection is often a recurrent lesion. Regional adenopathy and constitutional symptoms can occur with both primary and recurrent disease, but are very uncommon with the latter. The strains of virus affecting each location are not mutually exclusive and may indicate oral–genital sexual practices or may be spread through primary inoculation from one active lesion site to another anatomic location in the same individual. Patients should be made aware of the possibility of autoinoculation to other locations. Presence of primary or recidivans genital herpes in a child should always raise suspicion of sexual molestation. If cultures grow HSV-1, autoinoculation from another site is a possibility, and careful investigation is warranted. Recovery of HSV-2 makes molestation a very worrisome concern.

Both recidivans forms of herpes simplex recur in a cyclical fashion. The cyclical pattern and the anatomic locations are important clues to the true etiology. This historical information is particularly important if patients present between attacks or present with lesions that are so advanced that definitive diagnosis is not possible. Cyclical recurrences may occur for years and may be so frequent that the victim faces constant discomfort and embarrassment. With time, the recurrences become less frequent and eventually stop. The timing of these events is unpredictable, and the lesions may reactivate on a cyclical basis after years of apparent quiescence.

A special form of herpes recidivans is herpetic whitlow. This is an uncommon, but not rare variant that is disabling and difficult to diagnose. Recurrent and often very painful lesions erupt on a cyclical basis on the palmar surface of the hand, on the distal finger pad, or on the periungual skin. The thick palmar skin masks the true nature of the infection that was acquired by primary inoculation. Careful inspection of an active lesion will show deep-seated grouped vesicles or pustules, and the anatomic localization and cyclical pattern should suggest the diagnosis. Treatment with episodic or chronic suppressive antiviral medication is indicated as outlined in the therapy section. Medical professionals are particularly prone to this infection (*see* Photo 7).

Complications of herpes recidivans include the following:

1. **Ocular involvement:** Primary or recidivans herpes simplex can be spread to the eye by rubbing and autoinoculation. Rapid injury and blindness can occur. When there are active lesions on the periocular skin without signs or symptoms of eye involvement, prophylactically protecting the eye with an antiviral agent is indicated. One drop of trifluridine 1% ophthalmic solution QID is recommended. If there are any signs or symptoms of ocular inflammation, immediate ophthalmologic evaluation is essential (*see* Photo 8).
2. **Postherpetic erythema multiforme:** Herpes labialis in certain victims is regularly followed in 10 to 14 days by an attack of erythema multiforme. This almost always takes the form of the minor variant, but can be uncomfortable and interfere with work. If frequent, this is an indication for chronic suppressive antiviral treatment, as outlined in the therapy section.
3. **Eczema herpeticum:** This dread complication of herpetic infection usually occurs with primary infection of HSV-1 in a host with a preexisting skin disorder, most commonly atopic dermatitis. Some cases have followed recurrent herpes labialis. Dissemination of the herpetic lesions to widespread sites occurs and there is usually a dramatic flare of the preexisting skin condition. This can progress to systemic infection with severe sequelae and even death. Immediate dermatologic consultation is indicated, and once the diagnosis is confirmed, aggressive systemic antiviral therapy is indicated.
4. **Chronic edema:** Facial edema has been reported to follow recurrent attacks of HSV-1. This is due to progressive lymphatic fibrosis from the recurrent viral lymphangitis.

Evolution of Skin Lesions

Recurrent HSV-1 and HSV-2 produce skin lesions of identical morphology and evolution. In both types, reactivation may be heralded by an aura of tingling, burning, or hyperesthesia. This aura may precede the lesions by a few hours or as much as a few days. The earliest physical lesion is a red urticarial plaque, usually solitary, that occurs at the same site or very close to the same site each time. Abortive attacks may not progress beyond this phase. In most instances, within a matter of hours the urticarial base develops discrete papules that rapidly become clear, tense vesicles 1 to 3 mm across. The vesicles may remain discrete or become confluent and cover the entire base. Over several days the vesicles become umbilicated, then pustular, and rupture, leaving discrete bases that are often recognizable even in late lesions. Lesions normally regress in 10 to 14 days, and usually heal without scarring. Constitutional symptoms and regional adenopathy may be present but are uncommon.

Provoking Factors

Ultraviolet light exposure, especially acute sunburn of the lip area, is the most common trigger for herpes labialis attacks. Other commonly mentioned provoking factors include febrile illness, minor physical trauma, lip or oral surgery, neural surgery, dermabrasion, face peel procedures, and emotional stress. Herpes genitalis is occasionally reported to activate after resumption of vigorous sexual activity. This association is uncommon and is probably related to the physical trauma involved. Premenstrual recurrences of herpes labialis and genitalis have been reported.

Self-Medication

Self-treatment is not a significant problem. The OTC products for herpes labialis produce symptomatic relief but do not interfere with diagnosis or definitive therapy. Patients seldom treat genital lesions without seeking a medical opinion.

Supplemental Review From General History

When active genital lesions are present, or cultures suggest oral–genital contact, a history should be obtained regarding contacts and to warn the individual about high-risk behavior. Delayed healing, atypical lesions, or progressive lesions may indicate immunologic compromise, as with concomitant HIV infection. Appropriate general history review is indicated.

Dermatological Physical Exam

Primary Lesions

1. Erythematous urticarial plaque, usually solitary in recidivans lesions (*see* Photo 9).
2. Grouped 1- to 3-mm vesicles on the plaque that may umbilicate (*see* Photos 10,11).
3. Pustules that replace vesicles in late lesions (*see* Photo 11).

Secondary Lesions

1. Erosions as the blisters rupture (*see* Photo 12).
2. Crusting with secondary infection (*see* Photo 12).

Distribution

Microdistribution: None.

Macrodistribution: Herpes labialis tends to occur on the upper or lower lip, and may be on the vermilion or outer lip skin. Mucous membranes are spared in recurrent disease. Recurrent facial lesions are also common around the nose and periocular skin.

Herpes genitalis in men is most common on the penile shaft. It is also seen on the fore-skin and on the skin at the base of the penis. In women, lesions may occur on the vulva, within the vaginal vault, or on the cervix. Lesions are also common on the proximal thigh and buttock skin from primary inoculation. In homosexual and bisexual patients, perianal and anal lesions are seen.

Configuration

Grouped configuration. This refers to the arrangement of the vesicles on the urticarial base (*see* Photos 9–11).

Indicated Supporting Diagnostic Data

In most instances, herpes simplex recidivans can be diagnosed clinically from the historical data and a typical skin lesion. There are occasions however, where special circumstances make laboratory confirmation desirable.

Tzanck Smear

A smear of material from a fresh, ruptured blister base is placed on glass slide and immediately stained with Giemsa or some similar stain. A positive smear will show herpesvirus effect by the presence of keratinocytes with balloon nuclei and multinucleated giant cells with similar changes (*see* Photos 13,14). This test is rapid, inexpensive, and can be performed with equipment that is readily accessible. Sensitivity in experienced hands using material from a fresh vesicle approaches or exceeds 70%. In pustular lesions, sensitivity diminishes. This test does not distinguish between HSV-1, HSV-2, or herpes zoster virus.

Biopsy

Biopsy of a herpetic lesion shows pathognomonic features, but is usually done only to investigate a lesion that is clinically atypical. Biopsy does not distinguish HSV-1 from HSV-2 or herpes zoster virus (HZV), and adds nothing if the lesions are clinically diagnostic.

Complement Fixation Tests

These titers rise rapidly during primary infection and are valuable if acute and convalescent titers are obtained. In recurrent disease, titers show little change and are of no value. Western blot and enzyme-linked immunoassay tests, if available, are sensitive and will distinguish one virus from the other.

Viral Culture

Culture from fresh blister material can be very sensitive (80% +) and will distinguish HSV-1 from HSV-2 and HZV. Culture is indicated to confirm the diagnosis in unusual cases, to distinguish HSV-1 infection from HSV-2, and for medical–legal reasons in cases of rape and child molestation. In otherwise clinically typical cases, culture is unnecessary and the diagnosis can usually be confirmed by Tzanck smear or RIF test. Cultures are expensive and slow, and must be obtained from fresh lesions or their sensitivity falls precipitously.

Rapid Immunofluorescence Test for Herpes

This test employs a monoclonal antibody system and exhibits a sensitivity of about 65%. In addition to speed, this test can distinguish among HSV-1, HSV-2, and HZV. The specimen consists of a smear from a blister. The test is practical and reproducible. Results are available within 1 hour or less after receiving the specimen.

Polymerase Chain Reaction (PCR)

PCR testing performed from blister specimens shows a sensitivity of 83%, which is equivalent to culture. This test is rapid and can distinguish HSV-1 from HSV-2 and HZV. In addition, the test is positive when performed from crusts and with material from involuting lesions where culture, Tzanck, and RIF results are less reliable. The technology is expensive and not universally available at present. PCR should be reserved for atypical cases or unusual circumstances. HSV and HZV can be distinguished within 6 hours, and HSV types by 24 hours.

Additional Tests

Because sexually transmitted diseases are occasionally transmitted concurrently, a serologic test for syphilis should be done when herpes genitalis is diagnosed. Authorization should also be requested to run serologies for HIV.

Therapy

Prevention

Herpes labialis recurrences can often be avoided by simple measures, especially when history reveals specific triggers. Many cases are provoked by sunburn or intense ultraviolet exposure without a visible burn. Common sense regarding sun exposure and the use of a lip pomade and sunscreen of SPF 30 or greater will often prevent recurrent attacks, even without systemic treatment.

Avoidance of direct contact of active clinical lesions in the transmission of HSV infections is fairly obvious. There is, however, potential for transmission during asymptomatic periods of viral shedding, especially in genital herpes. Up to 70% of cases may be transmitted in this way; therefore, counseling regarding prevention is essential. This is also a good argument for chronic suppressive systemic antiviral therapy, especially in the first 12 months after acquired infection when asymptomatic shedding is highest.

Topical Therapy

Acyclovir ointment 5% has limited value in the treatment of primary HSV infections of skin and mucous membranes and a modest effect on recidivans lesions in immunocompromised patients. In controlled studies, there was no benefit in recurrent HSV lesions of otherwise healthy persons. There is some evidence linking the topical use of acyclovir to viral-resistant strains.

Penciclovir cream 1% is approved for topical treatment of recurrent orolabial herpes without regard to the patient's immune status. It must be started as early as possible in the course of a lesion and is applied every 2 hours while awake (approximately nine times daily). Symptoms were shortened by 1/2 day, as was total healing time. The period of viral shedding was also shortened.

A small study showed an apparent suppressive effect with zinc sulfate poultices at a concentration of 0.025 to 0.05% solution in patients with recurrent HSV-1. The proposed mechanism is inhibition of viral replication via an effect on viral DNA polymerase.

Silver sulfadiazine cream 0.01% has also been reported to have antiviral properties and, when used topically, seems to abort or shorten the course of recurrent lesions for some patients. It must be applied several times daily and can cause difficult-to-remove stains on apparel and bed linens.

Several OTC products are available for the treatment of herpes labialis. These provide symptomatic relief, dry the vesicles, and reduce secondary infection. Those containing phenol probably reduce viral shedding.

Systemic Therapy

Acyclovir has been in use for more than a decade, and has proven efficacy and safety in the treatment of HSV infections. Central nervous system (CNS) and renal side effects have been reported but are usually associated with high-dose intravenous therapy. Some resistant strains have been isolated, although these have been primarily encountered in patients with concomitant HIV infection. Safety in children under 2 years and during pregnancy has not been established. Doses listed are for adult patients, and pediatric doses should be adjusted accordingly. Doses of acyclovir and valacyclovir should be adjusted for patients with diminished renal function. Potentially fatal side effects have been reported with high-dose valacyclovir in immunologically compromised persons.

Therapeutic treatment of primary orolabial or genital infection is as follows:

1. Acyclovir: 200 mg five times a day or 400 mg three times a day for 7 to 10 days, *or*
2. Valacyclovir: 1 g twice daily for 7 to 10 days, *or*
3. Famciclovir: 250 mg three times a day for 5 to 10 days.

Topical acyclovir and penciclovir can be used, but require application every 2 hours and have marginal efficacy.

For abortive or episodic therapy of recurrences, treatment is as follows:

1. Acyclovir: 200 mg five times a day or 400 mg three times a day or 800 mg twice daily for 5 days, *or*
2. Valacyclovir: 500 mg daily for 3 to 5 days or 1 g/day for 5 days, *or*
3. Famciclovir: 125 mg twice daily for 5 days.

Medication must be started at the first sign of an attack; patients who have an antecedent aura should initiate dosing even in the absence of a clinical lesion. They must always have a supply of medication on hand since even a few hours' delay can reduce the effectiveness of this treatment. Abortive therapy is sometimes effective in the prevention of postherpetic erythema multiforme. For other patients, however, chronic suppressive treatment is required. Once erythema multiforme is clinically evident, acyclovir treatment is of no value.

Another indication for abortive treatment is a prior history of eczema herpeticum. For this indication, and in other immunocompromised hosts such as those with concomitant HIV infection, a larger dose of acyclovir, 400 mg five times a day for 7 to 14 days, is recommended.

Chronic suppressive therapy is administered as follows:

1.   Acyclovir: 400 mg twice daily, *or*
2.   Valacyclovir: 500 to 1000 mg daily, *or*
3.   Famciclovir: 250 mg twice daily.

Long-term suppressive therapy with acyclovir has been very effective for both oro-labial and genital lesions, and long-term studies do not reveal any significant side effects. Indications for this approach include frequent recurrences (six or more attacks per year), patients who have attacks without an aura, patients who cannot effectively initiate abortive therapy, or attacks with complications such as ophthalmic involvement, chronic lymphedema, disabling herpetic whitlow, or postherpetic erythema multiforme not controlled by abortive treatment. Chronic suppressive therapy should also be considered in the first 12 months after a diagnosis of primary genital herpes when the incidence of asymptomatic viral shedding is the highest. Appropriate doses reduce the incidence of viral shedding by 95%.

Once-daily 500 mg valacyclovir has been shown to significantly reduce the risk of transmission of herpes genitalis. Valacyclovir has been approved by the FDA for chronic suppression of HSV at a dose of 1 g daily. Since it is a prodrug of acyclovir, one would anticipate similar indications, effectiveness, and side effects. It has been effective in chronic suppression at a dose of 500 mg daily.

Famciclovir is approved for chronic suppressive therapy at 250 mg twice daily. It has been reported to effectively suppress genital herpes at that dose, but was ineffective when given once daily. Despite a similar mode of action, there have been reports that some acyclovir resistant strains of HSV remain sensitive to famciclovir. Treatment of acyclovir-resistant strains with foscarnet has also been reported.

Conditions That May Simulate Herpes Simplex Recidivans

Impetigo (Nonbullous)

Both diseases are common in the central facial region, and both begin with small clear vesicles on an inflammatory base. Herpetic lesions tend to remain fixed and discrete, and the vesicles are small, 1 to 2 mm across, tightly grouped, and persist for longer periods. Facial HSV occasionally develops secondary impetigo, causing some diagnostic confusion. A smear with a Gram stain will often show bacteria with cases of impetigo. A Tzanck smear of a blister base will show herpes virus cytopathic effect with herpes labialis. RIF test is also positive with herpes. Bacterial and viral cultures are expensive and are seldom justified.

Bacterial Paronychia and Whitlows

Differentiation of herpetic and bacterial lesions in periungual locations requires a high index of suspicion. The thick epidermis in these acral areas disguises the morphology of the herpetic lesion, which usually presents as an acute inflammatory pustule. Viral lymphangitis is common. Clear unilocular or multilocular vesicles should suggest herpes. Recurrent symptoms on the same digit in a cyclical pattern should immediately raise suspicion. Tzanck smear, RIF test, and viral cultures may be necessary.

Chancroid

Recurrent herpes genitalis can usually be distinguished from other venereal ulcers on the basis of history, inspection, and testing of a typical lesion. Early solitary lesions of chancroid (*H. ducreyi*) could cause confusion. Herpes lesions, unless secondarily infected, show evidence of multilocular vesicles even while regressing. Healing is usually evident at 5 to 7 days, and the lesions are almost always single. Chancroid lesions progress and become undermined. Progressive adenopathy with bubo formation is common. Adenopathy with herpes genitalis is uncommon, transient, and tends to resolve in a fashion that parallels the skin lesion. A smear from a chancroid lesion stained with Giemsa, Gram, or methyl green pyronine will reveal the bipolar organisms in half of the cases. Tzanck smear from HSV will show herpes virus cytopathic effect in a high percentage of cases and is negative in chancroid. RIF testing will increase diagnostic sensitivity. Herpes cultures are readily obtained. Cultures for chancroid are difficult and fresh material is essential. In rare cases, biopsy of an ulcer margin with special stains for *H. ducreyi* may be helpful. Remember, the two diseases may be simultaneously present in the same patient.

ANSWERS TO CLINICAL APPLICATION QUESTIONS

History Review

A 45-year-old man seeks your advice regarding lesions on the penile shaft that have recurred four times over the preceding 6 months. He is recently divorced and has participated in unprotected sexual activity with two partners. He is concerned about possible genital herpes. Exam reveals a single lesion on the left mid-penile shaft with what appear to be dry crusted vesicles on an erythematous base. Regional lymph nodes are normal.

1. **How is history helpful in the diagnosis?**

   Answer: In addition to information regarding sexual activity and cyclical recurrences, specific questions establish the following facts:
   a. Onset is heralded by an aura of itching and burning 12 hours before a visible lesion.
   b. Lesions have recurred at approximately the same site each time.
   c. The patient clearly describes an evolution from a red welt to bumps, blisters, and crusts.
   d. Evolution of each episode is about 10 days from start to finish.
   e. Lesions are described as irritable and uncomfortable, but not painful.

   This history supports a diagnosis of herpes genitalis and does not fit the course of other venereal diseases.

2. **You advise the patient that although the lesion present is in a late phase and is not diagnostic, the overall picture is consistent with genital herpes. He desires a definitive diagnosis if possible. What lab tests are indicated?**

   Answer: Tzanck smear, biopsy, and viral cultures will have very low sensitivity on a crusted involuting lesion. Complement fixation titers are of no value in recurrent disease. Since Tzanck smears are inexpensive, an attempt is not unreasonable; however, a negative smear at this stage offers no reassurance. The most specific and cost-effective test in this case is a rapid immunofluorescence (RIF) test for herpes performed on a smear of crusted material. A serologic test for syphilis should be done, and authorization requested for HIV titers.

As testing by polymerase chain reaction becomes universally available and less expensive, it may replace RIF testing.

3. The RIF test for herpes is positive and confirms the presence of HSV-2, but a serologic test for syphilis is negative, as are the HIV titers. What counseling will you give the patient regarding future sexual activity?

Answer: The latent nature of the infection and the concept of asymptomatic viral shedding with the possibility of transmission between active episodes must be explained with sensitivity. Use of barrier protection with a condom should be urged. Despite embarrassment, the patient should be strongly encouraged to discuss the problem frankly with any past, current, or future sex partners.

4. What treatment is indicated for this patient?

Answer: His attacks are preceded by a distinct aura. He will probably do well symptomatically with abortive (episodic) antiviral therapy. Since his attacks are frequent and there is a significant risk of asymptomatic viral shedding, chronic suppressive antiviral therapy makes sense. In addition, the freedom from symptomatic recurrences will help the patient deal with a difficult emotionally charged issue. Treatment for this specific episode is too late to be of value.

5. If the clinical findings included one or more small painful ulcers and regional adenopathy, what would be the most likely diagnosis?

Answer: Chancroid.

35 Herpes Zoster *(Shingles)*

INTRODUCTION

Herpes zoster is the recidivans form of varicella-zoster virus infection. The primary infection varicella or chickenpox most commonly occurs as an acute childhood exanthem. Widespread introduction of a vaccine for this exanthem will alter the incidence of varicella, but it is uncertain what the long-term effect will be on the incidence of zoster. The virus establishes latent infection in sensory ganglia at the base of the brain and spinal column. As the cell-mediated immune response conferred at the time of primary infection wanes, the disease increases in incidence. Certain provoking factors and concomitant illness are associated with attacks.

CLINICAL APPLICATION QUESTIONS

A 75-year-old man in good general health presents at your office regarding a blistering rash on the right face and nose of 48 hours' duration. Lancinating pain was noted for 2 or 3 days before the rash. He also complains of diminished visual acuity in the right eye. You diagnose herpes zoster of the ophthalmic division of the trigeminal nerve.

1. What are the primary lesions of herpes zoster?
2. What secondary lesions occur in herpes zoster?
3. What specific physical finding should you be alert for in this case?
4. What laboratory tests are needed to confirm the diagnosis?
5. What treatment would you recommend in this case?

APPLICATION GUIDELINES

Specific History

Onset

Zoster attacks may occur in children and young adults, but are quite rare. The incidence starts to climb during the fifth decade of life and peaks in the seventh and eighth decades. Severe or prolonged attacks, especially in young persons, should raise concern about concomitant illness and immune status. An attack usually confers lifelong immunity in an otherwise healthy person.

Evolution of Disease Process

Most cases of herpes zoster present with pain that is variously described as shock-like or a continuous burning sensation with hyperalgesia. Other patients experience less

From: *Current Clinical Practice: Dermatology Skills for Primary Care: An Illustrated Guide*
D.J. Trozak, D.J. Tennenhouse, and J.J. Russell © Humana Press, Totowa, NJ

intense but equally uncomfortable crawling or pruritic parasthesias, and find that even fabric touching the area is intolerable. Within 2 or 3 days, and rarely as long as a week, skin lesions develop within the anatomic area of the involved nerve segment. These lesions, like those of herpes simplex virus (HSV), consist of tightly grouped vesicles on an erythematous, urticarial base. The lesions are usually more extensive than those of HSV and may be continuous or, more often, exhibit skip areas within the neurologic segment. Mild constitutional symptoms of fatigue and lassitude may precede the skin lesions, but fever is rare.

Uncomplicated zoster in children usually is mild and often painless. It can run its entire course in 2 weeks or less, and normally clears without sequelae. In young adults, the average course is 2 to 3 weeks long, pain is mild to moderate, and sequelae are rare. Elderly, debilitated, or immunologically compromised patients often have a course of 3 to 4 weeks or longer, and are more prone to complications. In uncomplicated cases, the involution of the skin lesions and resolution of sensory symptoms parallel each other. On occasion, painful zoster may occur without skin lesions. This variant is called *zoster sine eruptione*, and has been responsible for exploratory laparotomies when abdominal segments and visceral nerve branches were involved. Cutaneous lesions without accompanying pain are referred to as *zoster sine neuralgia*.

Although most cases are unilateral, bilateral zoster does occur. The following anatomic locations are most frequently involved:

Thoracic dermatomes	53%
Cervical dermatomes	20%
Trigeminal nerve	15%
Lumbosacral dermatomes	11%

Special forms of herpes zoster include the following:

Trigeminal zoster: Any of the three divisions of the fifth cranial nerve may be affected (*see* Fig. 3). On rare occasions more than one branch is simultaneously involved. The ophthalmic division is most often attacked, and this site increases in frequency with advancing age. Lesions may occur on the eyelids, forehead, and anterior scalp, and if the nasociliary branches are affected, severe ocular sequelae may result. Zoster lesions on the distal nasal sidewall or nasal tip (Hutchinson's sign; *see* Photo 15) should immediately raise concern about the eye. Uveitis, keratitis, conjunctivitis, ocular muscle paralysis, scleritis, retinal vascular occlusion, and paralysis of the pupil may follow. Any ocular symptoms should prompt an immediate ophthalmologic examination. Consultation is recommended with severe cases, even in the absence of eye symptoms.

Involvement of the maxillary division is associated with vesicles on the tonsil and uvula. Mandibular zoster causes lesions on the buccal mucosa, floor of the mouth, and the anterior part of the tongue. Nerve damage may lead later to loss of teeth.

Ramsay-Hunt syndrome: The classic description includes the following triad of findings: (1) zoster lesions on the pinna (*see* Photo 16), meatus, and canal or tympanic membrane of one ear, (2) severe ear pain, and (3) an ipsilateral facial nerve palsy (*see* Photo 17). Vestibular symptoms and sensorineural hearing loss may also occur. The facial paralysis is usually complete and the recovery rate is low. Taste and lacrimation may also be affected.

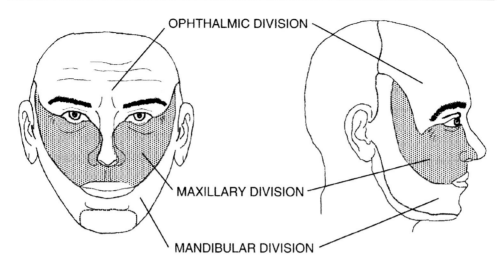

OPHTHALMIC DIVISION

MAXILLARY DIVISION

MANDIBULAR DIVISION

Figure 3: Major division of the trigeminal nerve.

Sacral zoster with motor involvement: Though we think of zoster as a sensory nerve problem, motor fibers are involved in about 5% of cases. When sacral segments are involved, fecal retention or bladder disturbances may occur. Hemorrhagic cystitis and incontinence have been reported. In one case, an elderly man was hospitalized with unexplained lower abdominal pain and acute urinary retention. Studies revealed an adynamic bladder. On the fifth hospital day, zoster lesions became evident in a sacral dermatome distribution (*see* Photo 18 for an example of sacral zoster).

Complications of herpes zoster include the following:

Generalized zoster: In addition to the problems associated with the special forms reviewed above, one of the most serious complications is generalized herpes zoster. Many patients will develop a few scattered lesions that are out of the primary neurologic segment. When extensive lesions occur along with fever and systemic toxicity, however, it is an indication of general viremia. **Fatalities can occur.** Elderly, debilitated, and immunologically compromised patients are most often affected. Early routine administration of antiviral agents for zoster should reduce the sequelae of this dread complication (*see* Photo 19).

Postherpetic neuralgia (PHN): Acute neuritis associated with a segmental zoster attack is uncommon in children and young adults who are otherwise in good health. The incidence of severe neuritis increases after age 40, as does the incidence of postherpetic neuralgia. This complication (persisting pain and/or altered sensation in the affected nerve segments after healing of the skin lesions) occurs in more than 50% of cases in some series reported. It is the most common complication of herpes zoster. The incidence peaks in patients in their sixth and seventh decades, probably due to more severe attacks and lowered capacity to regenerate after nerve injury. Most patients without long-term neurologic sequelae note clearing of the neurologic symptoms before or concurrently with healing of the skin lesions. Pain or altered nerve function persisting more than 30 days after the onset of skin lesions is considered PHN. Of those with persisting pain or altered sensation, a large number gradually improve and clear over several months. Some patients have permanent symptoms. Lancinating pain, hyperalgesia, and crawling dysesthesias are most common. These symptoms may be severe enough to be physically disabling or may be a source of chronic depression.

Other rare complications: Encephalitis, myelitis, cranial/peripheral nerve palsies, delayed contralateral hemiparesis, and acute retinal necrosis have been associated with herpes zoster.

Evolution of Skin Lesions

Zoster lesions begin with an urticarial plaque that is at first bright-red in color. Abortive lesions may simply regress. In most instances, however, tightly grouped papules develop within several hours to a few days. These rapidly evolve into vesicles and then into flaccid pustules. In uncomplicated cases, the eruption peaks in 4 to 5 days, stabilizes, then heals over a period of 2 to 3 weeks. Lesions should remain well localized to the involved nerve segment. Regional nodes may be reactive. As the pustules dry, crusts form, which are shed over several days. Even uncomplicated zoster lesions may leave long-standing postinflammatory hyperpigmentation. Hemorrhagic lesions are more frequent in patients with underlying disease (*see* Photo 20). Elderly and debilitated patients are prone to deep, slow-healing, necrotic, or gangrenous lesions that leave substantial scarring and pigmentation (*see* Photo 15).

Provoking Factors

Immunosuppression, whether iatrogenic or secondary to disease, predisposes to herpes zoster. Hemorrhagic zoster lesions or zoster of unusual severity in a young host should raise suspicion of underlying disease such as lymphoma, hematologic malignancies, or HIV disease.

Physical trauma to infected sensory ganglia, and occasionally to peripheral nerves, can trigger attacks. Radiation therapy of solid tumors and spinal manipulation are among the other common causes.

Self-Medication

Self-treatment is seldom a problem in herpes zoster.

Supplemental Review From General History

Whenever zoster is atypical, generalized, hemorrhagic, gangrenous, or unusually prolonged, a careful general history and exam should be done for evidence of an underlying lymphoma, leukemia, solid tumor, or possible HIV disease. In many instances, the atypical course can be explained by existing treatments.

Dermatologic Physical Exam

Primary Lesions

1. Erythematous urticarial plaque or plaques within a dermatome segment or contiguous dermatomes (*see* Photo 21).
2. Grouped 3- to 5-mm vesicles that evolve and often umbilicate (*see* Photo 22).
3. Pustules that replace vesicles as the lesions mature (*see* Photo 23).

Secondary Lesions

1. Erosions as blisters and pustules rupture (*see* Photos 16,19).
2. Crusting as pustules dry and shrink or due to secondary infection (*see* Photos 16,19).
3. Hemorrhage into vesicles (*see* Photo 20).
4. Necrosis and gangrene in severe lesions having an active vascular component (*see* Photo 15).
5. Postinflammatory hyperpigmentation, common even in uncomplicated zoster.
6. Scarring, more common in older patients or in zoster that is associated with underlying systemic disease.

Distribution

Microdistribution: None.

Macrodistribution: Follows a dermatome segment or contiguous neural segments.

Configuration

Zosteriform, in the shape of a girdle.

Indicated Supporting Diagnostic Data

In most instances, herpes zoster can be diagnosed clinically on the basis of the skin lesions and associated symptoms. There are times, however, when special circumstances make laboratory confirmation desirable.

Tzanck Smear

A smear of material from a fresh ruptured blister base is placed on a glass slide and immediately stained with Giemsa or some similar stain. A positive smear will show herpesvirus effect by the presence of keratinocytes with balloon nuclei and multinucleated giant cells with similar changes. This test is rapid and inexpensive, and can be performed with equipment that is readily accessible. Sensitivity, in experienced hands, from a fresh vesicle approaches or exceeds 70%. In pustular lesions, sensitivity diminishes to about 55%. This test does not distinguish HZV from HSV-1 or HSV (*see* Photo 24).

Biopsy

Biopsy of a zoster lesion shows pathognomonic features, but is usually done only to investigate a lesion that is clinically atypical. Biopsy does not distinguish HZV from HSV-1 or HSV-2, and adds nothing if the lesions are clinically diagnostic.

Complement Fixation Tests

These titers rise rapidly following onset, and are useful in atypical infections.

Viral Culture

Although culture is very specific and will distinguish HZV from HSV-1 and HSV-2, sensitivity is low (50% or less). Cultures may be used to confirm the diagnosis in unusual cases. In otherwise clinically typical cases, culture is unnecessary and the diagnosis can usually be confirmed by Tzanck smear or RIF test.

Rapid Immunofluorescence Test (RIF) for Herpes

This test employs a monoclonal antibody system and exhibits a sensitivity of about 65%. In addition to speed, RIF can distinguish among HZV, HSV-1, and HSV-2. The specimen consists of a smear from a blister, and the test is practical and reproducible. Results are available in 1 hour or less after receiving the specimen.

Polymerase Chain Reaction (PCR)

PCR testing performed from blister specimens shows a sensitivity of 97%, which is superior to culture. PCR is rapid and can distinguish HZV from HSV-1 and HSV-2. In addition, it is positive when performed from crusts and material from involuting lesions where culture, Tzanck, and RIF results are less reliable. The technology is expensive and not universally available at present. PCR should be reserved for atypical cases or unusual circumstances. With PCR, HZV and HSV can be distinguished within 6 hours.

Therapy

Acute Herpes Zoster

Prevention: Suppressive doses of acyclovir have been reported to reduce the incidence of zoster attacks in immunosuppressed patients following bone marrow transplantation. A live attenuated vaccine reduced the incidence and severity of varicella in a population of pediatric leukemia patients, but failed to alter the incidence of herpes zoster.

Topical therapy: During the acute attack, topical therapy should be directed at minimizing secondary infection of the blistered areas and providing whatever symptomatic relief is possible. While the blisters are fresh and intact, calamine lotion with 0.5% to 1.0% phenol will help to speed crust formation, ease itching and dysesthesia, and reduce the risk of secondary bacterial infection. These are available OTC or can be easily compounded. Products with benzocaine, diphenhydramine, or other topical sensitizers should be avoided. In necrotic or gangrenous lesions, or when the blisters break down and rupture, applications of Polysporin® ointment or 0.01% silver sulfadiazine cream are soothing and reduce secondary infection.

Systemic therapy: Relief of pain during the acute attack is an important part of the recovery process. The type and strength of pain medication will depend on the circumstances. In some instances, strong narcotics may be needed for short periods of time. Because discomfort may be prolonged, medications with any potential for physical dependency must be monitored. Choice of analgesics in elderly patients must be carefully tailored to the patient's degree of discomfort, agility, level of orientation, and amount of local support in the home environment.

Three antiviral agents are currently approved for the treatment of acute herpes zoster: acyclovir, famciclovir, and valacyclovir. Famciclovir and valacyclovir have more convenient dosing schedules and are more effective in the acute phase and for decreasing the incidence of postherpetic neuralgia (PHN) at 6 months. In head-to-head studies, they appear to be equally efficacious. They are now the preferred agents. To be optimally effective, treatment should be started within 48 to 72 hours of onset and should be continued for 7 days. Longer courses have no apparent additional benefit. All three drugs inhibit HZV replication which shortens viral shedding and also speeds healing of the skin lesions by about 2 days. For treatment of herpes zoster, use one of the following:

1. Valacyclovir: 1000 mg three times a day for 7 days, *or*
2. Famciclovir: 500 mg three times a day for 7 days.

Antiviral therapy should be reserved for specific situations and should not be routinely used for every case of zoster. In an otherwise healthy host where neurologic symptoms are minimal or absent, uncomplicated zoster should be treated with topical therapy only. The risk of long-term neurologic sequelae under these circumstances is minimal, and the modest effect of these systemic medications on healing time and viral shedding does not warrant the expense. The major indications for antiviral therapy are the following:

1. Patients aged 60 or older who present with symptoms of moderate to severe acute neuritis.
2. Patients in any age group presenting with severe acute neuritis.
3. Patients who present with extensive areas of skin involvement.
4. Patients with ophthalmic zoster. Early antiviral therapy has been shown to significantly reduce the incidence of ocular complications.
5. Patients with early hemorrhagic or necrotic lesions. Late treatment is usually ineffective.
6. Patients with chronic or progressive lesions. Intravenous treatment may be required.
7. Special forms of zoster where there is a high risk of postherpetic neuralgia, motor involvement, or injury to the eyes or ears (such as Ramsay-Hunt syndrome and low sacral zoster).
8. Generalized zoster. If the disease is mild with minimal toxicity, oral regimens can be used. If fulminant, or if progressive on the oral regimen, then intravenous dosing is indicated with acyclovir at a dose of 10 mg/kg every 8 hours for 7 days.
9. Patients who have significant immune suppression either from medication or preexisting disease, or who have a prior history of generalized zoster, should be placed on the therapeutic oral schedule listed above. If the onset of their zoster is unusually severe, iv administration should be considered.

Systemic steroids have been used for two decades in the treatment of herpes zoster. Studies clearly show substantial reductions of the symptoms of acute neuritis and the total time required to heal the skin lesions. Studies of their effect on the incidence of postherpetic neuralgia have given conflicting results. A criticism of some of the negative studies is their failure to compare patients in the seventh and eighth decades, where this complication is most common. The main indications are reduction of acute neurologic symptoms or where there is a high risk of post-zoster nerve damage. Systemic steroids are usually given in the form of 40 to 60 mg per day oral prednisone in a single morning dose for 10 to 14 days and then tapered gradually over the next 3 weeks. Despite initial fears about dissemination of the infection, this has not been a problem in otherwise healthy persons. Use of steroids in debilitated or immune-suppressed patients carries a high risk of dissemination and is not recommended. Steroid side effects do occur and should be anticipated. The major indications for steroid therapy are the following:

1. Patients aged 60 or older who present with symptoms of moderate to severe acute neuritis.
2. Patients in any age group presenting with severe acute neuritis.
3. Special forms of zoster where there is a high risk of postherpetic neuralgia, motor involvement, or injury to the eyes or ears (such as Ramsay-Hunt syndrome, ophthalmic zoster especially with nasociliary nerve distribution, and low sacral zoster).

There is no evidence of an effect of either antiviral agents or systemic steroids on postherpetic neuralgia once the acute zoster episode is over. Neither drug should be administered late for that purpose.

Postherpetic Neuralgia

Prevention: *See* the preceding discussions of systemic antiviral agents and systemic steroids.

Topical therapy: Topical treatment of postherpetic neuralgia should be instituted only after the acute skin lesions have healed. Use on partially healed acute lesions would be irritating and uncomfortable, and would increase the risk of allergic contact dermatitis. Capsaicin 0.025%, 0.075% cream, and 0.025% gel are available OTC for topical application. Patients need very specific instructions on proper application to avoid side effects. They must be warned about the initial stinging sensation, which is to be expected, and must also be advised about the gradual onset of relief. The product is applied three to four times daily to the affected skin segment. Use around eyes, mucous membranes, and intertriginous areas is not recommended. Compliance is often a problem, but improvement in some cases is gratifying. An alternative topical agent is a lotion composed of 650 mg (two 5-grain tablets) of aspirin dissolved in 15 to 30 mL of chloroform. This lotion, when applied to the affected skin, provides analgesia within 5 to 10 minutes and lasts 2 to 4 hours. Most patients have relief with three to four applications per day. The lotion leaves a chalky deposit, and occasional mild stinging is reported. This lotion should also not be used on mucous membranes and intertriginous skin.

The following systemic medications have been reported to reduce the discomfort of postherpetic neuralgia:

Agent	Initial Dose	Comments
Gabapentin	300 mg PO/day	Wide dosing range. Titrate according to patient response over 4 weeks
Pregabalin	150–300 mg PO/day	Dose may be titrated to 600 mg/day according to response and tolerance
Tricyclic antidepressants (nortriptyline, desipramine)	10–25 mg PO response	Titrate dose according to patient
Lidocaine (5% patch)	Apply to affected site. Maximum: three patches per application for 12 hours	Warn regarding overuse and systemic toxicity

Other drugs used for PHN include amitriptyline, carbamazepine, clonazepam, phenobarbital, and phenytoin. Intractable PHN should be referred to a neurology or pain management consultant.

Conditions That May Simulate Herpes Zoster

Herpes Simplex

HSV in a linear distribution may be clinically impossible to distinguish from herpes zoster. Linear lesions are more common in children and with HSV on the extremities. Groups of lesions in different stages of evolution and pain or dysesthesia favor zoster. Culture, RIF, and PCR testing will distinguish the two.

Toxicodendron (Rhus) Dermatitis

Vesicular poison oak (ivy, etc.) can be very similar to early zoster with minimal acute neuritis. Both may be linear and segmental, both may itch, and the morphology of the primary lesions is virtually identical. Pain or lack of pruritus favors zoster. Satellite lesions outside the primary dermatome or at distant sites favor rhus dermatitis. Tzanck smear helps to rapidly distinguish many cases, but it is not infallible. If the Tzanck smear is negative, RIF testing is indicated.

ANSWERS TO CLINICAL APPLICATION QUESTIONS

History Review

A 75-year-old man in good general health presents at your office regarding a blistering rash on the right face and nose of 48 hours' duration. Lancinating pain was noted for 2 or 3 days before the rash. He also complains of diminished visual acuity in the right eye. You diagnose herpes zoster of the ophthalmic division of the trigeminal nerve.

1. What are the primary lesions of herpes zoster?

Answer:
a. Single or multiple erythematous urticarial plaques.
b. 3- to 5-mm vesicles or pustules, often umbilicated.

2. What secondary lesions occur in herpes zoster?

Answer:
a. Erosions.
b. Crusts.
c. Hemorrhage into vesicles.
d. Necrosis.
e. Gangrene.
f. Scarring.
g. Postinflammatory hyperpigmentation.

3. What specific physical finding should you be alert for in this case?

Answer:
a. Involvement of the distal nasal sidewall or nasal tip (Hutchinson's sign).
b. Ocular muscle paralysis, indicating involvement of other cranial nerves.
c. Lack of accommodation or pupil light reflex.
d. Diminished visual acuity or evidence of ocular inflammation.

4. What laboratory tests are needed to confirm the diagnosis?

Answer: This case is typical from a clinical standpoint, and lab confirmation is not indicated. If desired, a simple, inexpensive Tzanck smear should suffice.

5. What treatment would you recommend in this case?

Answer:

    a. An analgesic of sufficient potency to allow rest and recovery.

    b. Seven days of antiviral therapy with oral famciclovir or valacyclovir.

    c. A 10- to 14-day burst of single-dose morning prednisone at 40 to 60 mg/day, provided there are no other contraindications.

    d. Immediate ophthalmologic referral for evaluation of decreased visual acuity.

    e. Close follow-up in 10 days or less until it is clear the acute process is resolved, and observation for possible postherpetic neuralgia.

36 Acne Vulgaris *(Acne, Zits)*

INTRODUCTION

This common disease of young persons can be physically and socially devastating. Any practitioner who wishes to treat acne should be prepared to deal with it in a serious and sensitive fashion. To many teenagers and young adults, this disease marks the end of a previously idyllic existence with their physical being and self-image. For the first time, they confront the fact that their bodies are vulnerable and imperfect. All practitioners should understand that acne vulgaris is a serious problem with a potential for very severe permanent cosmetic injury. Active disease and the resultant scarring can interfere with social development, mental health, and the victim's job opportunities. **Because it is so common, consider acne the most important dermatologic disease you treat.**

CLINICAL APPLICATION QUESTIONS

A shy 14-year-old girl accompanied by her mother presents for treatment of acne of 1 year's duration.

1. What historical information will assist in staging her disease and in the choice of appropriate treatment?
2. What should you look for on physical exam?
3. What general treatment measures other than medication should you institute?
4. The patient has fairly dense acne of the face and mid-upper back. Her chest, shoulders, neck, and lower back are spared. Her lesions are predominantly noninflammatory papules, open comedones, and a few inflammatory papules and pustules. Her mother has read about isotretinoin therapy. How would you grade her acne, and what would be an appropriate treatment regimen?
5. What would you change in your management if her acne also involved her chest, shoulders, and lower back?

APPLICATION GUIDELINES

Specific History

Onset

Acne most often begins in an insidious fashion with the accumulation of noninflammatory papules and blackheads. This phase is often ignored, especially by male patients, and may progress for months or years before the lesions become clinically inflammatory and are no longer easily ignored. Changes may be evident as early as ages 8 to 9 years;

From: *Current Clinical Practice: Dermatology Skills for Primary Care: An Illustrated Guide*
D.J. Trozak, D.J. Tennenhouse, and J.J. Russell © Humana Press, Totowa, NJ

however, the peak incidence occurs during the teens, ages 14 to 19 years. Adult onset is almost entirely limited to female patients who often remark that they never had acne as teenagers.

Evolution of Disease Process

In most patients, noninflammatory lesions accumulate over varying periods of time. This early phase may remain as such, and when it occurs without a significant number of inflamed lesions, is referred to as *comedonal* or grade I acne. Even this mildest type is usually associated with heavy oil secretion or seborrhea.

Some patients will transition gradually to inflammatory acne, or this change may occur suddenly in an explosive fashion. If the inflammatory lesions are small and superficial, this phase is referred to as *papulopustular* or grade II acne, and for the first time, there is a significant risk of permanent scarring. The disease, if untreated, can remain papulopustular or a deeper form may evolve, with deep nodules, cysts, fistulas, and sinus tracts. This is referred to as *nodulocystic* (conglobate) or grade III acne. Without prompt intervention, severe scarring is virtually certain to develop.

A very specific rare form of acne vulgaris is called *acne fulminans*. This may develop, acutely or may evolve during the course of severe nodulocystic acne. Immense areas of hemorrhagic acne develop associated with constitutional symptoms of leukocytosis, elevated sedimentation rate, and crippling inflammatory arthralgias of the sacroiliac, and large joints. Occasionally there are also ocular, skeletal, and renal abnormalities. The mechanism appears to be an immunologically driven small-vessel vasculitis. At least one fatal case has been reported in the literature. This is a rare but serious emergency that requires immediate dermatologic referral.

In whatever form it takes, acne can produce permanent emotional and physical scarring. Acne that seems relatively inconsequential to the practitioner may be socially devastating to the victim. It is here that the art and sensitivity of medical practice are of paramount importance. While most male patients recover by their late teen years or mid-20s, many female victims continue to have symptoms well into adult life. Adult acne in women in their fourth and fifth decades is not at all unusual. Another typical pattern in women is activity during the mid-teens with an apparent remission, only to be followed by an exacerbation during the mid-third to fourth decade.

Evolution of Skin Lesions

Acne is a disease that takes many clinical forms, depending on when the practitioner enters into the process. Occasional cases present monomorphic disease with a preponderance of papular lesions or inflammatory nodules. Most, however, show a spectrum of primary lesions in varying stages of evolution from early noninflammatory to varying degrees of inflammation. In long-standing cases, the full spectrum of secondary change may also be present. The practitioner's challenge is to classify the victim's level of activity and initiate a program of therapy to control the problem without resorting to medications that are needlessly costly or risky.

Since there is a natural progression in most acne patients from nonscarring, noninflammatory lesions to inflammatory, potentially scarring disease, a major aim of therapy in grade I disease is the elimination of the early lesions before they progress. In established grades II and III cases, the major objective is rapid control of the inflammatory component responsible for the permanent injury, then to obtain gradual control of the early papular component that is driving it.

Provoking Factors

Acne is a disease with a strong genetic linkage, and is triggered by the somatic maturation that occurs during puberty. Other extrinsic factors also affecting the disease include the following:

1. Regular premenstrual changes. These cause flaring, probably from the androgenic effects of progestins on a sensitized terminal hair follicle.
2. Humidity, especially tropical climates, that can markedly exacerbate acne. Hydration of the follicular opening is a possible mechanism. Exercise that regularly induces heavy perspiration and hot packs applied to the skin have a similar effect.
3. Comedogenic substances in some cosmetics. These can cause flaring.
4. Environmental factors affecting fast-food employees. They note regular flares, possibly due to heat and humidity or to the cooking oil exposure that is unavoidable.
5. Stress, especially with lost sleep. This can exacerbate acne primarily by inducing increased disease activity, and also secondarily by increasing the degree to which the patient picks at and excoriates the lesions.
6. Natural sunlight. This has a beneficial effect on most cases. There are, however, some rare patients who are distinctly worse during times of heavy solar exposure.
7. The following general classes of medication have been reported to exacerbate existing acne vulgaris: corticosteroids, hormones with anabolic or androgenic effect, halogens, analeptics, and tuberculostatic medications.
   Foodstuffs are probably not a major factor. There is at present no body of evidence to validate dietary treatment or even indicate which foodstuffs should be avoided. Chocolate, long held as a prime culprit, appears to have no adverse effect.

Self-Medication

Self-treatment with over-the-counter medications will occasionally control mild grade I disease. Grades II and III acne will not respond to proprietary medicines. In fact, when combined with improper advice, these products may aggravate the disease. The major drawbacks to self-treatment are the tendency for the patient to defer professional treatment until substantial permanent injury has developed, and interference with an ongoing therapy program.

Supplemental Review From General History

A general system review would be indicated only in cases of acne fulminans where other diseases would enter into the differential diagnosis. Careful review of other concurrent medications is important so that interactions with systemic acne medications can be avoided.

Dermatologic Physical Exam

Primary Lesions

1. 1- to 3-mm white or yellow-white noninflammatory papules (closed comedones, whiteheads) (*see* Photos 25,26).

2. 1- to 3-mm black or blue-black noninflammatory follicular papules (open comedones, blackheads) (*see* Photo 27).
3. 1- to 5-mm inflammatory follicular papules that may or may not show an evident comedo (*see* Photos 27,28).
4. 1- to-5 mm inflammatory follicular pustules (*see* Photo 28).
5. Inflammatory nodules that approach or exceed 1 cm in size (*see* Photo 29).
6. Inflammatory nodules that coalesce to form large cysts and sinus tracts (*see* Photos 30,31).

The first two primary lesions listed above predominate in grade I acne. The middle two primary lesions predominate in grade II acne. The last two primary lesions predominate in grade III acne. A spectrum of lesions in different stages of evolution is present in grades II and III.

Secondary Lesions

1. Macular hyperpigmentation, which may consist of short-lived erythema or longer-lasting postinflammatory melanin deposits (*see* Photo 32).
2. Hemorrhagic crusts (*see* Photo 31).
3. Eschars (*see* Photo 31).
4. Atrophic, ice-pick-like hypertrophic or keloidal scarring (*see* Photos 26,29–31,33).

Distribution

Microdistribution: Acne is a disease of the terminal or sebaceous hair follicle, which occurs in the anatomic locations listed below.

Macrodistribution:

1. Face (most common: over 95%) (*see* Photos 31,34).
2. Posterior neck and upper back (next most common: 60%) (*see* Photo 35).
3. Central chest (less common: 15%) (*see* Photo 36).
4. Lower back, arms, and forearms (uncommon) (*see* Fig. 4).

Configuration

None.

Indicated Supporting Diagnostic Data

Generally, laboratory data are unnecessary for the diagnosis of acne vulgaris. Laboratory work is indicated to monitor certain systemic medications, such as the retinoids. Connective tissue disease screens may be indicated in rare cases of acne fulminans. When acne becomes refractory to systemic medication, or clinical features suggest the possibility of a Gram-negative folliculitis, bacterial cultures with sensitivity studies are indicated.

Therapy

The treatment of acne involves skillful use of medications, avoidance of provoking factors, physical evacuation of cysts and comedones, and in some cases intense emotional support. Therapy must be tailored to each case and must be adjusted regularly as condi-

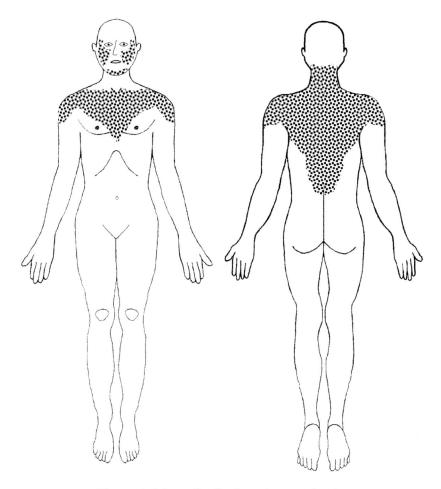

Figure 4: Macrodistribution of acne vulgaris.

tions change. In general, grade I and mild grade II acne can be treated with topical regimens. Moderate to severe grade II and grade III disease usually requires systemic agents combined with topical medication.

General Measures

From the specific history, the treating practitioner should point out to patients any extrinsic factors that may be provoking their disease so that these can be modified or avoided.

Cosmetics: Patients should be advised to avoid greasy, oil-based cosmetics and should receive specific advice on what is allowed. We ask our patients to use a foundation that is labeled "oil-free" and recommend a loose or pressed-powder blush, but allow complete latitude in the choice of lipsticks and eye cosmetics. Recommended sunscreens are clear gel-based products with an SPF of at least 30. Caution patients to avoid face masks, toners, and astringents, as these products may interfere with the treatment regimen. It is best to warn patients that disease flaring within a few months of initiating a new cosmetic makes that product a suspected aggravating factor.

Cleansing should be done gently two or three times daily, and we emphasize that although good hygiene is important, excessive hygiene can have a negative effect. For oily-skinned patients, a mild glycerin-based acne bar, warm (not hot) water, and gentle cleansing without undue pressure in the morning and evening are effective. For patients with dry or sensitive skin, a lipid-free lotion cleanser (such as Cetaphil Cleansing Lotion®) used in the same gentle fashion is more satisfactory. Abradant cleansers are harsh and encourage scrubbing with excess pressure that can precipitate deeper, more scarring acne. These are to be avoided. Steam packs aggravate the disease.

Picking and manipulation of acne lesions should be discouraged. This subject can be a touchy area and must be approached cautiously after patient and practitioner have developed rapport. Some patients are aware of their habit, while others completely deny doing it. These latter patients often have deep-seated emotional reasons for the habit and may find direct discussion quite threatening.

Diet has no clearly demonstrable effect on acne. For patients who insist on dietary advice, simply recommend avoidance of any food the patient feels has a repeated adverse effect.

Regular **rest** ("beauty rest") is important. Patients who are "burning the candle at both ends" usually experience flare-ups that resolve without other measures when a normal schedule is resumed.

Acne Surgery

Manual removal of whiteheads and blackheads, and the gentle evacuation of inflammatory papules, pustules, and cysts is an established and integral part of acne treatment. Properly done on a regular schedule, this procedure speeds recovery and prevents scarring. Although there are occasional patients without demonstrable comedo formation, most patients need active removal to achieve a satisfactory result. Several styles of comedo extractors are available. This procedure should be done only by a skilled operator, preferably the treating practitioner. Allowing patients or family members to perform this procedure usually leads to increased scarring or less than optimal improvement.

Ultraviolet Light

Modest amounts of natural sunlight or artificial UVB therapy are beneficial in most cases. The benefit is mainly due to removal of comedones. Because of the long-term aging and carcinogenic effects, use of this modality should be limited and it should be reserved as an adjunct to the primary treatment program.

Intralesional Steroids

Deep nodules and cysts can be rapidly improved with intralesional injection of small amounts of triamcinolone acetonide diluted to a concentration of 2.5 to 5.0 mg/cc in physiologic saline. Injection is best done using a control syringe with a 30-gage needle. Care should be taken to keep the solution within the lesion to prevent atrophy of the adjacent skin. Used appropriately, these injections will rapidly resolve painful nodules and cysts and minimize permanent scarring. By limiting the total dose to 10 mg or less in any

1-month period, and restricting usage to times of absolute need, the risk of systemic side effects is negligible.

Topical Therapy

Topical antibiotics: During the past several decades, the safety and value of topical antibiotic therapy in mild, minimally inflammatory acne have been well established. These are seldom used as monotherapy, but are combined with a retinoid or a benzoyl peroxide preparation. Products that contain erythromycin or clindamycin are available in an array of solutions, lotions, pledgets, and gel bases in concentrations of 1 to 2%. The choice of base depends on the patient's degree of oiliness and acceptance. Gel bases and high-alcohol vehicles seem to suit oily-skinned patients. Patients with dry or sensitive skin prefer vehicles with some degree of lubrication and lower alcohol content. The feel of the product can greatly affect compliance. Combination products, with erythromycin or clindamycin and benzoyl peroxide all in one, are also available. Some of these require refrigeration, which diminishes their shelf life and patient compliance. Teenagers dislike having to run to the refrigerator to apply an ice-cold medication. Newer combination products avoid this problem.

A topical antibiotic preparation should be used for 6 to 8 weeks before judging its effectiveness. Instruct patients to apply these products once daily in the morning. They may be worn under makeup, and should be reapplied after showering, swimming, and the like. Antibiotics are applied alone at a different time than other topicals, such as retinoids or benzoyl peroxides, that are used at bedtime. Side effects and allergic reactions have been rare. If these products are applied to wet skin immediately after cleansing, transient stinging and irritation may occur. This can be avoided by simply waiting 5 to 10 minutes.

Rare reports of allergic sensitization to erythromycin and clindamycin are recorded, and there have been rare reports of pseudomembranous colitis with topical clindamycin. Some practitioners use systemic and topical antibiotics concurrently. This is a wasteful practice and with the demonstrated antagonism between erythromycin and clindamycin, it could be self-defeating. Topical antibiotics are less effective in the deeper, more inflammatory types of acne. Occasionally, however, topicals can be very beneficial in patients who, for one reason or another, refuse systemic treatment.

Azelaic acid in a 15% gel or 20% cream preparation is also available as an alternative to traditional topical antibiotics. This agent has an antibacterial effect, modest comedolytic activity, and may also speed the resolution of postinflammatory hyperpigmentation. It has more potential for irritation than traditional topical antimicrobials.

Topical benzoyl peroxide preparations: These products are commonly available in concentrations ranging from 2.5 to 10% in a variety of lotion, pledget, gel, and hydrogel bases. Benzoyl peroxide loosens comedones, has a separate antibacterial effect, and suppresses excessive oil secretion. Hydrogel preparations tend to be less irritating. Irritation, dryness, and visible peeling are not essential to achieve the beneficial effects. Initiate this type of topical as a night lotion in conjunction with systemic antibiotics or the morning application of a topical antibiotic. The strength and vehicle are chosen based on the patient's visible oiliness, history, and reactivity to any previously used topicals. For patients with large amounts of comedonal acne, add a topical retinoid later, instructing the patient to use the two products on alternate evenings.

Benzoyl peroxide will bleach clothing and bed linens if used in cavalier fashion. It is important to warn the patient about this. Also instruct the patient to wait 5 to 10 minutes after washing before application. Otherwise, stinging and burning may occur and irritancy may be increased. Contact allergy to benzoyl peroxide is fairly common and, once present, eliminates this medication from the armamentarium. If a reaction occurs, document whether the reaction is true hypersensitivity or just irritation so that this important topical is not needlessly lost. Many generic benzoyl peroxide products are available. If a generic product is prescribed, make certain the pharmacy is consistent with one generic. The efficacy and irritancy of these generic products varies markedly with the composition of the vehicle, and can produce inconsistent treatment results. Although there is little evidence that higher concentrations of benzoyl peroxide have increased theraputic effect, the more concentrated preparations help to supress the excessive oiliness that some acne victims find very distressing. It is for this reason these more concentrated preparations remain on the market.

Topical retinoids: Tretinoin (also known as *trans*-retinoic acid or vitamin A acid) has become a mainstay of topical acne treatment. Use of tretinoin requires skill and close monitoring. It is manufactured in four strengths and is available in three vehicles: (1) 0.025%generic cream, (2) 0.025% gel, and (3) Retin A Micro® which comes in 0.04 and 0.1% concentrations in an optimized, microsphere gel base, which greatly reduces irritating side effects while maintaining efficacy.

Skin irritation manifested by dryness, redness, and peeling is a common side effect, and the drug must be started carefully after proper patient instruction. Failure to do this or to properly monitor the early side effects will result in low patient compliance. After a period of use, the epidermis "hardens" to the medication and stronger concentrations and more frequent applications are tolerated. The microsphere gels are the least irritating, followed by the cream and then the gel vehicles.

A second problem with tretinoin is its tendency to rapidly release comedones to the surface, causing an apparent flare of more inflammatory acne. This is particularly discouraging in the early stages of treatment, when the patient is seeking signs of remission and has yet to establish a trusting relationship with the practitioner. Proper instruction, reassurance, and careful selection as to the timing of entry of this medication into the regimen will lead to better results and a more satisfied and compliant patient. A simple explanation that the flaring is a prelude to long-term improvement is reassuring, and tells the patient that the practitioner understands the medication.

Tretinoin is particularly useful in the treatment of comedonal (grade I) acne and papulopustular (grade II) disease. In cases that are essentially comedonal, introduce tretinoin into the initial regimen by using it on an alternate-evening basis with a benzoyl peroxide hydrogel. The benzoyl peroxide hydrogel helps to control excessive oiliness and the inflammatory flare that can occasionally follow introduction of tretinoin. Try to use the tretinoin microsphere gel vehicle because of the lower irritancy and greater choice of concentrations. Start low and increase the concentration of the product as hardening occurs.

In papulopustular (grade II) disease, tretinoin must be introduced more cautiously or significant inflammatory flaring can occur. Start these patients on a regimen of a systemic or topical antimicrobial combined with bedtime applications of a benzoyl peroxide hydrogel. Once the inflammatory component of the acne settles, carefully introduce tretinoin, using a microsphere gel vehicle at what appears to be an appropriate strength. Alternate the tretinoin with the benzoyl peroxide product, or use it every third night in very sensitive cases. Concentration and frequency of application may then be gradually increased.

Tretinoin is generally ineffective in nodulocystic (grade III) acne unless there is a significant comedonal component. Even when comedones are present, the deep inflammatory component predominates and may be aggravated by tretinoin. Usage in nodulocystic disease should be very cautious and only after control of inflammation is achieved.

Adapalene is a topical retinoid introduced as an alternative to topical tretinoin. It is used and introduced in a similar fashion, but appears less irritating and less prone to cause early treatment flares than tretinoin. Adapalene is supplied as a 0.1% cream, gel, or solution. The cream is the least irritating and the solution the most. Unlike tretinoin, adapalene is not photosensitizing. Head-to-head comparative studies with tretinoin preparations are needed.

A third topical retinoid is tazarotene, which is marketed as a 0.05 and 0.1% cream or gel. This preparation tends to be more irritating than the other retinoids and carries a category X pregnancy warning. It is approved for mild to moderate acne.

Retinoids are teratogenic and fetotoxic in lower animals. Although there are no documented reports of problems to date, use during pregnancy and breastfeeding is not recommended. Tretinoin is also photosensitizing and has been reported to increase the tumerogenic effects of ultraviolet light in lower animals. For these reasons, patients should be instructed to wash the medication off before outdoor activities, avoid intense sun exposure, and wear a sunscreen with an SPF of 30 or greater on a daily basis. The generic tretinoin gel vehicle has been reported to be flammable. Warn patients about use around any open flame.

Other topicals: There also exists an extensive array of alternative proprietary and prescription topicals for acne. There are three in particular that may be useful.

In patients allergic to benzoyl peroxide or where heavy perspiration seems to be a factor, a prescription lotion of 6.25% aluminum chloride hexahydrate in 96% anhydrous ethyl alcohol (Xerac A-C®) can be quite effective. It is used as a night lotion, and comes with an applicator-topped bottle.

Extensive nodulocystic acne on the back and shoulders, and patients allergic to benzoyl peroxide, benefit from a lotion that contains 0.5% salicylic acid and 5% resorcin in a vehicle of 70% isopropanol. This inexpensive preparation can be easily compounded by the pharmacist and is simple and convenient to use.

Also effective as adjunctive therapy or monotherapy in mild cases is a clear prescription lotion of 10% sodium sulfacetamide (Klaron Lotion®). This may also be used in patients allergic to benzoyl peroxide, but must be avoided in patients with sulfonamide and sulfite sensitivity.

Systemic Therapy

Antibiotics: Tetracycline has been used since the mid-1950s for the treatment of inflammatory acne, and its efficacy and safety are well-established. Treatment is usually initiated at a dose of 250 mg QID and is tapered once adequate control is achieved. The main drawback to this medication is the frequency of dosing and adverse effect on its absorption by food, especially dairy products and iron. Single doses of 500 mg or daily dosing above 1 g/day have a high incidence of GI side effects. Photosensitivity can be a problem in sunny climates; however, this is uncommon and usually occurs only at maximal doses. Effectiveness of tetracycline or other antimicrobials should not be judged until 6 to 8 weeks after the start of treatment.

Erythromycin is also effective, and is usually administered in a divided starting dose of 500 to 1000 mg/day. It is more compatible with food, but has a greater potential for interaction with other medications (such as theophylline and some nonsedating antihistamines). Erythromycin is not photosensitizing. It seems to cause about the same amount of GI intolerance as tetracycline. Like tetracycline, it has an established safety record with chronic administration. The starting dose depends on the quality and extent of the inflammatory component. Both drugs are inexpensive.

A third inexpensive oral agent, frequently overlooked but often effective, is ampicillin. This antimicrobial is usually well tolerated by patients who experience GI intolerance to tetracycline and erythromycin. Dosing should start at 500 to 1000 mg/day in a divided dose depending on inflammatory activity. Amoxicillin may be used in a similar fashion.

The three antibiotic agents described above are usually used for initial treatment of mild to moderate grade II acne and mild grade III disease. Severe grade II and moderate to severe grade III acne are best treated with either doxycycline or minocycline.

Doxycycline is moderately priced, has a convenient BID dosing schedule, and can be quite effective. Drawbacks include occasional GI distress and a fairly high incidence of photosensitivity. Efficacy seems to fall between tetracycline and minocycline. Initial dose is usually 100 mg BID. It is indicated in moderate to severe grade II acne.

Minocycline is distinctly more rapid in onset and more effective in severe grade II and grade III acne. Minocycline is also helpful in patients who are prone to vaginal moniliasis. In severe acne disease, it is initiated at a dose of 100 mg BID. In less severe cases, 100 mg/day is often effective and is an appropriate maintenance dose once control is achieved. Because of high cost, appropriate dosing is essential. In severe cases, however, the drug can be very cost-effective by reducing the frequency of follow-up and by minimizing the long-term sequelae of the disease. Photosensitivity can occur, but is quite rare. An annoying idiosyncratic side effect is vertigo, which may occur many months after the start of treatment. This rapidly reverses upon withdrawal of the medication, but recurs with readministration. Another rare side effect is reversible liver toxicity. Minocycline can be administered with food but should not be taken at the same time as iron or iron-containing vitamin preparations. GI intolerance is rare. An additional rare side effect is the precipitation of connective tissue disease (lupus and rheumatoid arthritis) in a small number of patients.

Other antimicrobials used for resistant acne include trimethoprim/sulfamethoxazole and amoxicillin/clavulanic acid preparations. These resistant cases should be referred for dermatologic follow-up.

For patients with extensive mild to moderate inflammatory acne who are prone to vaginal yeast infections or are otherwise concerned about long-term use of antibiotics, a subantimicrobial regimen has been reported effective consisting of doxycycline 20 mg BID. This dose does not appear to alter skin, oral, bowel, or vaginal flora.

Female patients of childbearing age should be warned to stop systemic treatment in the event of a pregnancy or when breast-feeding.

Isotretinoin (13-*cis* retinoic acid): Because of the high cost, the significant potential for side effects, the risk of severe developmental defects if used during pregnancy, and the temporary but annoying side effects during usage, the decision to use isotretinoin should be based on proper indications that are well established. In addition, it should be administered only to a committed and reliable patient. Isotretinoin is indicated in cases of severe nodulocystic acne that are unresponsive to conventional therapy. Treatment should be initiated at a dose of 1.0 mg/kg of body weight or slightly higher. Lower dosing schedules will produce an initial response, but have a much higher incidence of relapse. In general, the incidence of side effects is dose-related. Treatment should continue for 16 to 20 weeks. It is important to complete at least a 4-month course. Treatment failures are higher in patients who fail to achieve a cumulative dose of 120 mg/kg of body weight. Many cases clear during the treatment period; however, some cases continue to improve after the regimen is complete. If disease activity persists, a second course may be initiated after a 2-month hiatus. Many patients will have a total remission, while others will convert to acne that is readily responsive to more conventional measures. As more experience is gained with isotretinoin, it is apparent that late recurrences several years posttreatment may occur. Even these are usually mild compared to the original disease.

Other factors besides isotretinoin dosage that are associated with a high recurrence rate include the following:

1. Papulopustular (grade II acne) without nodules or cysts.
2. Female patients with microcystic acne and signs of endocrine disease (such as irregular or absent menses, obesity, or hirsutism).
3. Predominantly truncal acne of any type.
4. Female patients greater than 25 years of age.

When these factors are present, conventional therapy may be more effective, safer and more cost-effective. The most serious side effects include photosensitivity, alopecia (both temporary and permanent), severe birth defects, hyperglycemia and aggravation of existing diabetes, reversible episodes of inflammatory bowel disease, xerophthalmia and reduced night visual acuity that may be permanent, pseudotumor cerebri, muscle injury with enzyme elevations usually triggered by sustained vigorous physical strain, reversible chemical hepatitis, and cases of acute pancreatitis (with triglyceride elevations).

A great controversy has arisen regarding possible linkage of this drug to suicidal depression. At the present time available evidence favors no connection, but the press coverage and legislative hearings have created a charged atmosphere. Patients should be screened for a history of depression and use in those with a positive history is not recommended.

When initiating systemic isotretinoin, all other systemic acne medicines should be suspended (especially tetracycline derivatives and vitamin products containing vitamin A). Patients should be warned to expect dry skin, fissured lips, increased sun sensitivity, and occasional muscle cramps. Existing deep acne may exacerbate during the first 4 to 6 weeks of treatment. Emollient skin lotions and lip pomades should be encouraged. Regular use of a sunscreen with an SPF of at least 30 is recommended, and even with the sunscreen, caution should be exercised when in the sun. CBC, liver functions, and lipid levels should be monitored every 2 weeks for the first 6 weeks of therapy and compared to a baseline study.

Isotretinoin treatment should be avoided in patients who plan periods of sustained vigorous physical exercise.

Female patients should be warned about the high risk and severity of possible birth defects, and should practice an effective form of pregnancy prevention for at least 1 month before and after treatment. Practitioners who use isotretinoin should be familiar with and follow the manufacturer's stringent guidelines in regard to pregnancy prevention. A pregnancy test prior to beginning treatment is essential.

Patients on isotretinoin should be warned to promptly report the following symptoms: visual changes, abdominal pain, rectal bleeding, and diarrhea. Diabetics should report any consistent change in blood sugar levels. Contact lens users should suspend or limit the use of those appliances. Blood donors should not donate during and for 1 month after completing treatment.

Isotretinoin is a marvelous medication for a group of acne victims for whom we once had little to offer. Use of this drug involves an in-depth familiarity with the disease process and the medication. The decision to proceed carries a heavy burden of responsibility for both physician and patient.

Systemic steroids: Occasionally patients present with nodulocystic acne that is so severe and extensive that isotretinoin is initially contraindicated. These cases must be initially handled with a combination of traditional treatment and moderate to high doses of oral prednisone. These patients should be promptly referred to a dermatologic consultant.

Emotional Support

Emotional support may be a major factor in the successful treatment of acne, and is especially important in the early stages when significant clearing is not yet evident. Patients who pick or manipulate their lesions need constant gentle prodding and support. The severity of the physical disease is not a measure of the emotional impact on the victim.

Scarring

Once the disease process comes under control, the patient's attention turns to the injury that has occurred. Most patients are anxious and prematurely pessimistic in this regard. Advise them that absolute control is the first essential step. Reassure them that much of what they see will soften or disappear, and that this process will continue for up to a year after good control has been achieved. If significant scarring remains at that point, a dermatologic consultation is indicated.

Conditions That May Simulate Acne Vulgaris

Rosacea

Papulopustular rosacea may resemble acne, but usually occurs on a backdrop of flushing and telangectasia. Comedones and cysts are absent except in rare cases when both diseases occur simultaneously. Most rosacea lesions are on the face.

Perioral Dermatitis

This localized eruption is almost exclusively limited to female patients. It presents with a localized papular and eczematous eruption with tiny pinpoint pustules in the perioral, perinasal, or periocular areas of the face. It superficially resembles acne, but lacks comedones, nodules, and cysts. Topical acne medications will exacerbate the condition.

Acne-Like Drug Eruptions

A long list of medications can cause an acne-like eruption. Hormones (especially systemic steroids), halogen-containing medications, tuberculostatic agents, and antiepileptic drugs are the major classes of drugs. These eruptions consist of sheets of fragile pustules, which are not limited to sebaceous locations. Comedones, nodules, and cysts are absent.

Gram-Negative Folliculitis

This is a complication of long-term antimicrobial therapy for acne. A patient who had achieved good control suddenly deteriorates. Multiple painful follicular pustules with or without nodulocystic lesions suddenly appear. Culture reveals Gram-negative pathogens. Appropriate antibiotics or isotretinoin are the treatment.

Pseudofolliculitis Barbae

Ingrown hairs of the chin and lateral neck areas are common in many young males, especially those of African-American background. These lesions are painful and respond only partially to acne medications. Observation of trapped hairs, looped hairs, and characteristic distribution establish the diagnosis. Shaving instructions are indicated.

ANSWERS TO CLINICAL APPLICATION QUESTIONS

History Review

A shy 14-year-old girl accompanied by her mother presents for treatment of acne of 1 year's duration.

1. What historical information will assist in staging her disease and in the choice of appropriate treatment?

Answer:
   a. Levels of activity. Acne is a disease of cyclical intensity. Establish the maximum level of activity compared to today's appearance.
   b. Provoking factors. Review the effect of menstrual phase, cleansing practices, exercise, cosmetic use, and occupation.
   c. Acne medications. Review any current prescribed or self-prescribed acne medication. These may have a profound effect on your acne program.
   d. Other systemic medications. Review other medications to avoid interactions, and identify any that may exacerbate existing acne.

2. What should you look for on physical exam?

Answer:
   a. The extent and distribution of the lesions.
   b. The degree of oiliness or seborrhea.
   c. The relative mixture of noninflammatory papules, inflammatory papules, pustules, nodules, cysts, and sinus tracts in each area.
   d. The degree of scarring in each involved area.

3. What general treatment measures other than medication should you institute?

Answer:

    a. Explain the general nature and course of the disease, and the need for a certain level of maintenance treatment once control is achieved.

    b. Review use of cosmetics.

    c. Review appropriate cleansing practices.

    d. Discourage picking and manipulation of lesions. The first visit is not always the best time for this discussion.

    e. Discuss diet and rest.

    f. Explain to the patient why you have chosen the program she is going to follow. This improves compliance.

4. The patient has fairly dense acne of the face and mid-upper back. Her chest, shoulders, neck, and lower back are spared. Her lesions are predominantly noninflammatory papules, open comedones, and a few inflammatory papules and pustules. Her mother has read about isotretinoin therapy. How would you grade her acne, and what would be an appropriate treatment regimen?

Answer:

    a. Grade I acne.

    b. Medication consisting of a topical antibiotic each morning and a topical retinoid every other night alternating with a benzoyl peroxide product tailored to her degree of oiliness.

    c. Regularly scheduled follow-up visits for acne surgery, medication adjustment, and to assess progress.

5. What would you change in your management if her acne also involved her chest, shoulders, and lower back?

Answer: A systemic antibiotic would be more cost-effective.

37 Rosacea *(Acne Rosacea)*

CLINICAL APPLICATION QUESTIONS

A 50-year-old woman is seen in your office for facial discoloration that has been very persistent for the past 2 months. She also complains of frequent styes and constant gritty eye discomfort with lid granulation each morning. Initial observation shows a striking butterfly erythema.

1. What items in the specific history would help you distinguish rosacea from lupus erythematosus (LE)?
2. What physical findings would help you to distinguish rosacea from LE?
3. What laboratory data are indicated?
4. Assuming that physical findings and lab results are consistent with rosacea, what is the most appropriate treatment for this patient?

APPLICATION GUIDELINES

Specific History

Onset

Rosacea is a disorder that presents most typically in the third, fourth, and fifth decades of life. It is seen occasionally in younger adults, and there are uncommon reports of otherwise typical rosacea in childhood. Presentation in adult patients beyond the fifth decade is fairly common. Women seem more frequently affected than men. This preference may be misleading, however, because of male machismo that prevents seeking help for skin disorders. Men are subject to the more severe and deforming variants. Although heritage is not an absolute protection, rosacea is rare in heavily pigmented skin types, whereas western Europeans, especially those of Celtic ancestry, are especially vulnerable. Onset may be explosive and may follow exposure to one of the provoking factors listed below. Most cases start insidiously, but inexorably worsen without medical intervention. Many patients will state on the initial visit, "I have watched this change for months (or years) and I finally have to do something about it." The earliest and most persistent symptoms are erythema and fine telangiectasias distributed symmetrically over the central face, but sparing the eyelids, upper forehead, and lips.

Evolution of Disease Process

The erythema and telangectasia of rosacea initially wax and wane from day to day, but gradually become more conspicuous and more persistent. The disease may retain this morphology throughout the course of the patient's life. This is referred to as *erythematous*

From: *Current Clinical Practice: Dermatology Skills for Primary Care: An Illustrated Guide*
D.J. Trozak, D.J. Tennenhouse, and J.J. Russell © Humana Press, Totowa, NJ

telangiectatic rosacea. In a significant number of cases, the course is punctuated by attacks of dusky rose-red papules that occur within the areas of erythematous skin. About 20% of cases will show pustules replacing some of the papules. The pustules are usually not tender and, except in rare instances of concurrent acne vulgaris, comedones are absent. These acute exacerbations are often associated with acute edema that is visible and palpable. This stage is referred to as *papulopustular rosacea.*

A small number of cases progress to large nodular lesions with permanently thickened skin, coarse pores, sebaceous gland hyperplasia, and persistent facial edema. This uncommon but deforming variant almost exclusively affects men and is called *glandular hyperplastic rosacea.*

During acute exacerbations, many patients complain of an uncomfortable suffused feeling of the facial skin and, in the case of nodular lesions, overt tenderness. Many also remark after treatment that because of the insidious onset, they failed to appreciate how uncomfortable the skin areas had become.

Without therapy, most patients have persisting symptoms punctuated by acute exacerbations often triggered by identifiable environmental factors discussed below. With medication, almost all rosacea patients can be controlled, and a substantial number go into complete remission. In one study, after adequate systemic treatment with oral tetracycline, 31% of patients remained free of disease during a 4-year follow-up. The other 69% relapsed, most within the first 6 months. Some patients with early rosacea remained asymptomatic without treatment for several years after complete control was achieved with systemic medication.

Special forms of rosacea include the following:

Disseminated rosacea: In rare cases, other locations such as the hairless scalp, V of the chest, upper mid-back, and wrists may be involved with otherwise typical lesions. However, the central face is the most constant and characteristic site.

Lupoid/granulomatous rosacea: Widespread red-brown papules and nodules appear on a background of dusky erythema. With diascopy using a glass slide, the lesions show the apple-jelly nodule change seen also with lesions of lupus vulgaris. Areas that are usually spared in common rosacea (such as the eyelids and perioral skin) are affected in lupoid rosacea. Biopsy shows granulomatous histology.

Complications of rosacea may include:

Ocular rosacea: Eye symptoms occurred in more than 50% of cases in one study. Practical experience suggests that the actual incidence is about 10% or less. In most cases, findings are those of a low-grade conjunctivitis manifest by tenderness, a gritty discomfort, lid granulations, and conjunctival injection. Other eye complications reported include meibomianitis, trichiasis, episcleritis, chalazion, and hordeolum. Rosacea-associated keratitis can cause corneal scarring and blindness. Any rosacea patient with pain, photophobia, or altered visual acuity should have an ophthalmologic evaluation and prompt systemic treatment for the rosacea. The ocular complications respond to systemic rosacea medication provided corneal scarring has not yet occurred.

Rhinophyma: A progressive alteration of the nose develops in some male rosacea patients. Contrary to popular belief, this is not a sign of alcoholism. Deformity and coarseness of the nasal skin with enlarged patulous follicles begins on the distal nose and gradually spreads. The hypertrophy may be asymmetric, causing marked distortion. On rare occasions, the tip of the chin and the earlobes may be similarly affected. Treatment with standard systemic medication for rosacea will improve the color and control inflammatory lesions, but has no effect on the thickening or deformity. A dermatologic referral is appropriate. Surgical revision can dramatically improve the changes.

Rosacea lymphedema: A persistent nonpitting edema of the forehead, cheeks, chin, or (on rare occasions) the earlobes develops during the course of chronic rosacea. Color varies from mild to intense erythema. Standard medications have little effect on this complication.

Evolution of Skin Lesions

The intensity of the erythema, telangectasia, and edema varies from day to day. However, over long time periods, they become progressively more persistent and widespread. The papular and nodular lesions are often quite chronic, and advanced lesions may require several weeks to resolve even with systemic treatment. A certain number of the papular lesions in some cases develop a dome-shaped pustule at their apex. Some pustules are quite small and can be best discerned with the aid of a hand lens. As the pustules deteriorate, they form a small hemorrhagic crust. The papular and nodular lesions of rosacea, in contrast to those of acne vulgaris, do not scar.

Provoking Factors

Patients who develop rosacea are almost universally flushers and blushers. Environmental factors that stimulate this vasomotor instability will aggravate the disease and may precipitate the initial attack and subsequent acute exacerbations. Chronic sun-induced degenerative changes in the connective tissue that supports the dermal blood vessels also appears to play a permissive role in the onset of the disease. Common environmental triggers include the following:

1. Acute sunburn with its attendant erythema.
2. Ingestion of piping-hot liquids, irrespective of their content.
3. Persistent diet of hot or spicy foods.
4. Regular use of alcoholic beverages.
5. Medications that produce vasodilation have become increasingly important in this regard over the last quarter-century. β-blocking agents, acetazolamide, nitrates, and psoralens have all been reported to exacerbate the disease. Any medication that produces prolonged vasodilation should be considered suspect, especially if there is a temporal relationship between its introduction and increased rosacea activity.

Self-Medication

In contrast to acne, self-treatment is not a significant problem with rosacea patients.

Supplemental Review From General History

A review of prescription and proprietary medications, dietary habits, and alcoholic beverage use is indicated. Questions regarding any ocular symptoms or visual changes are also important. Otherwise, rosacea does not have any systemic manifestations.

Dermatologic Physical Exam

Primary Lesions

1. Patches of pink to dusky-red erythema covered with a network of fine dilated (telangiectatic) blood vessels (*see* Photo 37).
2. Dusky-red inflammatory papules (*see* Photo 38).
3. Dusky-red inflammatory nodules (*see* Photo 39).
4. Dome-shaped pustules (*see* Photo 40).

Secondary Lesions

1. Acute palpable edema of the facial skin that is present during attacks and resolves during periods of control (*see* Photo 41).
2. Chronic persistent edema of the involved skin that is unresponsive to treatment.
3. Chronic noninflammatory papules and nodules seen in glandular hyperplastic rosacea.

Although they are usually primary lesions, here papules and nodules may occur as secondary lesions.

Distribution

Microdistribution: None.

Macrodistribution: Central forehead, nose, chin, and butterfly-flush area of the face (*see* Fig. 5). The upper forehead, lips, and eyelids are spared except in the lupoid variant and in cases of topical steroid-induced rosacea. Other locations may be involved in the uncommon disseminated variant.

Configuration

Grouped papules, nodules and/or pustules on a background of telangiectatic erythema.

Indicated Supporting Diagnostic Data

In most instances, rosacea is a clinical diagnosis. On rare occasions, biopsy may be indicated when individual lesions simulate other conditions or when there is a question of rosacea versus cutaneous lupus erythematosus. In these instances, a dermatologic consultation is indicated. The skills of the dermatologist in physical examination may avoid needless expense and manipulation of the patient.

Therapy

Rosacea is a disease that, if left untreated, can progress through a continuum of change to a point where irreversible damage occurs. This potential, plus the emotional and actual physical discomfort, make rosacea treatment more than just cosmetic.

Prevention

Avoiding sunburn, extreme environmental heat, prolonged hot baths, ingestion of piping-hot liquids, hot spicy meals, and alcoholic beverages will minimize the attacks. Once good control of the disease is achieved, occasional dietary relaxation can usually be allowed. If a medication such as a β-blocking agent is implicated, the medication should be changed.

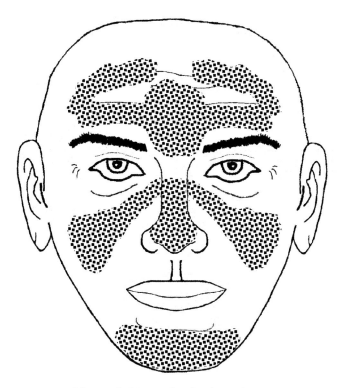

Figure 5: Macrodistribution of rosacea.

Systemic Therapy

Oral tetracycline has been recognized as a safe and effective treatment for rosacea for more than 30 years. The mechanism of action in this disease is not known. Most cases respond to an initial dose of 250 mg BID and can be maintained on a single capsule daily. The disease shows no tendency to become resistant to this medication and, if increased activity is noted in a patient, other external provoking factors should be sought. Tetracyclines are often combined initially with a nonfluorinated group VI or group VII steroid cream or lotion (*see* Chapter 4, Table 1). Desonide 0.05% and 2.5% hydrocortisone are common examples. Fluorinated corticosteroids, however, are contraindicated. Topical steroids alone are not effective monotherapy. In severe or disseminated rosacea, higher doses of 250 mg tetracycline QID or use of doxycycline or minocycline may be indicated. Minocycline is also helpful in patients with GI intolerance to tetracycline and in female patients who are prone to vaginal candidiasis. Systemic tetracyclines control the ocular complications of rosacea provided irreversible injury has not occurred. Systemic metronidazole is also effective, but has never been used on a chronic basis because of concerns regarding side effects. Severe or recalcitrant rosacea will respond to isotretinoin. These cases should be referred to a dermatologic consultant.

Topical Therapy

Topical metronidazole is available as a 0.75 to 1% cream, 0.75% gel, or lotion for the treatment of rosacea. All are effective as monotherapy in mild to moderate erythematous telangiectatic rosacea, and can be used in more advanced cases with systemic tetracycline to induce remissions and then maintain control while the systemic medication is withdrawn. Equally effective are premade prescription products containing sodium sulfacetamide. They are available in clear and tinted formulations. Patients with chronic renal disease, or sulfonamide or sulfite sensitivity, should not use these products. Azaleic acid gel 15% has also been approved for treatment of mild to moderate rosacea. In a head-to-head study it was superior to 0.75% metronidazole gel.

Conditions That May Simulate Rosacea

Acne Vulgaris

The two diseases may occur concurrently. Otherwise, their clinical features distinguish them. Acne does not have the background of erythema and dilated blood vessels. Comedones and inflammatory cysts are present with acne (features not seen in rosacea). Acne frequently involves the central chest and back, and often leaves scars.

Perioral Dermatitis

This localized eruption presents with pinpoint papules and pustules in the perioral and perinasal areas, and is seen almost exclusively in females. The lesions are so small that a hand lens is often required to appreciate their morphology. The background skin is eczematous.

Discoid and Systemic LE

Both discoid and systemic lupus erythematosus can be confused with the erythematous telangiectatic variant of rosacea. Papules and pustules do not occur, so there should be no confusion with the other forms of rosacea. Neither form of LE waxes and wanes dramatically from day to day as does rosacea. Lesions of both forms of lupus tend to extend beyond the usual distribution of rosacea and, with discoid lupus, the scaling, atrophy, scarring, and pigmentary changes help to distinguish it. Biopsy may help in difficult cases; however, direct immunofluorescence gives false-positive results and should not be used.

Steroid Rosacea

Although topical steroids have been used as adjunctive treatment in rosacea for years, fluorinated topical steroids can aggravate active rosacea and can produce a rosacea-like eruption in persons without a previous problem. The drug-induced form initially shows erythema and telangectasia, but can progress to a papulopustular phase. Involvement of the entire forehead, lips, and eyelids (areas normally spared in spontaneous rosacea) is an important clue.

ANSWERS TO CLINICAL APPLICATION QUESTIONS

History Review

A 50-year-old woman is seen in your office for facial discoloration that has been progressive for the past 6 months. She also complains of frequent styes and constant gritty eye discomfort with lid granulation each morning. Initial observation shows a striking butterfly erythema.

1. **What items in the specific history would help you distinguish rosacea from LE?**

Answer:
   a. Gradual onset and progression.
   b. A history of remissions and exacerbations.
   c. Ocular symptoms.
   d. A history of blushing and flushing (vasomotor instability).
   e. Exacerbations when exposed to known provoking factors.

2. **What physical findings would help you to distinguish rosacea from LE?**

Answer:
   a. Dusky-red inflammatory papules and nodules.
   b. Dome-shaped pustules.
   c. An active conjunctivitis.

3. **What laboratory data are indicated?**

Answer: An antinuclear antibody (ANA) test would be appropriate because of the similarity between the two eruptions. Extensive serologic testing for LE is indicated only if other findings raise a significant suspicion that this is not rosacea.

4. **Assuming that physical findings and lab results are consistent with rosacea, what is the most appropriate treatment for this patient?**

Answer: Systemic therapy with tetracycline or a tetracycline-derivative antibiotic. This will control her ocular and cutaneous symptoms.

REFERENCES for Part VI

1. Champion RH, Burton JL, Ebling FJG. Textbook of Dermatology. 5th. Ed. Oxford: Blackwell Scientific Publications, 1992 pp. 965–968, 879–893, 999–1000,888–892, 716–743, 1699–1744, 1851–1863.
2. Braun-Falco O, Plewig G, Wolff HH, Winkelmann RK.Dermatology. Berlin-Heidelberg: Springer-Verlag, 1991 pp. 156–159, 22–36, 125–129, 32–36, 716–743, 730–736.
3. Darmstadt GL, Lane PT. Impetigo: An overview. Pediatric Dermatol 11: 293–303, 1994.
4. Drug Facts and Comparisons. St. Louis: Wolters-Kluwer Co. 2003 Ed.
5. Erlich KS, Mills J. Chemotherapy for Herpes simplex virus infections; Medical staff conference. West J Med 1985;143:648–655.
6. Lever WF, Schaumburg-Lever G. Histopathology of the Skin. 6th. Ed. Philadelphia: J B Lippincott Company, 1983, pp. 364.
7. Solomon AR. New diagnostic tests for Herpes simplex and varicella zoster infections. J Amer Acad Dermatol 1988;18:18–221.
8. Goodyear HM, Wilson P, Cropper L et al. Rapid diagnosis of Herpes simplex infections using specific monoclonal antibodies. Clin Exper Dermatol 1994;19:294–297.
9. Nahass GT Goldstein BA, Zhu WY et al. Comparison of Tzanck smear, viral culture, and DNA diagnostic methods in detection of Herpes simplex and varicella-zoster infection. JAMA 1992;268:2541–2544.
10. Brody I. Topical treatment of recurrent Herpes simplex and postherpetic erythema multiforme with low concentrations of zinc sulphate solution. Br J Dermatol 1981;104:191–194.
11. Busso M, Berman B. Antivirals in dermatology. J Amer Acad Dermatol 1995;32:1031–1040.
12. Chatis PA, Miller CH, Schrager LE, Crumpacker CS. Successful treatment with foscarnet of an acyclovir resistant mucocutaneous infection with Herpes simplex virus in a patient with acquired immunodeficiency syndrome. NEJM 1989;320:297–300.
13. Safrin S, Crumpacker C, Chatis P et al. A controlled trial comparing foscarnet with vidaribine for acyclovir resistant mucocutaneous Herpes simplex in the acquired immunodeficiency syndrome. NEJM 1991;325:551–55.
14. La Rossa D, Hamilton R. Herpes simplex infections of the digits. Arch Surg 1971;102: 600–603.
15. Sachs E, House RK. The Ramsay Hunt Syndrome. Neurol 1956;6:262–268.
16. Cockrell CJ. Cutaneous manifestations of HIV infection other than Kaposi's sarcoma: Clinical and histologic aspects. J Amer Acad Dermatol 1990;22:1260–1269.
17. Wood MJ, Johnson RW, McKendrick MW et al. A randomized trial of acyclovir for 7 days or 21 days with and without prednisolone for treatment of acute Herpes zoster. NEJM 1994;330:896–900.
18. Famciclovir for Herpes zoster. The Medical Letter 1994;36:7–98.
19. Kishore–Kumar R, Max MB, Schafer SC et al. Desipramine relieves postherpetic neuralgia. Clin Pharmacol Ther 1990;47:305.
20. Whitley JJ, Gnann JW. Acyclovir: A Decade Later. NEJM 1992;327:782–789.
21. Balfour HH. Acyclovir therapy for Herpes zoster: advantages and adverse effects. JAMA 1986;255:387–388.
22. King RB. Topical aspirin in chloroform and the relief of pain due to Herpes zoster and postherpetic neuralgia. Arch Neurol 1993;50:1046–1053.
23. Leider M, Rosenblum M. A Dictionary of Dermatological Words, Terms and Phrases. New York-Toronto-London-Sydney: Mc Graw-Hill, 1968, pp. 9.

From: *Current Clinical Practice: Dermatology Skills for Primary Care: An Illustrated Guide*
D.J. Trozak, D.J. Tennenhouse, and J.J. Russell © Humana Press, Totowa, NJ

24. Karvonen SL. Acne fulminans: Report of clinical findings and treatment of twenty-four patients. J Amer Acad Dermatol 1993;28:572–579.
25. Leyden JJ. The treatment and management of acne. J Internat Postgrad Med 1991;4:11–16.
26. Layton AM, Cunliffe WJ. Guidelines for optimal use of isotretinoin in acne. J Amer Acad Dermatol 27 #6 1992;part 2:S2–S7.
27. Lehucher-Ceyrac D, Weber-Buisset MJ. Isotretinoin an acne in practice: A prospective analysis of 188 cases over nine years. Dermatology 1993;186:123–128.
28. Stainforth JM, Layton AM, Taylor JP, Cunliffe WJ. Isotretinoin for the treatment of acne vulgaris: Which factors may predict the need for more than one course? Br J Dermatol 1993;129:297–301.
29. Layton AM, Knaggs H, Taylor J, Cunliffe WJ. Isotretinoin for acne vulgaris—10 years later: A safe and successful treatment. Br J Dermatol 1993;129:292–296.
30. Knight AG, Vickers CFH. A follow-up of tetracycline-treated rosacea. Br J Dermatol 1975;93:577–580.
31. Wilkin JK. Vasodilator Rosacea. Arch Dermatol 1980;116:98.
32. The guide to drug eruptions. 6 th. Ed. Amsterdam: Free University Amsterdam; File of Medicines, 1995, pp. 6.
33. Wilkin JK. Rosacea: Pathophysiology and treatment. Arch Dermatol 1994;130:359–362.
34. Mertz GJ, Loveless MA, Kraus SJ, et al. Famciclovir for the suppression of genital herpes. Proceedings of the 34th Interscience Conference on Antimicrobial Agents and Chemotherapy. Washington DC: American Society for Microbiology; 1994. Abs. H3.
35. Patel R, Crooks JR, Bell AR, and the International Valacyclovir Study Group. Once daily valacyclovir for the suppression of recurrent genital herpes—the first placebo controlled clinical trial. The First European Congress of Chemotherapy. Glasgow, UK; 1996. Abs.
36. Tyring S, Barbarash RA, Nahlik JE, et al., and the Collaborative Famciclovir Herpes Zoster Study Group. Famciclovir for the treatment of acute Herpes zoster: Effects on acute disease and postherpetic neuralgia. Ann Int Med 1995;123 #2:89–96.
37. Kost RG, Straus SE. Postherpetic neuralgia—pathogenesis, treatment, and prevention. NEJM 1996;335:32.
38. Leyden JJ. Therapy for acne vulgaris. NEJM 1997;336:1156–1162.
39. Adapalene for acne. The Medical Letter 1997;39:19–20.
40. Topical penciclovir for Herpes labialis. The Medical Letter 1997;39:57–58.
41. Genital Herpes Simplex Virus (HSV) Infection. Arch Dermatol 1998;134:650–652.
42. Langenberg AGM, Corey L, Ashley RL et al. A Prospective Study Of New Infections With Herpes Simplex virus Type 1 And Type 2. NEJM 1999;341:1432–1438.
43. Lautenschlager S, Eichman A. Urethritis: an underestimated clinical variant of genital herpes in men? J Amer Acad Dermatol 2002;46:307–308.
44. Brown TJ, Yen-Moore A, Tyring SK. An overview of sexually transmitted diseases. Part I. J Amer Acad Dermatol 1999;41:511–529.
45. Drugs For Non-HIV Viral Infections. The Medical Letter 2002;44:9–11.
46. Corey L, Wald A, Patel R et al. Once-Daily Valacyclovir to Reduce the Risk of Genital Herpes. NEJM 2004;350:11–20.
47. Gnann JW, Whitley RJ. Herpes Zoster. NEJM 2001;2002;347:40–346.
48. Wolverton SE. Comprehensive Dermatologic Therapy. W B Saunders Company.
49. Physicians Desk Reference. Thomson 58th. Ed., 2004.
50. Skidmore R, Kovach R, Walker C et al. Effect of Subantimicrobial-Dose Doxycycline in the Treatment of Moderate Acne. Arch Dermatol 2003;139:459–464.
51. Russell JJ. Topical Therapy for Acne. Am Family Physician 2000;61:357–366.
52. Elewski BE, Fleisher Jr. AB, Pariser DM. A Comparison of 15% Azaleic Acid Gel and 0.75%Metronidazole Gel in the Topical Treatment of Papulopustular Rosacea. Arch Dermatol 2003;139:1444–1450.
53. Kimberlin DW, Rouse DJ. Genital Herpes. NEJM 2004;350:1970–1977.

Appendix A: Table of Primary Lesions and Related Disorders

Bullae
    Erysipelas [Part III]
    Erythema multiforme [Part III]
    Fixed drug eruption [Part III]
    Impetigo [Part VI]
    Tinea (large, multiloculated) [Part III]
    Urticaria (bullae as secondary lesions) [Part III]
Macules
    Actinic keratosis (erythematous) [Part V]
    Atypical nevi [Part V]
    Common benign nevi (pigmented) [Part V]
    Ephelides [Part V]
    Erysipelas (erythematous) [Part III]
    Erythema multiforme (erythematous) [Part III]
    Erythrasma [Part III]
    Fixed drug eruption [Part III]
    Halo nevi [Part V]
    Impetigo (deep red) [Part VI]
    Lentigines [Part V]
    Malignant melanoma [Part V]
Nodules
    Acne [Part VI]
    Basal cell carcinoma (translucent, dome-shaped) [Part V]
    Keratoacanthoma (dome-shaped) [Part V]
    Malignant melanoma [Part V]
    Molluscum (dome-shaped umbilicated) [Part II]
    Rosacea (red) [Part VI]
    Squamous cell carcinoma (indurated) [Part V]
    Verruca vulgaris [Part II]
Papules
    Acne (with or without comedones) [Part VI]
    Atopic dermatitis [Part IV]
    Atypical nevi [Part V]
    Basal cell carcinoma (translucent, dome-shaped) [Part V]
    Developed dermal nevi (sharply defined) [Part V]
    DLE (sharply defined, raised, smooth, shiny) [Part IV]
    Early compound nevi (dome-shaped) [Part V]
    Erythema multiforme (erythematous) [Part III]

From: *Current Clinical Practice: Dermatology Skills for Primary Care: An Illustrated Guide*
D.J. Trozak, D.J. Tennenhouse, and J.J. Russell © Humana Press, Totowa, NJ

Halo nevi [Part V]
Keratoacanthoma (dome-shaped) [Part V]
Lichen planus (flat-topped, angular, polygonal) [Part II]
Malignant melanoma [Part V]
Mature compound nevi (sharply defined) [Part V]
Mature dermal nevi (pedunculated) [Part V]
Miliaria (small, erythematous) [Part II]
Molluscum (dome-shaped umbilicated) [Part II]
Pityriasis rosea (rosy red) [Part II]
Psoriasis (erythematous, scaling) [Part II]
Rosacea (red) [Part VI]
Scabies (papulovesicle at end of burrow) [Part II]
Seborrheic dermatitis (red-brown, follicular) [Part II]
Seborrheic keratosis [Part V]
SLE (sharply defined, may coalesce) [Part IV]
Squamous cell carcinoma (indurated) [Part V]
Striae distensae (yellow papules as secondary lesions) [Part IV]
Tinea (follicular) [Part III]
Verruca vulgaris [Part II]

Patches
Actinic keratosis (erythematous) [Part V]
Asteatosis [Part IV]
Atopic dermatitis [Part IV]
Erythrasma [Part III]
Malignant melanoma [Part V]
Rosacea (erythematous) [Part VI]
Seborrheic keratosis [Part V]
Senile purpura (purple) [Part IV]
Striae distensae (linear) [Part IV]
Tinea [Part III]
Toxicodendron dermatitis (linear) [Part IV]

Plaques
Actinic keratosis (thin) [Part V]
Atypical nevi [Part V]
Basal cell carcinoma [Part V]
Congenital melanocytic nevi (pigmented) [Part V]
Developed compound nevi [Part V]
DLE (sharply defined, raised, smooth, shiny) [Part IV]
Erysipelas (erythematous) [Part III]
Erythema multiforme (erythematous) [Part III]
Fixed drug eruption [Part III]
Herpes simplex (erythematous) [Part VI]
Herpes zoster (erythematous) [Part VI]
Impetigo (red) [Part VI]
Lichen planus (coalescing papules) [Part II]

    Malignant melanoma [Part V]

    Molluscum (tightly-grouped papules) [Part II]

    Pityriasis rosea (rosy red) [Part II]

    Psoriasis [Part II]

    SCLE (sharply defined) [Part IV]

    Seborrheic keratosis [Part V]

    SLE (edematous) [Part IV]

    Squamous cell carcinoma (indurated) [Part V]

    Tinea (indurated) [Part III]

    Toxicodendron dermatitis (linear) [Part IV]

    Urticaria (edematous) [Part III]

Pustules

    Acne [Part VI]

    Herpes simplex (late) [Part VI]

    Herpes zoster (late) [Part VI]

    Miliaria (as secondary lesions) [Part II]

    Rosacea (dome-shaped) [Part VI]

    Tinea (follicular) [Part III]

Vesicles

    Atopic dermatitis [Part IV]

    Erysipelas [Part III]

    Erythema multiforme [Part III]

    Fixed drug eruption [Part III]

    Herpes simplex [Part VI]

    Herpes zoster [Part VI]

    Impetigo (small, transient) [Part VI]

    Miliaria (crystalline, intra-dermal) [Part II]

    Scabies (papulovesicle at end of burrow) [Part II]

    Tinea (intra-dermal, small, grouped) [Part III]

    Toxicodendron dermatitis (linear) [Part IV]

Appendix B: Table of Secondary Lesions and Related Disorders

Atrophy
   DLE (epidermal and dermal) [Part IV]
   Lichen planus [Part II]
   SCLE (epidermal) [Part IV]
   Senile purpura (epidermal) [Part IV]
   SLE (epidermal and dermal) [Part IV]
Calcinosis
   SLE [Part IV]
Crusting
   Acne (hemorrhagic) [Part VI]
   Atopic dermatitis [Part IV]
   Atypical nevi (malignant change) [Part V]
   Basal cell carcinoma [Part V]
   Herpes simplex [Part VI]
   Herpes zoster [Part VI]
   Impetigo [Part VI]
   Malignant melanoma (very late) [Part V]
   Molluscum (on involuting lesions) [Part II]
   Scabies [Part II]
   Toxicodendron dermatitis [Part IV]
Cutaneous horn
   Actinic keratosis [Part V]
   Squamous cell carcinoma [Part V]
Erosions
   Actinic keratosis [Part V]
   Atypical nevi (malignant change) [Part V]
   Basal cell carcinoma [Part V]
   Congenital melanocytic nevi [Part V]
   Erysipelas [Part III]
   Erythema multiforme [Part III]
   Fixed drug eruption [Part III]
   Herpes simplex [Part VI]
   Herpes zoster [Part VI]
   Lichen planus [Part II]
   Malignant melanoma (very late) [Part V]
   Squamous cell carcinoma [Part V]
Eschar
   Acne [Part VI]
   Basal cell carcinoma (late) [Part V]

Excoriations
    Atopic dermatitis [Part IV]
    Congenital melanocytic nevi [Part V]
    Molluscum [Part II]
    Scabies [Part II]
    Toxicodendron dermatitis [Part IV]
Fissures
    Asteatosis [Part IV]
    Atopic dermatitis [Part IV]
    Psoriasis (intertriginous areas) [Part II]
    Seborrheic dermatitis (intertriginous areas) [Part II]
    Squamous cell carcinoma [Part V]
    Tinea (intertriginous areas) [Part III]
Gangrene
    Erysipelas [Part III]
    Herpes zoster [Part VI]
    SLE [Part IV]
Hyperpigmentation
    Acne [Part VI]
    DLE [Part IV]
    Erythrasma [Part III]
    Fixed drug eruption [Part III]
    Herpes zoster [Part VI]
    Impetigo [Part VI]
    Lichen planus [Part II]
    Psoriasis [Part II]
    Senile purpura [Part IV]
    SLE [Part IV]
    Tinea [Part III]
Hypopigmentation
    DLE [Part IV]
    Halo nevi (macular) [Part V]
    Impetigo [Part VI]
    Malignant melanoma [Part V]
    Pityriasis rosea (transient) [Part II]
    Psoriasis [Part II]
    SCLE [Part IV]
    SLE [Part IV]
    Tinea [Part III]
Hypertrichosis
    Common benign nevi [Part V]
    Congenital melanocytic nevi [Part V]
Impetiginization
    Asteatosis [Part IV]
    Erythema multiforme [Part III]

Miliaria [Part II]
Scabies [Part II]
Tinea [Part III]
Toxicodendron dermatitis [Part IV]
Lichenification
Scabies [Part II]
Erythrasma [Part III]
Atopic dermatitis [Part IV]
Necrosis
Erythema multiforme [Part III]
Herpes zoster [Part VI]
SLE [Part IV]
Papillomatosis
Compound nevi [Part V]
Squamous cell carcinoma [Part V]
Purpura
Erysipelas [Part III]
Erythema multiforme [Part III]
Urticaria [Part III]
Scale
Actinic keratosis (adherent scale) [Part V]
Asteatosis (white scale) [Part IV]
Atopic dermatitis (loose, white scale) [Part IV]
Atypical nevi (malignant change) [Part V]
Compound nevi (hyperkeratotic) [Part V]
DLE (white adherent scale) [Part IV]
Erythrasma (dry, velvety) [Part III]
Impetigo (loose, white scale) [Part VI]
Lichen planus [Part II]
Malignant melanoma [Part V]
Pityriasis rosea [Part II]
Psoriasis (loose and silvery) [Part II]
SCLE [Part IV]
Seborrheic dermatitis (loose scale) [Part II]
SLE (white adherent scale) [Part IV]
Squamous cell carcinoma (adherent scale) [Part V]
Tinea [Part III]
Toxicodendron dermatitis [Part IV]
Scarring
Acne [Part VI]
Atypical nevi (malignant change) [Part V]
Basal cell carcinoma [Part V]
DLE [Part IV]
Herpes zoster [Part VI]
Keratoacanthoma [Part V]

    Lichen planus [Part II]
    Molluscum (mild scarring) [Part II]
    Senile purpura (stellate) [Part IV]
    SLE [Part IV]
    Tinea [Part III]
Sclerosis
    Basal cell carcinoma [Part V]
    SLE [Part IV]
Telangectasia
    DLE [Part IV]
    Rosacea [Part VI]
    SCLE [Part IV]
    SLE [Part IV]
Ulceration
    Actinic keratosis [Part V]
    Atypical nevi (malignant change) [Part V]
    Basal cell carcinoma (central) [Part V]
    Congenital melanocytic nevi (benign or malignant change) [Part V]
    Erysipelas [Part III]
    Malignant melanoma (very late) [Part V]
    Squamous cell carcinoma [Part V]
Vegetation
    Keratoacanthoma [Part V]

Part I: Color Photographs

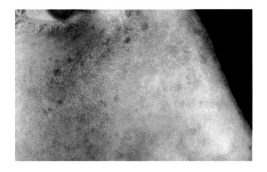

PHOTO 1

Ephelides (freckles), macules of melanin with pigment in the lower epidermis and basal cell layer. Note the lack of distortion of the skin lines.

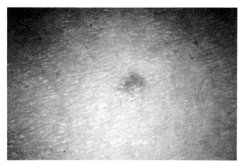

PHOTO 2

A blue 3 mm macule caused by a deposit of graphite in the dermis following a pencil jab. Note the lack of distortion of the skin lines.

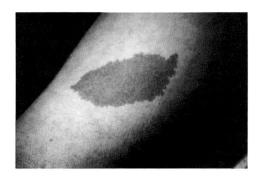

PHOTO 3

A "coast of Maine" spot, a patch of melanin pigment in the lower epidermis and basal cell layer. Note the lack of distortion of the skin lines.

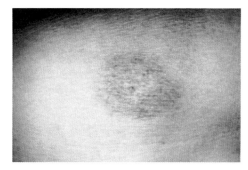

PHOTO 4

A patch of increased melanin in the upper dermis, the end result of a fixed drug reaction. Note the lack of distortion of the skin lines.

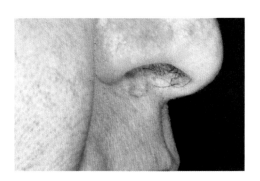

PHOTO 5

A papular wart of the upper lip. The elevation consists of proliferating epidermis. Note the normal skin lines are missing.

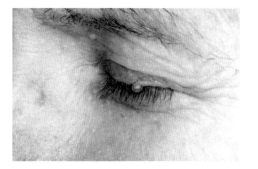

PHOTO 6

A papule of the upper lid margin that is caused by a benign cyst in the dermis. Note the shiny surface and effacement of the epidermis.

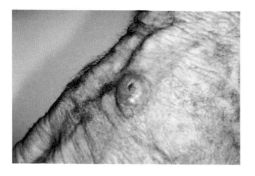

PHOTO 7

A nodular keratoacanthoma. The nodule consists of proliferating epidermal cells and the surface lines are effaced by the keratin debris in the central pit.

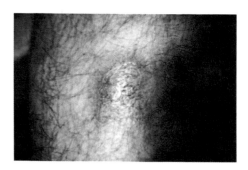

PHOTO 8

A nodule of erythema induratum on the shin. This lesion is caused by inflammation in the dermis and subcutis. Note although it is easily palpated, there is minimal visible elevation.

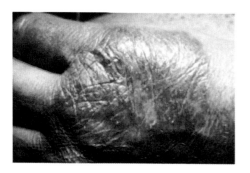

PHOTO 9

A plaque of mycosis fungoides caused by a malignant T-cell infiltrate in the dermis.

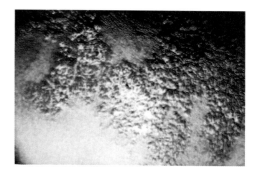

PHOTO 10

Scaling pebbly plaques of metastatic breast carcinoma formed by a confluence of papules.

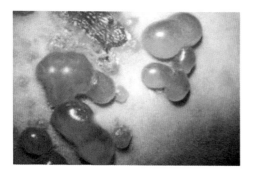

PHOTO 11

Pinpoint vesicles on the left evolving to tense bullae several centimeters in size in the center.

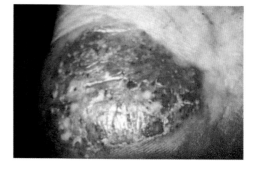

PHOTO 12

Flat intra-epidermal pustules on the heel in a case of pustular psoriasis.

380

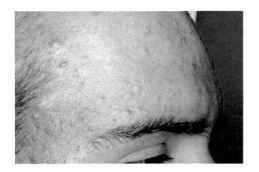

PHOTO 13

Adnexal pustules occur within adnexal skin structures. In acne the terminal hair follicle is affected.

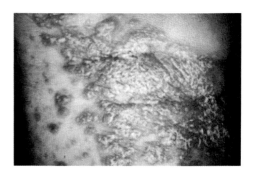

PHOTO 14

Adherent white scale in lichen planus.

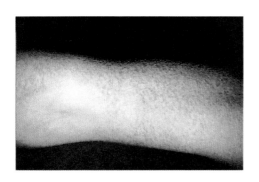

PHOTO 15

Adherent brown scale in ichthyosis vulgaris.

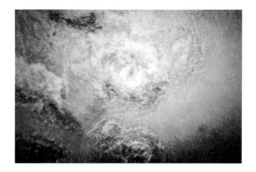

PHOTO 16

Silvery white, loosely adherent scale of psoriasis.

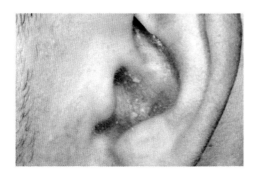

PHOTO 17

Greasy, yellow, loosely adherent scale of seborrheic dermatitis.

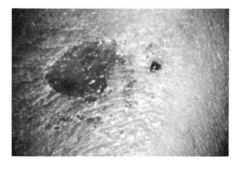

PHOTO 18

Moist eroded lesion of erythema multiforme.

381

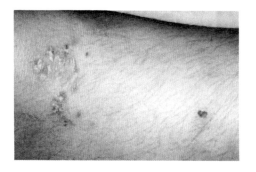

PHOTO 19

Crusted lesions of nonbullous impetigo.

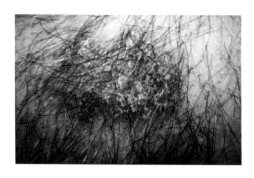

PHOTO 20

A moist impetiginized lesion of nummular eczema.

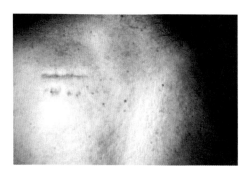

PHOTO 21

Sclerosis of the upper back in a case of scleredema. The sclerosis is due to an accumulation of mucopolysaccharide and edema fluid. Note the "orange-peel" surface and the accentuation of the old scar. The skin cannot be pinched.

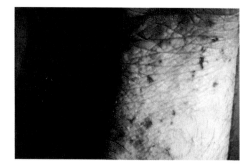

PHOTO 22

Excoriations on the wrist in atopic dermatitis. Note the accentuated skin markings: a change referred to as lichenification.

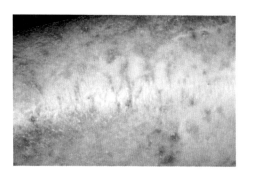

PHOTO 23

Linear canal-like fissures on the extremely dry skin of an elderly patient.

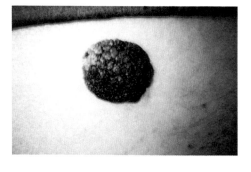

PHOTO 24

A large seborrheic keratosis with a papillomatous surface of epidermal origin.

382

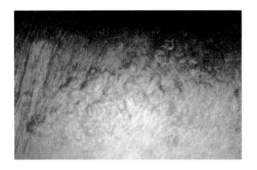

PHOTO 25

Lichen amyloidosis. Infiltrates of amyloid substance in the dermis push up and produce papillomatosis.

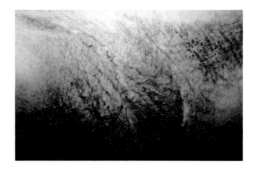

PHOTO 26

Acanthosis nigricans in the axilla. The surface projections of epidermis and dermis produce soft smooth vegetations in this condition.

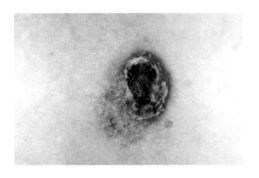

PHOTO 27

An eschar composed of scale, secretion and necrotic tissue on the central surface of a basal cell carcinoma.

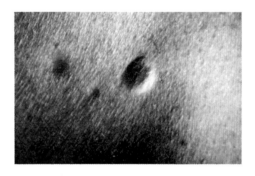

PHOTO 28

Dermal atrophy in malignant atrophic papulosis. The early papular lesions (left) evolve leaving dermal atrophy. At edge is a rim of normal dermis.

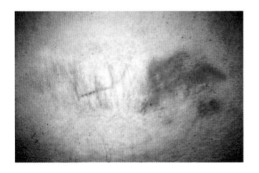

PHOTO 29

Atrophy of the subcutaneous fat allows visualization of a sizable vein at the base of this depressed lesion of panatrophy. Epidermal and dermal atrophy are also present.

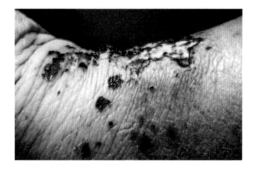

PHOTO 30

Ulcerations of the epidermis and upper dermis in a patient with a necrotizing vasculitis.

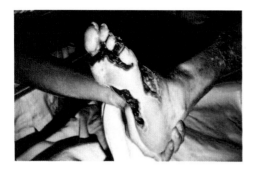

PHOTO 31

An elderly diabetic with wet streptococcal gangrene.

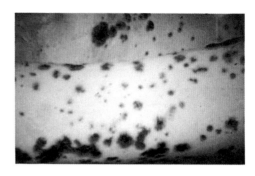

PHOTO 32

Dry gangrenous infarcts in a case of severe necrotizing vasculitis.

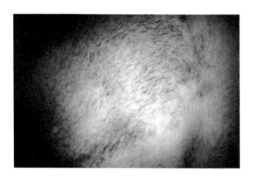

PHOTO 33

Hyperpigmentation from increased basal cell melanin in a lesion known as a Becker's nevus. The focal change in hair growth is called hypertrichosis.

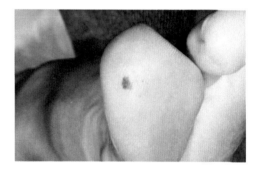

PHOTO 34

Hyperpigmentation, in this instance hemosiderin pigment free in the upper dermis from trauma on the toe of a jogger.

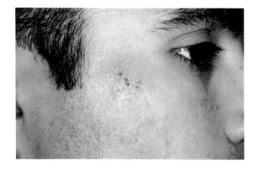

PHOTO 35

A patch of pityriasis alba. Surrounding the inflammatory center is a circular zone of partial pigment loss.

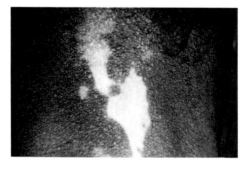

PHOTO 36

Segmental vitiligo on the posterior neck would show absent melanin with special stains.

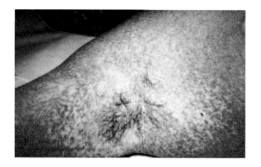

PHOTO 37

Poikiloderma atrophicans vasculare associated with an underlying lymphoma.

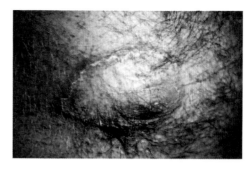

PHOTO 38

Annular tinea corporis, note the similarity to a solitary herald patch of pityriasis rosea.

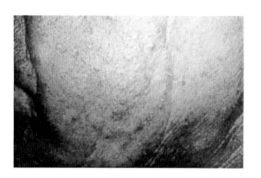

PHOTO 39

Arciform lesions of tinea faciale.

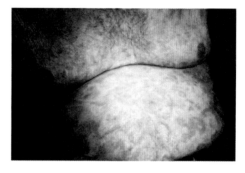

PHOTO 40

Polycyclic lesions in a patient with erythema gyratum repens.

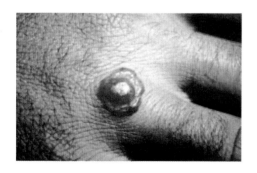

PHOTO 41

An iris lesion in a case of milker's nodules (paravaccinia virus infection).

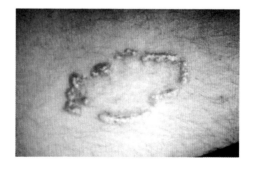

PHOTO 42

Serpiginous-shaped lesion of elastosis perforans serpiginosum.

385

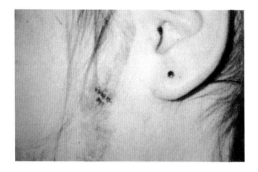

PHOTO 43

A linear birthmark on the preauricular skin.

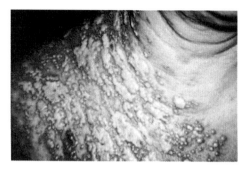

PHOTO 44

Herpes zoster of the right mid cervical and upper thoracic dermatome segments. Note the midline cutoff.

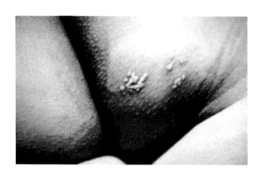

PHOTO 45

Two groupings of herpetic vesicles on the buttock skin.

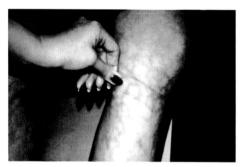

PHOTO 46

Netlike pigment deposition in erythema ab igne. Color fails to blanch with diascopy indicating pigment within tissue as opposed to blood in a vessel.

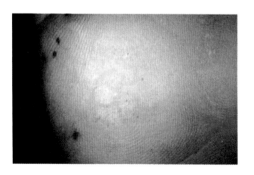

PHOTO 47

A corymbiform plantar wart.

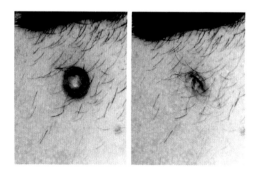

PHOTO 48

Pyogenic granuloma on the neck simulating a melanoma. Note the difference on the right after application of gentle pressure.

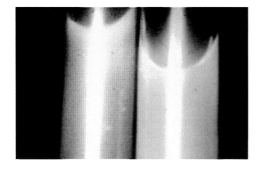

PHOTO 49

Wood's lamp exam: Pink urine of porphyria cutanea tarda, left; normal urine right.

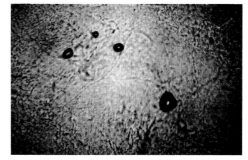

PHOTO 50

KOH slide showing the long branching hyphae of a dermatophyte fungal infection.

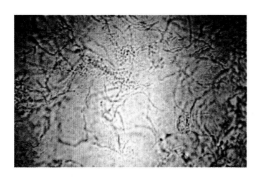

PHOTO 51

KOH slide showing the short club-shaped hyphae and clusters of spores in tinea versicolor.

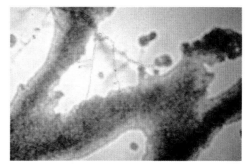

PHOTO 52

Segmented pseudohyphae and round chlamydospores of Candida albicans are occasionally seen in KOH preparations.

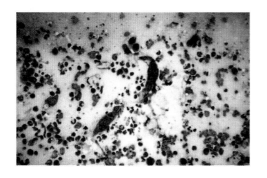

PHOTO 53

Tzanck smear from the base of a herpetic vesicle. Note the large multinucleated giant cells and epidermal cells with enlarged (ballooned) nuclei.

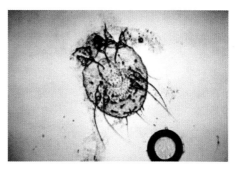

PHOTO 54

Scabies prep. shows a mature itch mite with a maturing ovum. These are easily identified under low power.

387

Part II: Color Photographs

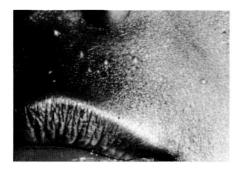

PHOTO 1

Grouped dome-shaped lesions of molluscum. Note the white central core.

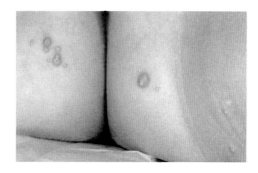

PHOTO 2

Grouped molluscum lesions on the buttocks of a child. Several lesions show a dimple and peripheral ridge. Mature lesion on the right shows distinct scale.

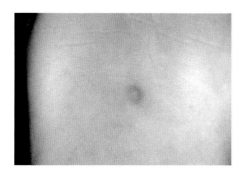

PHOTO 3

Dusky molluscum lesion which is starting to involute. Note the halo of inflammation at its base.

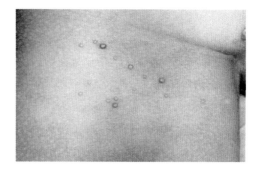

PHOTO 4

Typical grouping of molluscum lesions on an inner thigh.

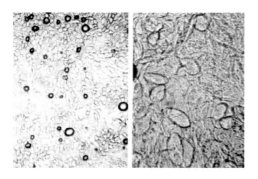

PHOTO 5

Molluscum smear, expressed contents of lesion floating in physiologic saline. Low and high power.

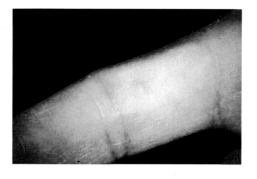

PHOTO 6

Early wart on the palmar surface of the finger interrupts skin lines.

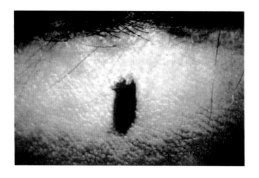

PHOTO 7

Pedunculated wart on forehead composed of filiform papules.

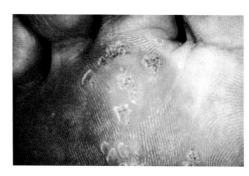

PHOTO 8

Plantar wart shows dome-shaped papules which interrupt skin lines. Note the fine scale and black ends of the thrombosed vessels.

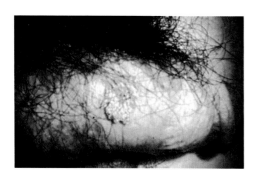

PHOTO 9

Large filiform wart on the penile shaft.

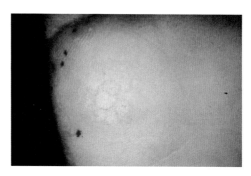

PHOTO 10

Corymbiform plantar wart.

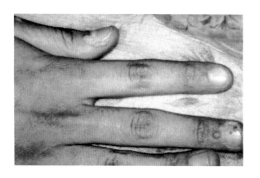

PHOTO 11

Warts on the hand and periungual tissue.

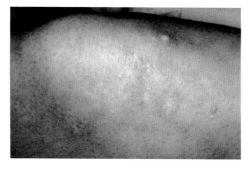

PHOTO 12

Clustered partially treated warts on the knee.

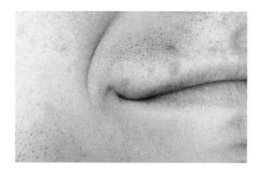

PHOTO 13

Verrucae of the beard area in a young adult man.

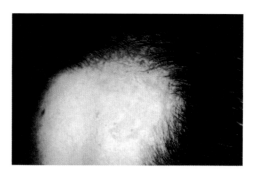

PHOTO 14

Dull red patches of seborrheic dermatitis along the scalp margin.

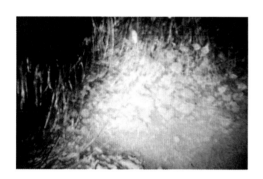

PHOTO 15

Yellow greasy scale at the scalp edge.

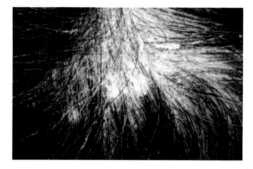

PHOTO 16

White loose scale in the scalp.

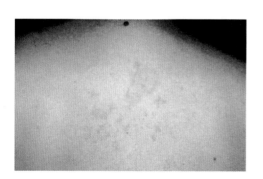

PHOTO 17

Petaloid patches of seborrhea on the mid back.

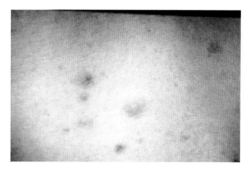

PHOTO 18

Early rosy-red papules of pityriasis rosea.

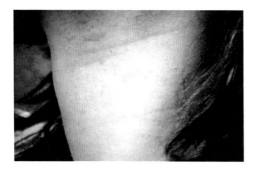

PHOTO 19

Rosy-red plaques of pityriasis rosea.

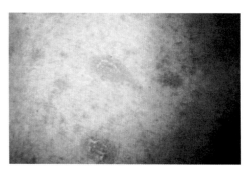

PHOTO 20

Scale with free edge turned toward the center of the lesion.

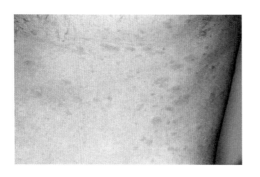

PHOTO 21

Oval lesions in linear configuration, long axes follow skin tension lines.

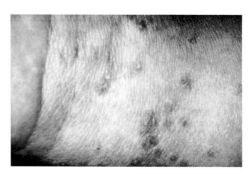

PHOTO 22

Early papules of psoriasis with loose silvery scale.

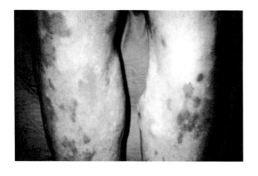

PHOTO 23

Plaques formed by centrifugal extension and confluence.

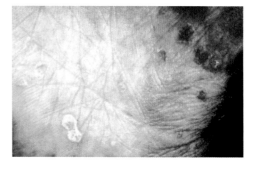

PHOTO 24

Plaques. Some show white mica-like scale.

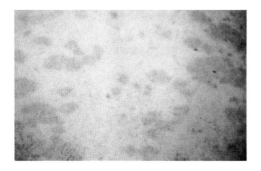

PHOTO 25

Macular hyperpigmentation at the sites of resolved plaques.

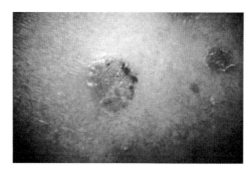

PHOTO 26

Positive Auspitz's sign. Bleeding points where scale has been removed.

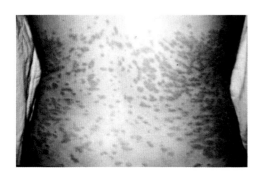

PHOTO 27

Guttate (small drop-like) lesions of psoriasis. Some have merged into plaques and others are becoming confluent.

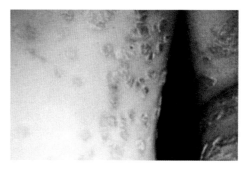

PHOTO 28

Nummular or coin-sized psoriasis lesions in a child.

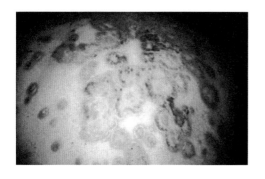

PHOTO 29

Annular, polycyclic psoriasis lesions.

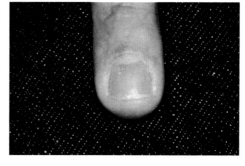

PHOTO 30

Linear nail pits strongly support a diagnosis of psoriasis.

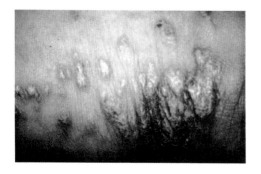

PHOTO 31

Violaceous, angular, flat-topped primary papules of lichen planus.

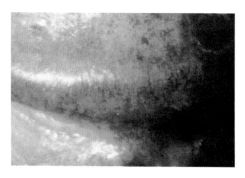

PHOTO 32

Wickham's stria in a mucosal lesion of lichen planus. Note the erosion on the right.

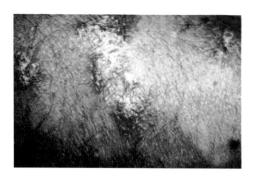

PHOTO 33

Hypertrophic lichen planus shows plaques with thick adherent white scale.

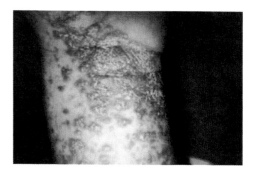

PHOTO 34

Plaques of lichen planus formed by coalescence of papules. Note the satellite papules at the periphery.

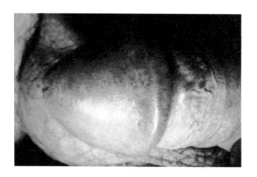

PHOTO 35

Mucosal lichen planus. Note the deep violaceous color, Wickham's stria, and the erosion on the top.

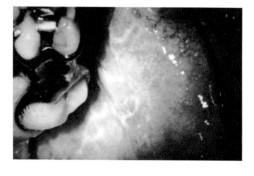

PHOTO 36

Lacy pattern of oral lichen planus. Note the erosions at the extreme upper and lower edges of the photo.

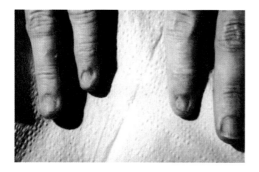

PHOTO 37

Permanent scarring due to lichen planus of the nail matrix.

PHOTO 38

Tiny crystalline vesicles of early miliaria.

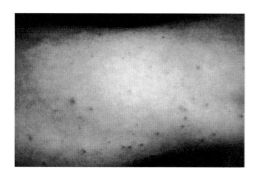

PHOTO 39

Red papules of miliaria rubra.

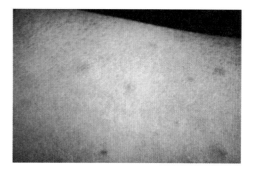

PHOTO 40

Early pustular lesions of miliaria rubra profunda.

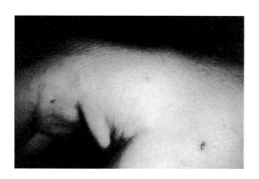

PHOTO 41

Track of scabies at the base of the forefinger. Note the vesicle.

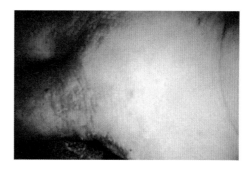

PHOTO 42

Linear scabies track at the base of the digit.

397

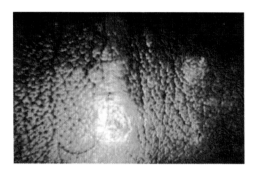

PHOTO 43

Linear scabies track. Note the point of entry at the bottom of the photo.

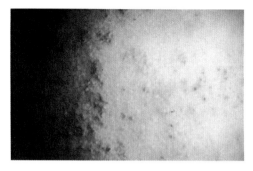

PHOTO 44

Secondary papular scabies lesions with excoriations, eczematization, and secondary infection.

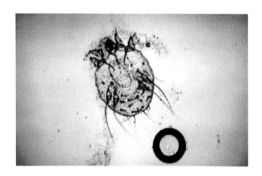

PHOTO 45

Ectoparasite prep., shows mature eight-legged itch mite with ova. Ova alone may also be seen.

Part III: Color Photographs

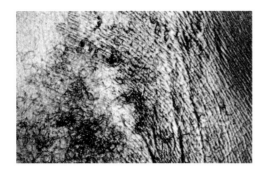

PHOTO 1

Erythrasma showing brown macules and patches in the inguinal crease area. Scale and early lichenification present.

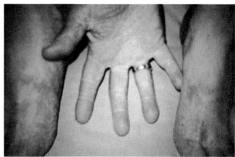

PHOTO 2

Tinea pedis and tinea manuum, so-called "two foot–one hand disease." Note the erythema and diffuse scale which is accentuated in the palmar creases. Also typical is the "moccasin" distribution on the lateral margins of the feet.

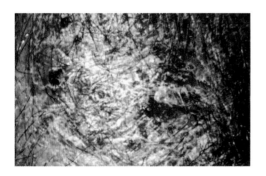

PHOTO 3

Inflammatory tinea of hair-bearing area. Note the partial alopecia, scale, broken hairs and follicular pustules.

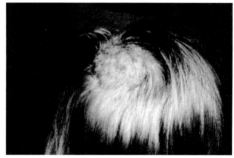

PHOTO 4

Thick, secondarily infected kerion. Cervical nodes were enlarged. Culture grew Microsporum canis.

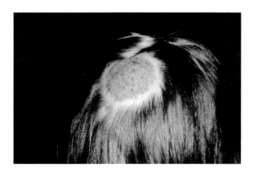

PHOTO 5

Kerion site after 10 days of combined broad spectrum antibiotics, prednisone and systemic antifungal therapy. Some scarring and permanent hair loss is expected.

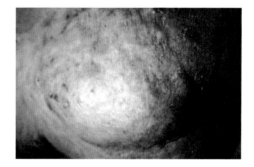

PHOTO 6

Chronic tinea barbae of the chin. Note the deep inflammatory character of the nodules and the scarring.

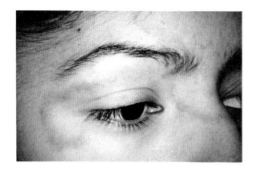

PHOTO 7

Tinea faciale with advancing scaling margin.

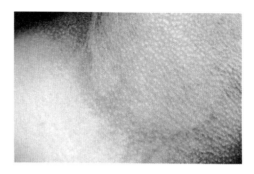

PHOTO 8

Tinea of the neck with a very subtle advancing margin. Color change is partially due to inappropriate use of a topical corticoid.

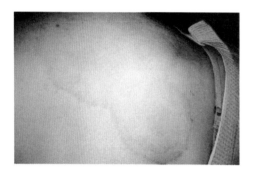

PHOTO 9

Extensive tinea corporis. Note the advancing margin and concentric margins at the lower edge.

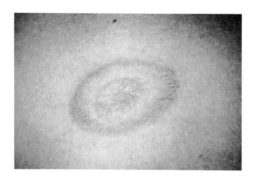

PHOTO 10

Tinea corporis showing the classic concentric lesions of ringworm.

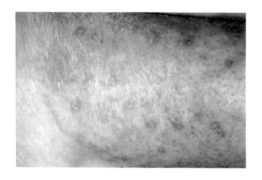

PHOTO 11

Tinea near the ankle. Note the subtle advancing margin, inflammatory pustules, papules and nodules.

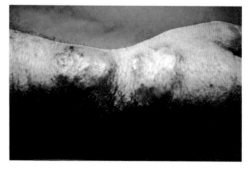

PHOTO 12

Boggy nodular tinea on the dorsum of the hand and wrist.

402

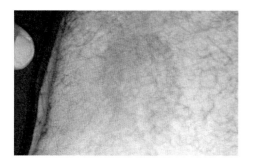

PHOTO 13

Tinea cruris with advancing margin extending from the inguinal crease onto the inner thigh.

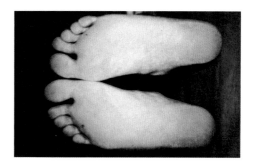

PHOTO 14

Diffuse tinea of the sole. Note the margin that extends in a moccasin-like fashion across the instep. Also note the scale and fissures at the base of the toes.

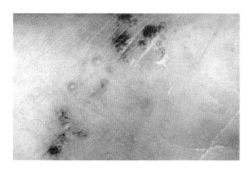

PHOTO 15

Deep-seated vesicles on the instep in a case of tinea pedis. KOH prep. was positive. Contact dermatitis can cause identical lesions which are KOH negative.

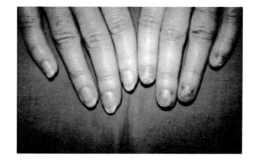

PHOTO 16

Tinea unguium causing distal separation, dystrophy and discoloration of the nail plate.

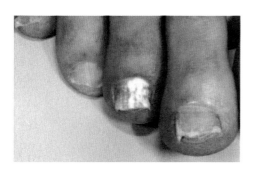

PHOTO 17

Tinea unguium showing white superficial onycho-mycosis of nail 3 and distal subungual involvement of nail 2.

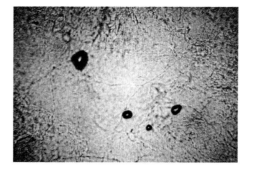

PHOTO 18

Positive KOH preparation. Long, refractile, branching hyphae.

403

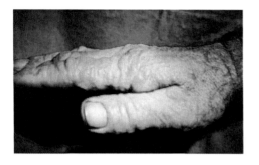

PHOTO 19

Vesicular id reaction on the hand caused by an inflammatory tinea pedis. These vesicles are KOH negative.

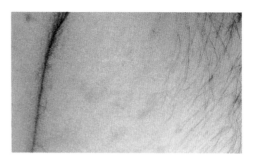

PHOTO 20

Wheals of common urticaria. The lesions vary in size, are palpably raised and the centers show a pink or white color depending on the degree of edema.

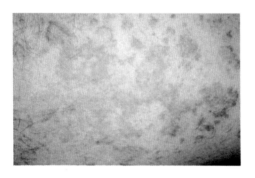

PHOTO 21

Common hives showing papules and confluent plaques. Some of the more edematous lesions have white centers.

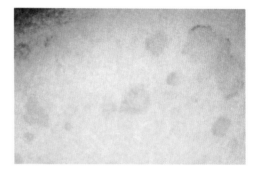

PHOTO 22

Hives with polycyclic borders.

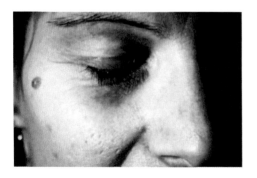

PHOTO 23

Early fixed drug eruption in the form of an indurated plaque of the eyelid and upper cheek.

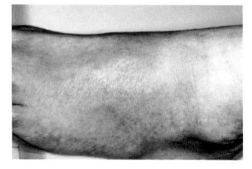

PHOTO 24

Fixed drug eruption in the form of a dusky, violet-brown plaque on the dorsum of the foot. Underlying tendons are not visible.

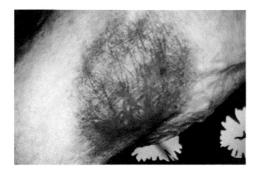

PHOTO 25

Acute bullous fixed drug reaction to sulfa.

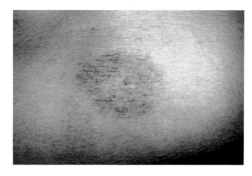

PHOTO 26

Persisting hyperpigmentation after resolution of the fixed acute drug reaction in photo 25.

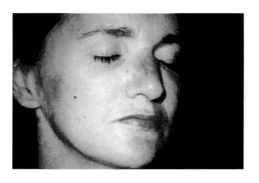

PHOTO 27

Plaque of sharply marginated, tender erysipelas in a classic location.

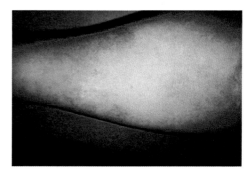

PHOTO 28

Cellulitis of the shin. Ill-defined patches of tender warm erythema.

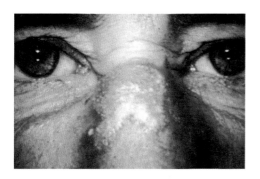

PHOTO 29

Erysipelas which has become vesicular.

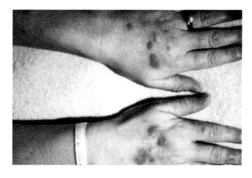

PHOTO 30

Erythema multiforme showing early papular and developing plaque lesions with dusky centers.

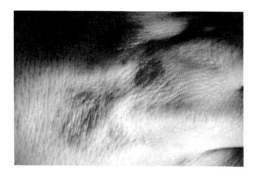

PHOTO 31

Enlarged view of erythematous plaque lesions showing early hemorrhage in the center.

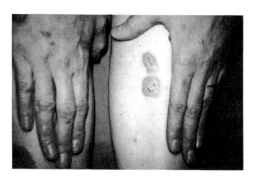

PHOTO 32

Vesiculobullous erythema multiforme.

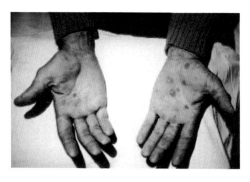

PHOTO 33

Target or iris lesions of erythema multiforme on the palmar skin.

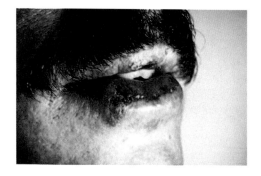

PHOTO 34

Hemorrhagic crusted lesions of the vermilion margin of the lips.

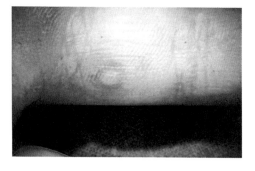

PHOTO 35

Close-up of a target lesion on the palmar surface of the digit.

Part IV: Color Photographs

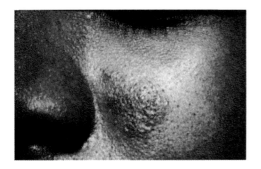

PHOTO 1

Early DLE. Photo shows a plaque with a papule above. The lesions are becoming confluent. Note the accentuation of the hair follicle openings, the loss of normal skin surface pattern and shiny surface.

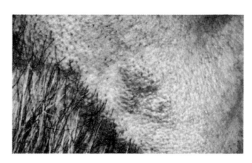

PHOTO 2

A discrete plaque of DLE near the sideburn. Early white scale is evident and in the center it shows a distinct follicular pattern.

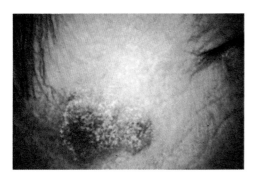

PHOTO 3

Developed plaque of DLE with thick adherent white scale. Central scale has become mounded and brownish-yellow.

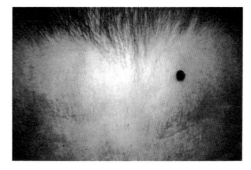

PHOTO 4

DLE of forehead at hairline shows an advancing indurated margin with telangiectatic vessels. Central area shows hypopigmentation where activity of disease has burned out.

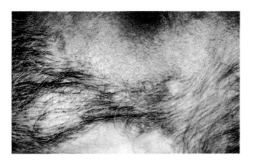

PHOTO 5

Pigmentary changes in chronic scarring DLE.

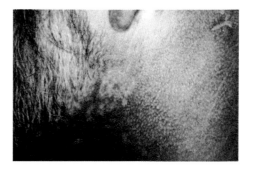

PHOTO 6

Hypopigmented scar at the hairline in chronic DLE.

409

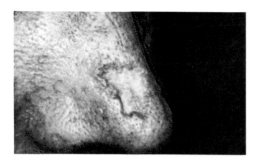

PHOTO 7

Punched out DLE scar. Note the typical white base with telangiectatic blood vessels.

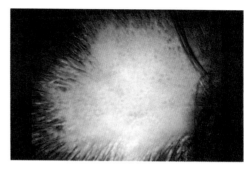

PHOTO 8

Scarring DLE of the scalp often results in permanent alopecia.

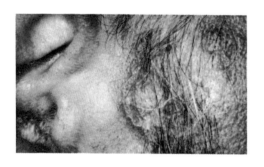

PHOTO 9

Discoid lesion in sideburn shows a margin with erythema and telangectasia, a white depressed center and peripheral scale.

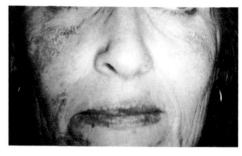

PHOTO 10

DLE lesions suggest a butterfly pattern, but are absent over the upper central face and show asymmetry on the upper lip.

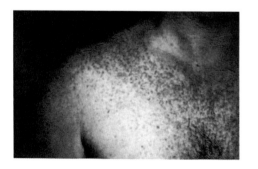

PHOTO 11

DLE flare following an acute sunburn.

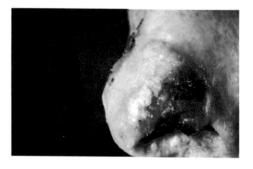

PHOTO 12

Squamous cell carcinoma of the nasal ala arising in a burned out DLE lesion.

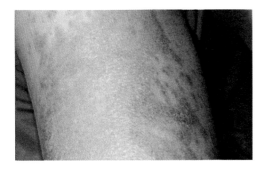

PHOTO 13

SCLE, extensive lesions were present on other light-exposed sites (*see* photo 17). Note the papulosquamous character and the mixture of sharply demarcated papules and plaques.

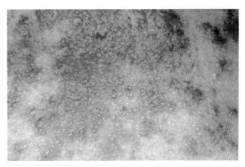

PHOTO 14

Close-up of lesions in photo 13. Note the sharp margins, mixture of papules and plaques, telangiectatic vessels and the loose central white scale.

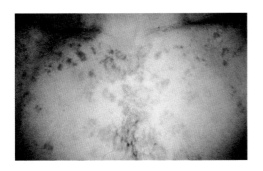

PHOTO 15

SCLE: Extensive chest lesions. Many are developing an annular configuration.

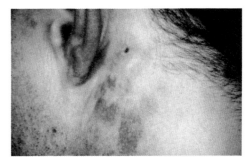

PHOTO 16

Sharply demarcated papules and plaques. Lesion with biopsy site exhibits areas of central gray-white hypopigmentation and atrophy.

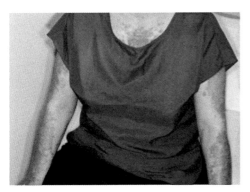

PHOTO 17

SCLE onset with skin lesions showing distinct photo-accentuation. Covered skin areas were clear.

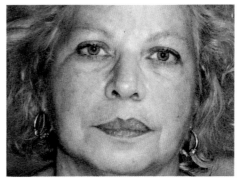

PHOTO 18

Butterfly rash of lupus. In this instance the patient has SCLE without evidence of systemic disease.

411

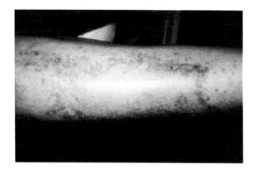

PHOTO 19

Pruritic papular eruption extensor surface of limb in a patient with SLE.

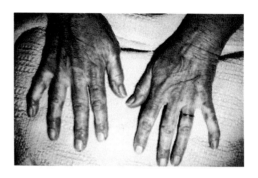

PHOTO 20

Papular erythema on the dorsum of the hands. Similar changes are seen in cases of dermatomyositis.

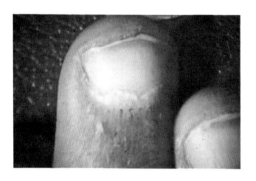

PHOTO 21

Ragged cuticle, opaque nailbed with absence of the lunula and prominent tortuous capillaries in the proximal nail fold. These changes are seen in SLE and other major connective tissue diseases.

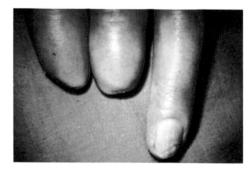

PHOTO 22

The results of severe peripheral vascular involvement in a case of SLE.

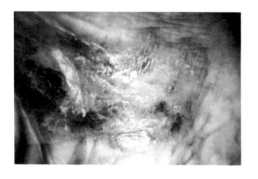

PHOTO 23

DLE-like lesion on the foot in a patient with SLE.

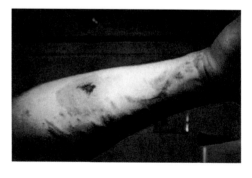

PHOTO 24

Linear plaques and patches of erythema typical of toxicodendron dermatitis.

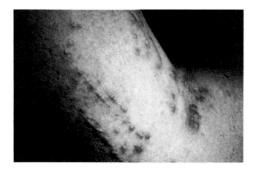

PHOTO 25

Linear streaks and patches of vesicles also typical of a plant-acquired allergic contact dermatitis.

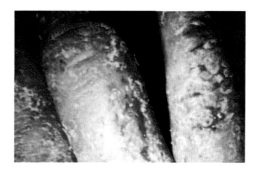

PHOTO 26

Secondary infection with honey-colored exudate, fissuring, scale and crusting. This can occur with any acute eczematous process.

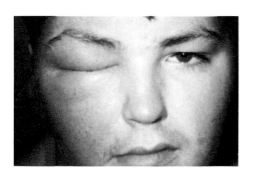

PHOTO 27

Confluent dermal edema common with secondary transfer or airborne exposure to the antigen.

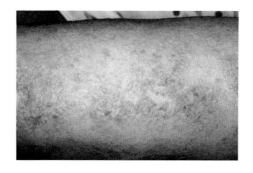

PHOTO 28

Early patchy linear toxicodendron dermatitis with vesicles can simulate early Herpes zoster with minimal neuritis.

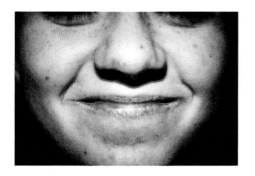

PHOTO 29

Perioral eczema in a young woman with atopic dermatitis. Note the mild wrinkling and lichenification laterally; also note the reaction is limited to an area reached by the tongue.

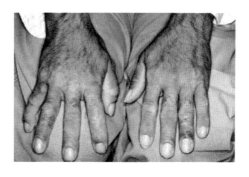

PHOTO 30

Eczema of the hands in a man with classic flexural atopic dermatitis. Note the focal lesions which began as rings of pruritic vesicles. Also note the lichenification, excoriations, painful fissures, crusting and paronychial involvement.

413

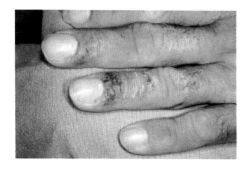

PHOTO 31

Eczema of the proximal nail fold. Note the edema, loss of the cuticle and the early rippling of the nailplates on digits 3 and 4.

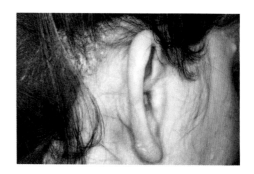

PHOTO 32

Scalp eczema shows erythema, white scale, excoriations and secondary impetiginization.

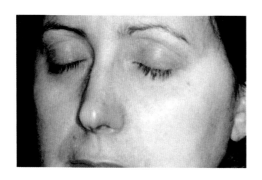

PHOTO 33

Allergic shiners.

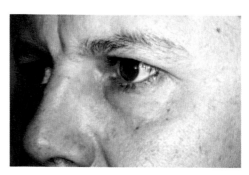

PHOTO 34

Morgan-Dennie's line of the lower eyelid.

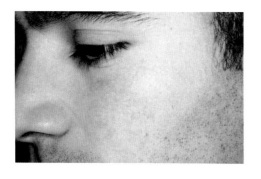

PHOTO 35

Pityriasis alba in the active phase as a scaling pink patch.

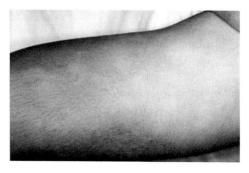

PHOTO 36

Pityriasis alba, the erythema has resolved leaving subtle pigment loss.

414

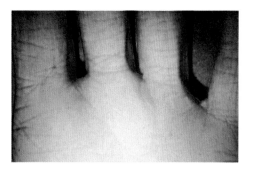

PHOTO 37

Atopic palmar markings.

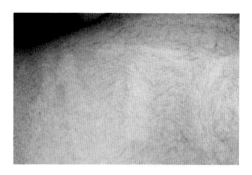

PHOTO 38

Delayed white dermographism in an area of active atopic dermatitis. Note the "A," "T," and partial "O."

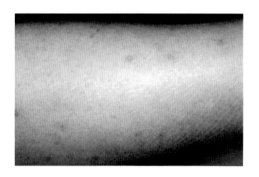

PHOTO 39

Ichthyosis, "like fish scale" on the shin of a patient with atopic dermatitis.

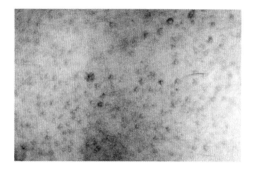

PHOTO 40

Keratosis pilaris on the arm of an atopic person.

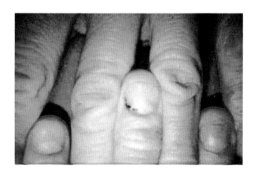

PHOTO 41

Buffed nails from scratching.

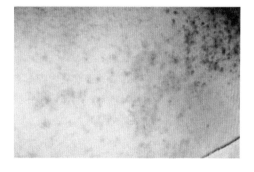

PHOTO 42

Early atopic dermatitis shows patches of erythema, papules and papulovesicles.

415

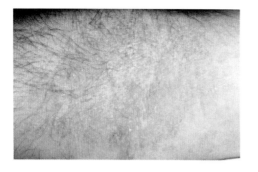

PHOTO 43

Lichenified eczema of the antecubital fossa. Note the indistinct margins and excoriations.

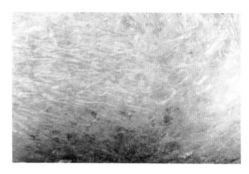

PHOTO 44

Xerotic skin is dull, scaly and shows fine wrinkling with focal areas of erythema.

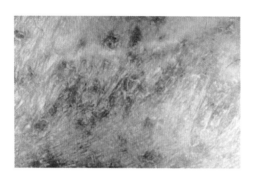

PHOTO 45

More severe xerosis with fissuring erythema and early impetiginization.

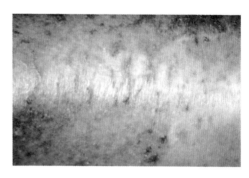

PHOTO 46

Long canal-like fissures with exudate in the base.

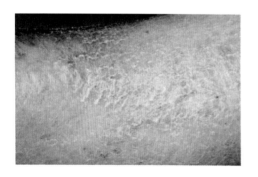

PHOTO 47

Craquelé or crazy-pavement pattern.

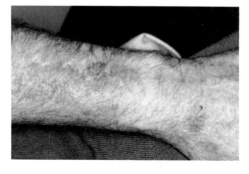

PHOTO 48

Irregular patches of purpura following minor trauma. Note also the epidermal atrophy from chronic solar damage. Patchy tan pigment is left from prior episodes.

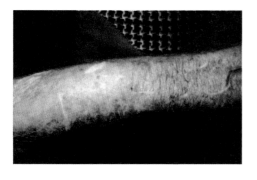

PHOTO 49

More advanced atrophy, small foci of purpura and white stellate scars from epidermal tears.

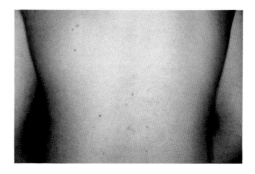

PHOTO 50

Light transverse stria in a teen-aged weightlifter.

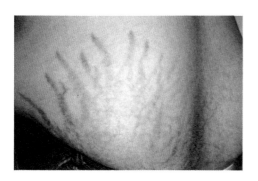

PHOTO 51

Extensive fan-shaped stria on the lower back in a patient on long-term, high-dose systemic steroids.

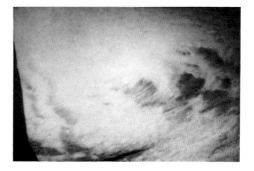

PHOTO 52

Dark wide stria from abuse of potent topical steroids.

Part V: Color Photographs

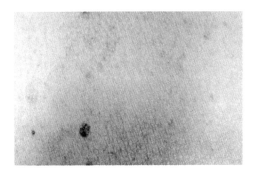

PHOTO 1

Field of early 1–4 mm seborrheic keratosis. Yellow-tan color, dull, stuck on, some show comedones on surface.

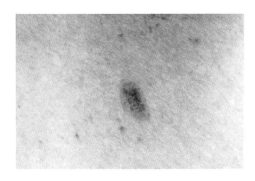

PHOTO 2

Seborrheic keratosis. Typical mature, "stuck on" yellow-tan lesion. Note multiple tiny early SKs in the field.

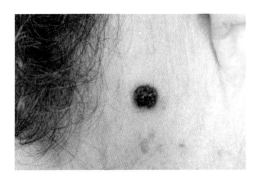

PHOTO 3

Developed brown-black seborrheic keratosis, stuck on with inflammation at the base. Contrast with smaller 1–3 mm yellow-tan SKs in field.

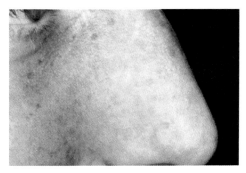

PHOTO 4

Typical ephelides in a teenager of Celtic heritage.

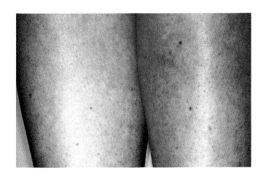

PHOTO 5

Non-solar lentigos. Individual lesions are clinically indistinguishable from junctional nevi.

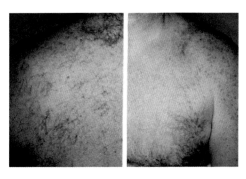

PHOTO 6

Front and back view of a man with extensive solar-induced lentigines. Note the scar on the left upper anterior shoulder where an *in situ* melanoma was discovered.

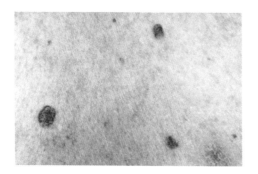

PHOTO 7

Junctional nevus, right lower corner, developed compound nevi right upper and left lower corners.

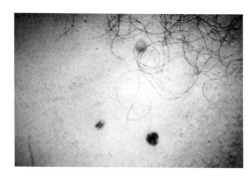

PHOTO 8

Early compound nevi lower center, mature compound or developed dermal nevus upper center.

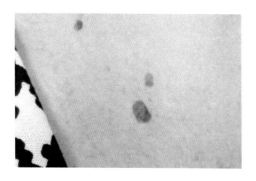

PHOTO 9

Mature pink-tan dermal nevi, center, contrast color and reflectance with several dull yellow and grey-tan SKs in the same field.

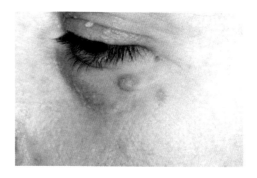

PHOTO 10

Mature soft dermal nevus lower eyelid. Compare with pedunculated SKs on the upper lid and outer canthus.

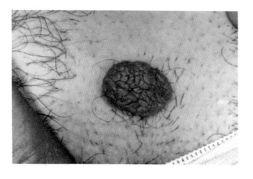

PHOTO 11

Large nevus with a mammillated cerebriform surface.

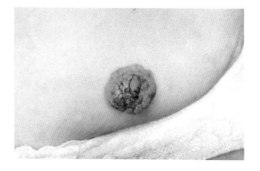

PHOTO 12

Mature benign compound or dermal nevus with scale.

422

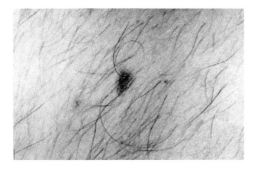

PHOTO 13

Mature compound nevus with long terminal hair growth.

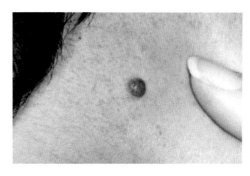

PHOTO 14

Mature compound nevus. The dark spots are keratotic plugs or comedones.

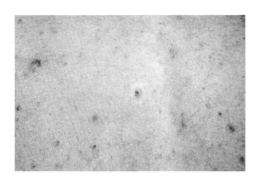

PHOTO 15

Halo nevus of Sutton. Note the central regressing pink-brown compound nevus with an achromic border.

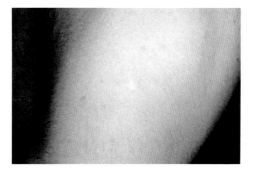

PHOTO 16

Depigmented macule at site of totally regressed nevus. Same patient as photo 15.

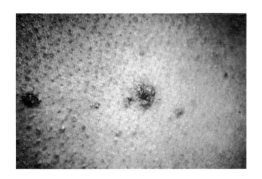

PHOTO 17

Primary lesion in patient with atypical mole syndrome. Irregular shape and color. Mammillated surface with an indistinct macular margin. Compare with other typical benign junctional moles in the same photo.

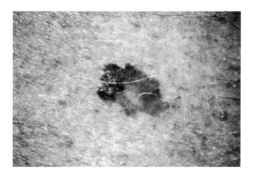

PHOTO 18

Atypical nevus close-up. Note the irregular shape, color and margins.

423

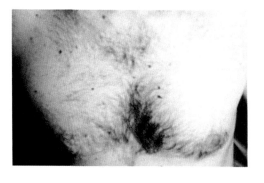

PHOTO 19

Atypical mole syndrome. Note the irregular and variable appearance of the nevi.

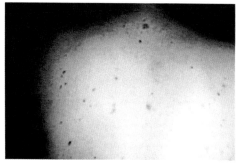

PHOTO 20

Atypical mole syndrome. Note the irregular and variable appearance of the nevi.

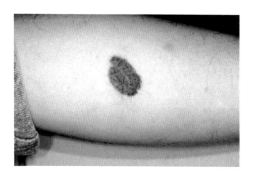

PHOTO 21

Medium-sized CMN. Note the mammillated surface, irregular but not truly notched border, dark terminal hair and speckling. Lesion is a uniform plaque.

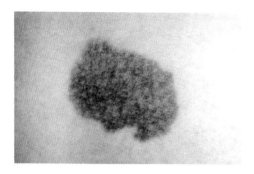

PHOTO 22

Medium-sized CMN. Note the speckled surface, distinct but irregular margins and the central pink-tan benign compound component.

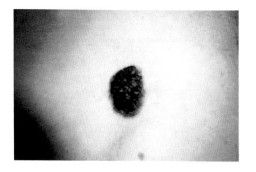

PHOTO 23

Congenital melanotic nevus, medium sized. Note the raised mammillated surface. Contrast with the 5 mm compound nevus at the bottom of the photo.

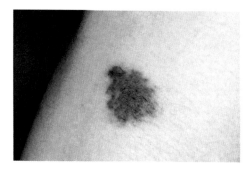

PHOTO 24

An acquired congenital pattern nevus.

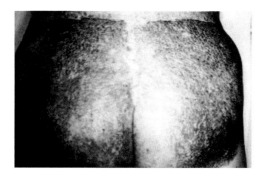

PHOTO 25

Giant congenital melanotic nevus (bathing trunk type). Note the speckled variable color and elevation.

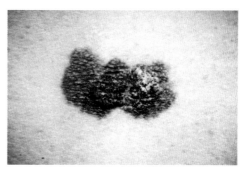

PHOTO 26

Superficial spreading malignant melanoma. Asymmetric, irregular border and color, size exceeds 6 mm. Note the central raised papule, a sign of invasion.

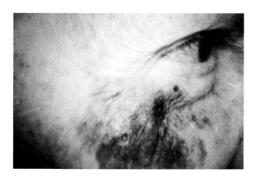

PHOTO 27

Lentigo maligna. Irregular pigmentation, irregular margins and the lesion is typically quite large. Entire surface is still macular and lesion is still *in situ*.

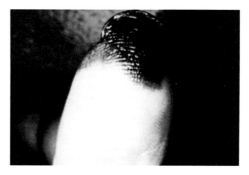

PHOTO 28

Acral lentiginous melanoma of the nail bed. Note the asymmetry and blush of lighter brown pigment at the periphery. Skin markings are still retained.

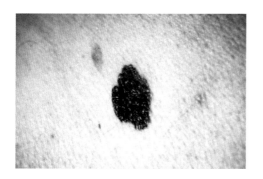

PHOTO 29

SSMM. Note the notched, pseudopod-like border. Lesion is asymmetric and size exceeds 6 mm. Contrast its highlighted surface with the dull yellow-tan SK immediately adjacent.

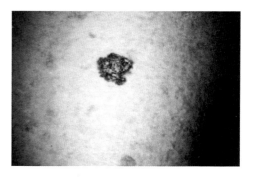

PHOTO 30

SSMM, shows loss of skin markings, irregular border, asymmetry and a developing central papular area. Compare with the mature dermal nevus at the bottom.

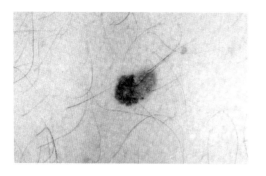

PHOTO 31

Early SSMM. Some asymmetry, speckling, dramatically contrasting color areas, early border notching. Size exceeds 6 mm.

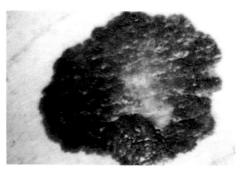

PHOTO 32

SSMM. Asymmetric, irregular notched border, color varies from white to pink to blue-grey to brown and brown-black. Nodule at lower edge indicates vertical growth.

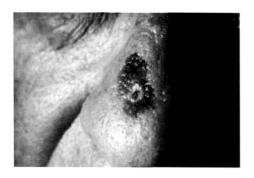

PHOTO 33

LMM of the nasal bridge. Note the asymmetry, size, irregular color and areas of speckling. Border is also notched.

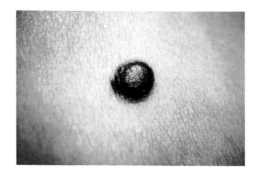

PHOTO 34

Nodular melanoma presenting as a deeply pigmented rapidly growing lesion with loss of skin lines. Deep color correlates with depth.

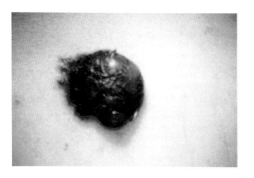

PHOTO 35

Nodular melanoma with irregular base.

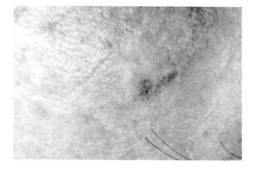

PHOTO 36

Erythematous actinic keratosis with a fine adherent yellow scale. Note the tiny bleeding point where scale has been removed. Lesion is easier to detect by palpation than by vision.

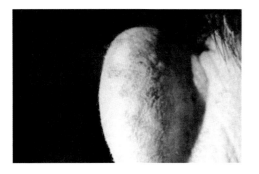

PHOTO 37

Actinic keratosis of helix shows focal erythema, adherent white and brown scale.

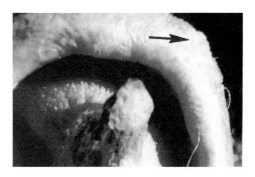

PHOTO 38

Cutaneous horn of antihelix. This one had a squamous cell carcinoma at the base. Note the thick white AK near the apex of the helix.

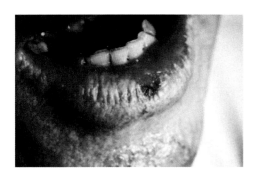

PHOTO 39

White actinic cheilitis of the lower lip with scale. Central area shows erosion and ulceration.

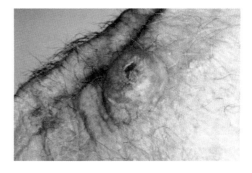

PHOTO 40

Keratoacanthoma on dorsum of hand. Note the dull central core and dilated surface vessels. Note also the adjacent AK with white scale and the chronic actinic damage.

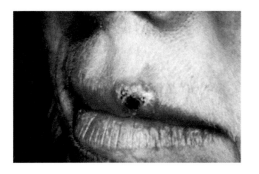

PHOTO 41

Keratoacanthoma of upper lip.

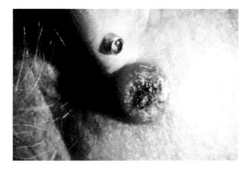

PHOTO 42

Nodular keratoacanthoma.

427

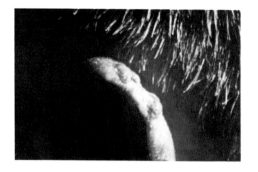

PHOTO 43

Depression and epithelial tags at the site of a regressing keratoacanthoma.

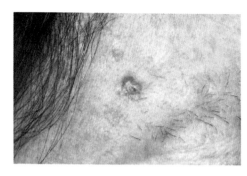

PHOTO 44

Translucent papular BCC of temple. Note the developing central dell and compare with the yellow-tan SK above.

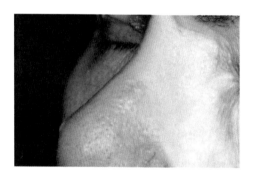

PHOTO 45

Translucent papular BCC of nasal bridge with dilated vessels.

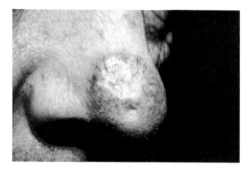

PHOTO 46

Nodular basal cell. Note the small erosions and depressed areas. Also note the translucent character and dilated surface vessels.

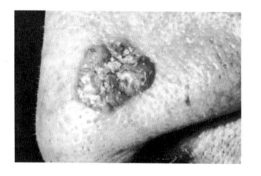

PHOTO 47

Nodular BCC with central erosion and prominent surface vessels.

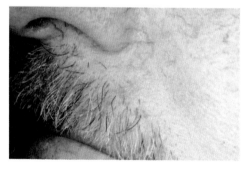

PHOTO 48

Yellow-pink scaling depression of upper lip is actually a sizable BCC.

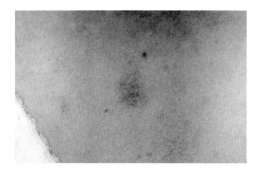

PHOTO 49

Subtle yellow-pink plaque with loss of skin markings is actually a superficial BCC.

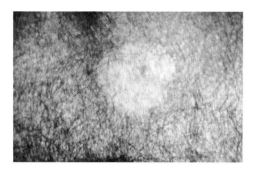

PHOTO 50

BCC presenting as a white plaque.

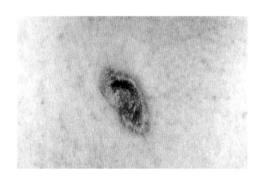

PHOTO 51

Red plaque BCC with central dell, raised thready border and erosion.

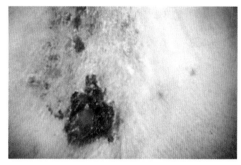

PHOTO 52

BCC presenting as a red plaque with loss of skin lines, surface erosions and scale.

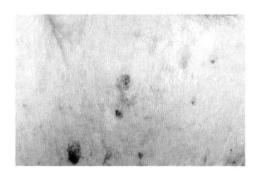

PHOTO 53

BCC with areas of regression and pigmentation.

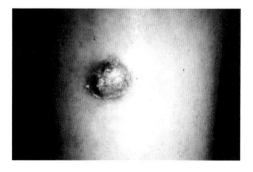

PHOTO 54

Nodular BCC with pigmented areas. Differential would include nodular melanoma.

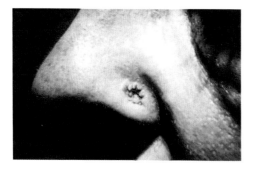

PHOTO 55

BCC which has ulcerated and spread peripherally.

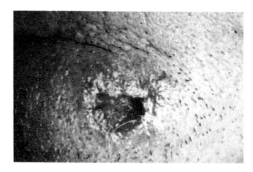

PHOTO 56

BCC with central rodent ulcer and peripheral extension.

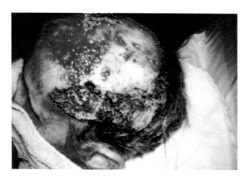

PHOTO 57

Neglected BCC covers most of the scalp and extends into bone. Shows erosions, ulceration, crusting, scarring and eschar formation.

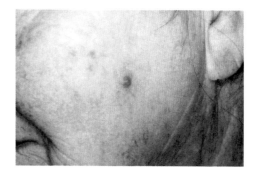

PHOTO 58

Early SCC. Note the deep indurated quality of the papule.

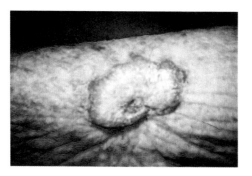

PHOTO 59

Large nodular ulcerating SCC.

430

Part VI: Color Photographs

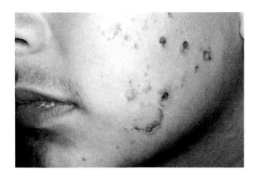

PHOTO 1

Non-bullous impetigo with early small vesicles (upper photo.) and older lesions which have ruptured, enlarged and coalesced.

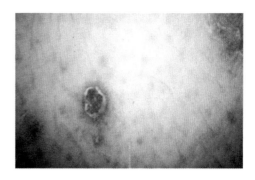

PHOTO 2

Ruptured vesicle leaving a moist burnished red base.

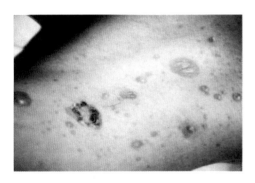

PHOTO 3

Bullous impetigo shows grouped vesicles of various sizes.

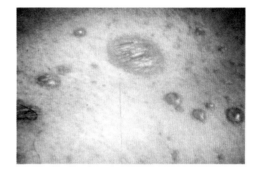

PHOTO 4

Impetigo. Early blisters are clear while the older central blister is clouding as inflammatory cells accumulate.

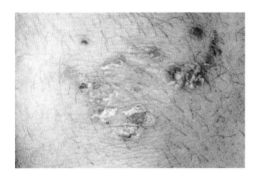

PHOTO 5

Scaling plaque of impetigo with areas of spontaneous resolution.

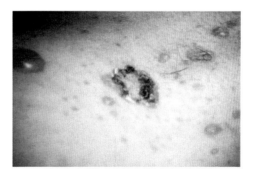

PHOTO 6

Lesion of bullous impetigo with a peripheral hemorrhagic crust.

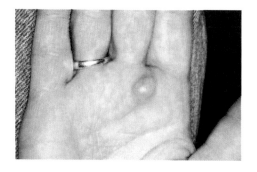

PHOTO 7

Herpetic whitlow that had been recurrent for over a decade before the diagnosis was made. Multiple hospitalizations and courses of antibiotics were given needlessly for the accompanying viral lymphangitis.

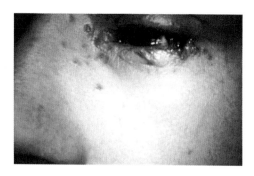

PHOTO 8

Periocular Herpes simplex.

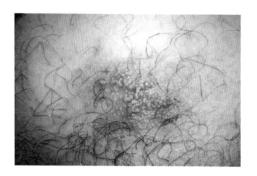

PHOTO 9

Herpes. Grouped umbilicated vesicles on an erythematous urticarial base.

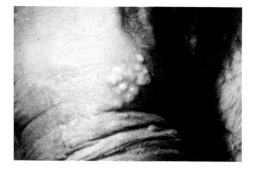

PHOTO 10

Solitary lesion of Herpes genitalis on the penile shaft. Note the two warts in the foreground.

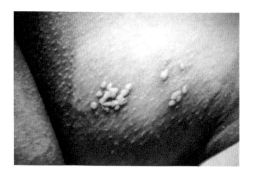

PHOTO 11

A typical location for Herpes genitalis in female victims. Lesions are clouding and becoming pustular.

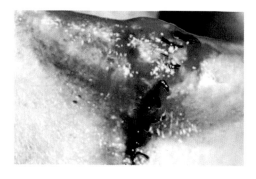

PHOTO 12

Eroded Herpes labialis triggered by lip surgery. Today this complication can be prevented with prophylactic antiviral therapy.

434

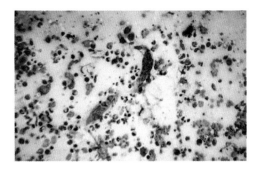

PHOTO 13

Tzanck smear shows multinucleated syncytial giant cells and epidermal cells with ballooned nuclei typical of herpes virus cytopathic effect.

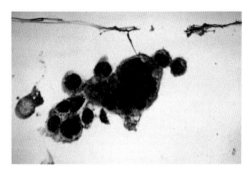

PHOTO 14

High power view of giant cell and keratinocytes with ballooned nuclei.

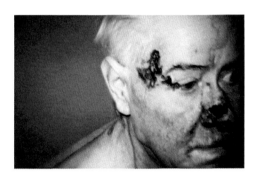

PHOTO 15

Hemorrhagic and necrotic zoster of the ophthalmic branch of the fifth cranial nerve. Note Hutchinson's sign is present and there is injection of the sclera of the right eye.

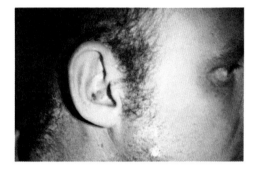

PHOTO 16

Ramsay-Hunt syndrome with vesicles in the concha accompanied by severe pain in the ear.

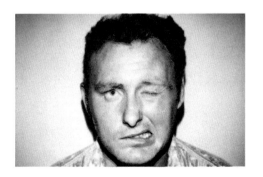

PHOTO 17

Ramsay-Hunt syndrome (same case) demonstrating a complete facial nerve paralysis on the same side.

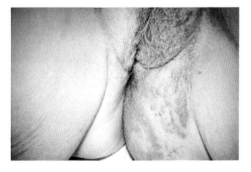

PHOTO 18

Sacral Herpes zoster of left segments S-2, 3, 4.

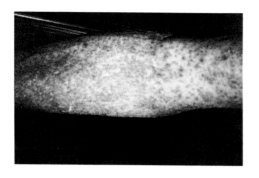

PHOTO 19

Generalized Herpes zoster in a patient with chronic lymphocytic leukemia.

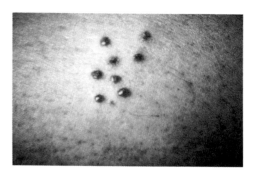

PHOTO 20

Hemorrhagic zoster in a patient with advanced myeloma. Suppression of the immune system is responsible for the absence of the inflammatory base.

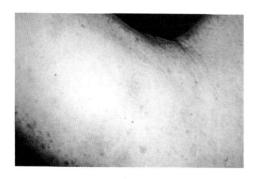

PHOTO 21

Groups of vesicle traveling down a nerve segment on the arm and forearm.

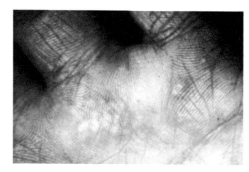

PHOTO 22

Herpes zoster in the same case as photo 21 with segmental lesions on the palm.

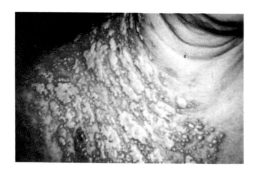

PHOTO 23

Segmental zoster with sharp midline cutoff. Umbilicated vesicle and pustules are present.

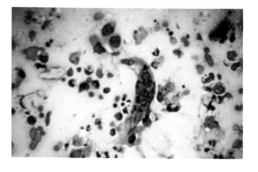

PHOTO 24

Positive Tzanck smear shows giant cells, balloon cells and acute inflammatory cells.

436

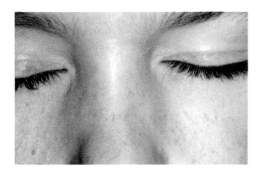

PHOTO 25

Early grade I comedonal acne. Closed comedones and occasional open comedones are present.

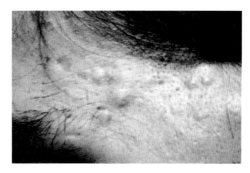

PHOTO 26

More advanced grade I acne with closed cysts, and open and closed comedones.

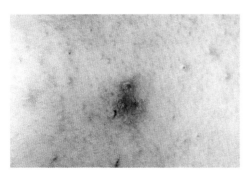

PHOTO 27

Open and closed comedones with a single inflamed papule in the center of the photo.

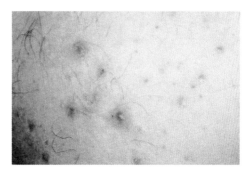

PHOTO 28

Early grade II acne also shows inflammatory follicular papules and pustules.

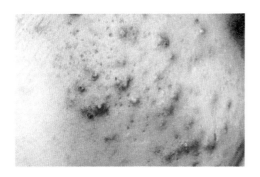

PHOTO 29

Inflammatory papules and pustules that are coalescing into nodules. Note also the appearance of ice-pick scarring.

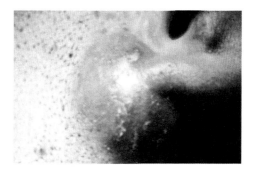

PHOTO 30

Nodules, cysts, and sinus tracts of grade III acne.

437

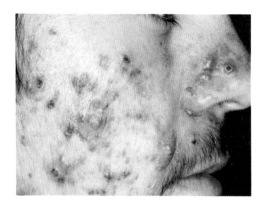

PHOTO 31

Grade III acne. Large inflammatory papules have become confluent to form cysts and sinus tracts. Note also scattered crusts and eschars.

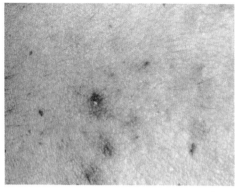

PHOTO 32

Post-acne pigmentation. The erythema component will fade within 3-4 months; the tan melanin component may take months or years to diminish.

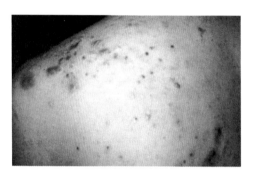

PHOTO 33

Acne of the upper back and shoulder causing hypertrophic scarring.

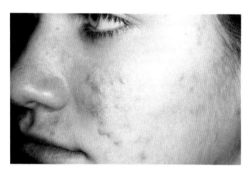

PHOTO 34

Typical facial acne, mild grade II.

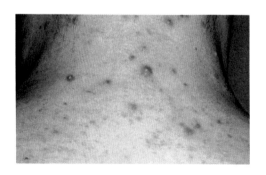

PHOTO 35

Moderate grade II acne of the upper back.

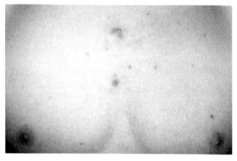

PHOTO 36

Mild grade II acne on the central chest.

438

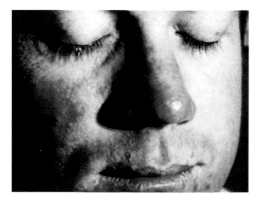

PHOTO 37

Erythematous telangiectatic rosacea; only occasional papules and pustules are evident. Erythema is the predominant finding.

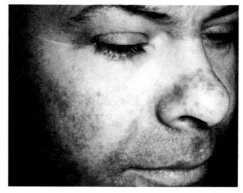

PHOTO 38

Papulopustular rosacea with a component of seborrheic dermatitis.

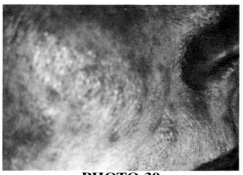

PHOTO 39

Severe rosacea with inflammatory nodules.

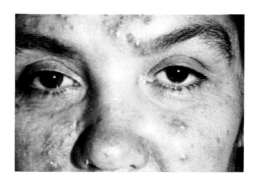

PHOTO 40

Severe papulopustular rosacea with dome-shaped pustules and nodules.

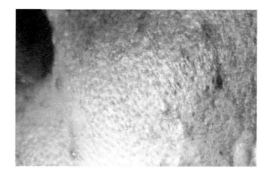

PHOTO 41

Rosacea. Edema causing a shiny orange-peel appearance to the upper cheek.

439

Index

Made in United States
Orlando, FL
27 October 2023

38301144R00263